Advanced Techniques in Dermatologic Surgery

BASIC AND CLINICAL DERMATOLOGY

Series Editors

ALAN R. SHALITA, M.D.
Distinguished Teaching Professor and Chairman
Department of Dermatology
SUNY Downstate Medical Center
Brooklyn, New York

DAVID A. NORRIS, M.D.
Director of Research
Professor of Dermatology
The University of Colorado
Health Sciences Center
Denver, Colorado

1. Cutaneous Investigation in Health and Disease: Noninvasive Methods and Instrumentation, *edited by Jean-Luc Lévêque*
2. Irritant Contact Dermatitis, *edited by Edward M. Jackson and Ronald Goldner*
3. Fundamentals of Dermatology: A Study Guide, *Franklin S. Glickman and Alan R. Shalita*
4. Aging Skin: Properties and Functional Changes, *edited by Jean-Luc Lévêque and Pierre G. Agache*
5. Retinoids: Progress in Research and Clinical Applications, *edited by Maria A. Livrea and Lester Packer*
6. Clinical Photomedicine, *edited by Henry W. Lim and Nicholas A. Soter*
7. Cutaneous Antifungal Agents: Selected Compounds in Clinical Practice and Development, *edited by John W. Rippon and Robert A. Fromtling*
8. Oxidative Stress in Dermatology, *edited by Jürgen Fuchs and Lester Packer*
9. Connective Tissue Diseases of the Skin, *edited by Charles M. Lapière and Thomas Krieg*
10. Epidermal Growth Factors and Cytokines, *edited by Thomas A. Luger and Thomas Schwarz*
11. Skin Changes and Diseases in Pregnancy, *edited by Marwali Harahap and Robert C. Wallach*
12. Fungal Disease: Biology, Immunology, and Diagnosis, *edited by Paul H. Jacobs and Lexie Nall*
13. Immunomodulatory and Cytotoxic Agents in Dermatology, *edited by Charles J. McDonald*
14. Cutaneous Infection and Therapy, *edited by Raza Aly, Karl R. Beutner, and Howard I. Maibach*

Advanced Techniques in Dermatologic Surgery

edited by

Mitchel P. Goldman
University of California
San Diego, California, U.S.A.
and
La Jolla Spa MD
La Jolla, California, U.S.A.

Robert A. Weiss
The Johns Hopkins University School of Medicine
Baltimore, Maryland, U.S.A.
and
Maryland Laser, Skin & Vein Institute
Hunt Valley, Maryland, U.S.A.

associate editors

Neil S. Sadick
Weill Medical College of Cornell University
New York, New York, U.S.A.

Alina A. M. Fratila
Jungbrunnen-Klinik Dr. Fratila GmbH
Bonn, Germany

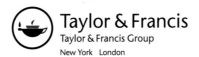

Taylor & Francis
Taylor & Francis Group
New York   London

Published in 2006 by
Taylor & Francis Group
270 Madison Avenue
New York, NY 10016

International Standard Book Number-10: 0-8247-5405-0 (Hardcover)
International Standard Book Number-13: 978-0-8247-5405-1 (Hardcover)
Library of Congress Card Number 2005052954

Library of Congress Cataloging-in-Publication Data

Advanced techniques in dermatologic surgery / edited by Mitchel P. Goldman, Robert A. Weiss.
    p. ; cm. -- (Basic and clinical dermatology ; 35)
    Includes bibliographical references and index.
    ISBN-13: 978-0-8247-5405-1 (Hardcover : alk. paper)
    ISBN-10: 0-8247-5405-0 (Hardcover : alk. paper)
    1. Skin--Surgery. 2. Lasers in surgery. I. Goldman, Mitchel P. II. Weiss, Robert A. III. Series.
    [DNLM: 1. Skin Diseases--surgery. 2. Cosmetic Techniques. 3. Laser Surgery--methods. 4. Reconstructive Surgical Procedures--methods. WR 650 A244 2005]

RD520.A38 2005
617.4'77--dc22
          2005052954

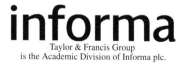

Taylor & Francis Group
is the Academic Division of Informa plc.

Visit the Taylor & Francis Web site at
http://www.taylorandfrancis.com

*To all of our authors and all of our hardworking, dedicated colleagues who have advanced the field of cosmetic dermatology and lasers.
And to my wife, Margaret, who puts up with my writing and editing way past normal bedtimes.*

Robert A. Weiss

*It is always a pleasure to work on a project that will help others. It is my hope that this text will not only help our patients but all cosmetic dermatologic surgeons in advancing and perfecting their techniques.
Another pleasure is to work with a close personal friend and brilliant colleague—"two heads are better than one."
Finally, it is wonderful to have a "Type A" wife, Dianne, who can tolerate long hours working at home most evenings and many weekends across the same desk while still having time to enjoy both our hard work as well as the other pleasures of life together.*

Mitchel P. Goldman

Series Introduction

During the past 25 years, there has been a vast explosion in new information relating to the art and science of dermatology as well as fundamental cutaneous biology. Furthermore, this information is no longer of interest only to the small but growing specialty of dermatology. Clinicians and scientists from a wide variety of disciplines have come to recognize both the importance of skin in fundamental biological processes and the broad implications of understanding the pathogenesis of skin disease. As a result, there is now a multidisciplinary and worldwide interest in the progress of dermatology.

With these factors in mind, we have undertaken this series of books specifically oriented to dermatology. The scope of the series is purposely broad, with books ranging from pure basic science to practical, applied clinical dermatology. Thus, while there is something for everyone, all volumes in the series will ultimately prove to be valuable additions to a dermatologist's library.

The latest addition to the series, volume 35, edited by Drs. Mitchel P. Goldman and Robert A. Weiss, is both timely and pertinent. The editors are well-known authorities in the fields of dermatological surgery and cosmetic dermatology. We trust that this volume will be of broad interest to scientists and clinicians alike.

Alan R. Shalita
Distinguished Teaching Professor and Chairman
Department of Dermatology
SUNY Downstate Medical Center
Brooklyn, New York, U.S.A.

Preface

The concept for this book arose from a need to provide an international approach to the latest in cosmetic dermatologic procedures from not only seasoned experts, but advanced thinkers. When we first approached the publisher, the concept of a CD or DVD accompanying a textbook displaying the procedures discussed was completely novel. It is now not only a reality found in many textbooks, but a necessity. We believe that combined with written text, an accompanying video becomes an observational and interactive learning experience which is almost as good as watching the procedure live. The authors have produced these videos to that end.

The topics covered in this text are the core of cosmetic dermatologic surgery: from botulinum toxin and fillers, to liposuction, non-ablative lasers, and the newest ablative lasers. What makes this text quite unique is the inclusion of the latest sclerotherapy techniques such as foam and endovenous procedures as well as the use of radiofrequency for skin tightening. For those of us versed in principles of dermatologic surgery, this text takes us to the next level. Designed to be procedure oriented but comprehensive as a reference, this book is well illustrated and designed to allow the reader to enter the realm of expert cosmetic dermatologic surgery.

Dr. Alina A. M. Fratila was a source of great inspiration for many of the topics covered in this text. Her relentless dedication to the success of many meetings of the International Society of Dermatologic Surgery of which she was President, provided the concept for a comprehensive international course on cosmetic dermatologic surgery. It is with this in mind that this text expands and updates the content but keeps true to the intent of Dr. Fratila in organizing an international team to explain and teach modern aspects of cosmetic dermatologic surgery. We are also indebted to Sonja and Gerhard Sattler, who organize live cosmetic dermatologic surgery symposia in Rosenpark every other year in which most of the procedures covered in this text can be observed live.

We truly hope that all the readers will gain insight into procedures they are already performing or add additional procedures to their armentarium. We also hope that you will enjoy the international exchange of techniques tweaked to maximize results and the sharing of cosmetic dermatology pearls.

Robert A. Weiss
Mitchel P. Goldman

Contents

Contributors

Murad Alam Section of Cutaneous and Aesthetic Surgery, Department of Dermatology, Northwestern University, Chicago, Illinois, U.S.A.

Kenneth A. Arndt SkinCare Physicians, Chestnut Hill, Massachusetts, U.S.A.; Department of Dermatology, Harvard Medical School, Boston, Massachusetts, U.S.A.; Department of Medicine (Dermatology), Dartmouth Medical School, Hanover, New Hampshire, U.S.A.; and Section of Dermatologic Surgery and Cutaneous Oncology, Department of Dermatology, Yale University School of Medicine, New Haven, Connecticut, U.S.A.

Janna Bentley University of Alberta, Edmonton, Alberta, Canada

Kimberly J. Butterwick Dermatology/Cosmetic Laser Associates of La Jolla, La Jolla, California, U.S.A.

Alastair Carruthers Division of Dermatology, University of British Columbia, Vancouver, British Columbia, Canada

Jean Carruthers Department of Ophthalmology, University of British Columbia, Vancouver, British Columbia, Canada

Jeffrey S. Dover Department of Medicine (Dermatology), Dartmouth Medical School, Hanover, New Hampshire, U.S.A.; Section of Dermatologic Surgery and Cutaneous Oncology, Department of Dermatology, Yale University School of Medicine, New Haven, Connecticut, U.S.A.; and SkinCare Physicians, Chestnut Hill, Massachusetts, U.S.A.

Alina A. M. Fratila Jungbrunnen-Klinik Dr. Fratila GmbH, Bonn, Germany

Paul M. Friedman Department of Dermatology, University of Texas Medical School, DermSurgery Laser Center, Houston, Texas, U.S.A.

Alessandro Frullini Studio Flebologico, Incisa Valdarno, Florence, Italy

Roy G. Geronemus Ronald O. Perelman Department of Dermatology, New York University School of Medicine, Laser and Skin Surgery Center of New York, New York, New York, U.S.A.

Adrienne S. Glaich   Department of Dermatology, DermSurgery Laser Center, University of Texas, Houston, Texas, U.S.A.

David J. Goldberg   Skin Laser & Surgery Specialists of New York & New Jersey, and Mount Sinai School of Medicine, New York, New York, U.S.A.

Mitchel P. Goldman   Department of Dermatology/Medicine, University of California, San Diego, California, U.S.A. and La Jolla Spa MD, La Jolla, California, U.S.A.

Te-Shao Hsu   SkinCare Physicians, Chestnut Hill, Massachusetts, U.S.A.

Carolyn I. Jacob   Northwestern Medical School, Department of Dermatology, Chicago Cosmetic Surgery and Dermatology, Chicago, Illinois, U.S.A.

Michael S. Kaminer   Department of Dermatology, Yale Medical School, Yale University, New Haven, Connecticut, U.S.A.; Department of Medicine (Dermatology), Dartmouth Medical School, Dartmouth College, Hanover, New Hampshire, U.S.A.; and SkinCare Physicians of Chestnut Hill, Chestnut Hill, Massachusetts, U.S.A.

Arielle N. B. Kauvar   New York University School of Medicine, New York, New York, U.S.A.

Suzanne L. Kilmer   Laser and Skin Surgery Center of Northern California, Sacramento, California, U.S.A.

Erick A. Mafong   University of California, San Diego, California, U.S.A.

Albert-Adrien Ramelet   Spécialiste FMH en Dermatologie et en Angiologie, Lausanne, Switzerland

Jaggi Rao   University of Alberta, Edmonton, Alberta, Canada

Neil S. Sadick   Weill Medical College of Cornell University, New York, New York, U.S.A.

Gerhard Sattler   Center for Cosmetic Dermatologic Surgery, Rosenparkklinik, Darmstadt, Germany

Steven Q. Wang   Department of Dermatology, University of Minnesota School of Medicine, Minneapolis, Minnesota, U.S.A.

Margaret A. Weiss   Department of Dermatology, The Johns Hopkins University School of Medicine, Baltimore, Maryland, U.S.A.

Robert A. Weiss   Department of Dermatology, The Johns Hopkins University School of Medicine, Baltimore, Maryland, U.S.A.

Brian D. Zelickson   Department of Dermatology, University of Minnesota School of Medicine and Skin Specialists Inc., Abbott Northwestern Hospital Laser Center, University of Minnesota, Minneapolis, Minnesota, U.S.A.

1

Topical Anesthesia

Paul M. Friedman
*Department of Dermatology, University of Texas Medical School, DermSurgery
Laser Center, Houston, Texas, U.S.A.*

Erick A. Mafong
University of California, San Diego, California, U.S.A.

Adrienne S. Glaich
*Department of Dermatology, DermSurgery Laser Center, University of Texas,
Houston, Texas, U.S.A.*

Roy G. Geronemus
*Ronald O. Perelman Department of Dermatology, New York University School of
Medicine, Laser and Skin Surgery Center of New York, New York,
New York, U.S.A.*

INTRODUCTION

With the emergence of new laser and surgical techniques, the need
for more effective topical anesthesia continues to grow. There are now
several topical preparations of local anesthetics that are being used prior
to various dermatologic procedures. Eutectic mixture of local anesthetics
(EMLA) is the most frequently used agent prior to dermatologic procedures; however, there has been a recent release of newer topical anesthetics claiming increased efficacy and faster onset of action. We review
and compare the efficacy of several commonly used topical anesthetics
and provide a glimpse into the future developments in this field.

Topical anesthetics are weak bases typically composed of three
important components: an aromatic ring, an intermediate length ester
or amide linkage, and a tertiary amine. The ester anesthetics have an ester
linkage, while the amide anesthetics have an amide linkage between the
aromatic ring and the intermediate chain (Fig. 1). Ester-type topical anesthetics are metabolized by plasma cholinesterase and other nonspecific
esterases, while the amide anesthetics are primarily metabolized in the
liver via the microsomal enzymes. Allergic contact reactions to the
ester group of anesthetics are common, while reactions to amide anesthetics, including lidocaine and prilocaine, are rare (1,2). The metabolite
p-aminobenzoic acid (PABA) formed by ester hydrolysis is capable of

1

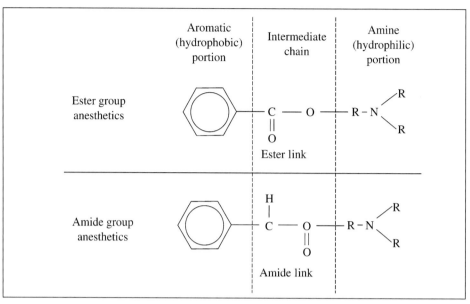

Figure 1
Chemical structure of ester and amide anesthetics.

causing allergic reactions in a small percentage of patients (3). Ester-linked anesthetics are contraindicated in patients with allergies to PABA, hair dyes, and sulfonamides.

Topical anesthetics prevent the initiation and transmission of nerve impulses and provide cutaneous analgesia by targeting free nerve endings in the dermis. Topical anesthetics block nerve impulse conduction by interfering with the function of sodium channels. By inhibiting sodium flux, the threshold for nerve excitation increases until the ability to generate an action potential is lost.

The stratum corneum is the main barrier in topical anesthetic delivery to the free nerve endings in the dermis (4). The aromatic portion is primarily responsible for the lipid solubility that allows diffusion across the nerve cell membrane, governing the intrinsic potency of these agents (5,6). Both the aromatic and the amine portion determine protein-binding characteristics, which are thought to be the primary agents of anesthesia duration (6).

Different methods for evaluating and comparing anesthetic efficacy have included venipuncture (7–13), pinprick testing (14), split-thickness skin graft donation (15–17), and laser pulses as pain stimuli. Laser-induced thermal pain stimuli are advantageous for comparing topical anesthetics by providing reproducible, quantifiable stimuli with minimal intraindividual variation (18–20). Laser pulses also provide selective activation of nociceptors, without interference from mechanosensitive receptors (19).

EMLA

EMLA cream is a 5% eutectic mixture of two local anesthetics, lidocaine and prilocaine (Astra USA, Westborough, Massachusetts). It was released in the United States in 1993 and is composed of 25 mg/mL of lidocaine and 25 mg/mL of prilocaine in an oil-in-water emulsion cream. A eutectic mixture is defined as a compound that melts at a lower temperature than any of its components (21). Using a eutectic system, Fredrick Broberg discovered that equal parts of lidocaine and prilocaine produced adequate analgesia after topical application to the skin (22). The formulation allowed for a concentration of 80% of the anesthetics in oil droplets. However, a low overall concentration of 5% was maintained in the vehicle, thus minimizing systemic toxicity associated with higher concentrations (23).

EMLA is the most widely used topical agent with proven efficacy from several clinical trials (7–19). Multiple studies have shown its usefulness in producing dermal analgesia in patients treated for molluscum contagiosum and venereal lesions, venepuncture in children, shave biopsies, dermabrasion in tattoo removal, and debridement of venous leg ulcers (7–13). Additionally, EMLA has provided sufficient analgesia for harvesting split-thickness skin grafts after a 90-minute application period (15). Lahteenmaki et al. (16) in a dose-finding study demonstrated that 15 gm of EMLA applied to each 100 cm^2 area with application times of two to five hours provided enough analgesia to perform split-thickness skin graft harvesting. More recently, Gupta and Sibbald (24) demonstrated that either EMLA cream or patch applied for two to three hours provided sufficient analgesia in 87% of the subjects for the performance of minor skin surgical procedures such as excisional biopsy or curettage and electrosurgery.

EMLA can also provide cutaneous analgesia for various laser procedures. Many studies have shown that EMLA is effective in reducing or eliminating pain associated with pulsed-dye laser treatments (25,26). Ashinoff and Geronemus (27) demonstrated that EMLA was a safe and effective topical anesthetic which could be used in the treatment of port-wine stains with the pulsed-dye laser. The use of EMLA did not interfere with the clinical efficacy of the pulse-dye laser, despite the fact that local vasoconstriction occurred in cutaneous blood vessels. EMLA has also been shown to provide effective anesthesia to laser-induced pain stimuli produced by the Q-switched Nd:YAG laser after a 60-minute application period (Figs. 2–4) (20).

EMLA produces dermal analgesia after application under an occlusive dressing for 60 minutes, with inadequate analgesia after application for only 30 minutes (28–30). Increased dermal analgesia is seen with up to two hours of occlusion (31). Dermal analgesia has been shown to continue and even increase for 15 to 60 minutes after its removal (18,20,28). This is likely due to a reservoir of anesthetic that accumulates in the stratum corneum during the occlusion period (18,28). After the anesthetic is removed, the diffusion continues from the stratum corneum to the sensory nerves located in the dermis. Arendt-Nielsen and Bjerring (18),

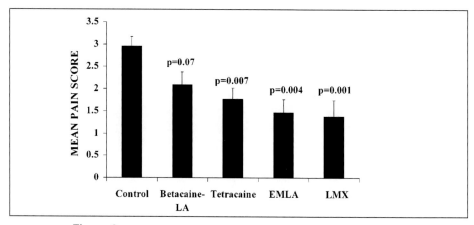

Figure 2
Mean pain scores after application of topical anesthetics for 60 minutes.
p-values represent comparisons of each anesthetic with the control. LMX®
was statistically superior to Tetracaine® and Betacaine-LA® at 60 minutes,
while EMLA was statistically superior to Betacaine-LA® at 60 minutes. *Abbreviations*: EMLA, Eutectic mixture of local anesthetics. *Source*: From Ref. 20.

based on their study, recommend application of EMLA cream under
occlusion one hour prior to laser treatment followed by its removal
prior to the procedure, thereby increasing its ability to reduce pain during
treatment.

The required application period of EMLA may vary depending on
the site of treatment. EMLA has been shown to be effective on the
face and thighs after as little as 25 minutes (32). On mucosal surfaces,

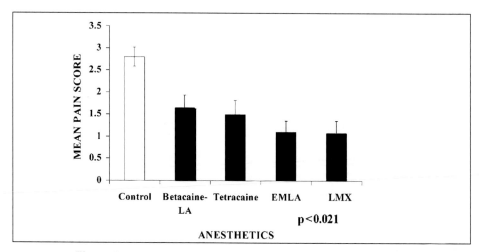

Figure 3
Mean pain scores 30 minutes after removal of the topical anesthetics. All anesthetics were superior to control. *Source*: From Ref. 20.

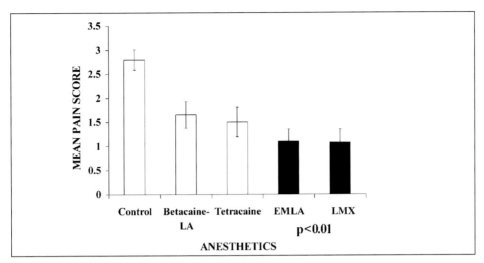

Figure 4
LMX® and EMLA were superior to Tetracaine® and Betacaine-LA® 30 minutes
after the 60-minute application period. *Source*: From Ref. 20.

analgesia can be obtained in as little as 5 to 15 minutes, given the lack of a
stratum corneum (33). In fact, the blood levels of lidocaine after application to mucosal surfaces have been shown to approach levels obtained
after parenteral administration (34). Therefore, caution must be exercised
in using topical anesthetics on mucosal surfaces. Due to the greatly thickened stratum corneum on the palms and the soles, EMLA is ineffective in
these areas despite long application period.

Adverse effects experienced with EMLA are generally transient and
localized. Blanching followed hours later by redness is commonly observed
in the area of application. The blanching is thought to be caused by peripheral vasoconstriction, which is maximal after 1.5 hours, and is followed by
vasodilatation after two to three hours (35). Other effects include pruritus,
burning, and the appearance of purpura.

Contact hypersensitivity is exceedingly rare, but has been reported in
a few cases. Both lidocaine and prilocaine belong to the amide group of
anesthetics. Allergic reactions are rarely encountered in this group, unlike
the ester group of anesthetics (e.g., procaine, benzocaine) (2,36,37). Cross-
reactivity among amide class anesthetics has been documented. However,
recent case reports of contact sensitivity specifically to EMLA cream have
clearly shown that the offending agent is indeed prilocaine alone, with the
patch test failing to implicate lidocaine.

The development of methemoglobinemia, a known complication of
prilocaine, is the most important systemic concern regarding the use
of EMLA cream. The development of methemoglobinemia involves the
oxidation of iron from the ferrous (Fe^{2+}) to the ferric (Fe^{3+}) state. This
renders the hemoglobin molecule unable to transport oxygen. Cyanosis
is evident when as little as 10% methemoglobin is present. At levels of

35%, breathlessness occurs, and toxicity occurs at levels in excess of 80%. Methemoglobinemia has been reported in a three month-old infant who became cyanotic after 5 gm of EMLA was applied for an extended period of five hours (38); the child was also on treatment with trimethoprim-sulphemethoxazole. The use of EMLA for pain relief in neonatal circumcision is becoming more prevalent. The neonate, and especially premature infants, may be vulnerable to this complication due to immaturity of the methemoglobinemia reductase pathway. Other people at risk are those with glucose-6-phosphate dehydrogenase deficiency. Caution should be taken when EMLA is used in patients with congenital methemoglobinemia or in patients less than 12 months of age and who are concomitantly receiving a medication known to exacerbate methemoglobinemia (39).

The development of methemoglobinemia with the use of EMLA is rare. Taddio et al. (40) found no increase in methemoglobin or adverse effects in 38 neonates who received 1 gm of EMLA cream 60 to 80 minutes prior to circumcision. In a study of 22 infants, EMLA was applied for four hours and plasma methemoglobin levels were measured for up to eight hours after the last application. The highest reported level of methemoglobin was 2%, well below toxic or clinically significant levels (41). Current guidelines recommend that in children weighing less than 10 kg, application should be limited to 2 gm and to an area smaller than 100 cm^2. In children weighing 10 to 20 kg, the maximum application of 10 gm should not be applied to an area greater than 100 cm^2 (Table 1).

Although most adverse effects noted with the use of EMLA are localized and transient, care must be taken when EMLA cream is used near the eyes. Sodium hydroxide is a component of the vehicle that imparts a pH of 9 to the product. This level of alkalinity is necessary to allow for proper penetration of the anesthetic. It is also sufficient to cause chemical eye injury in the form of corneal abrasions and ulcerations. Several cases have been reported, where eye injury occurred in association with the use of EMLA near the eye (42–44).

LMX®

LMX® (previously called ELA-MAX) contains either 4% or 5% (LMX® 5) lidocaine in a liposomal delivery system (Table 1), which uses multilamellar vesicles containing several lipid bilayers dispersed in an aqueous medium (Ferndale Laboratories, Ferndale, MI). LMX® 5 is marketed for temporary relief of anorectal pain; however there is no medical reason why it cannot be used as a skin anesthetic. Liposomes facilitate the penetration of anesthetic into the skin, carrying the encapsulated drug into the dermis and providing sustained release (45). Liposomes as drug carriers also protect the anesthetic from metabolic degradation, allowing prolonged duration of action (46). Prior studies have demonstrated the benefit of liposomal encapsulation in the delivery of topical anesthetics. As assessed by the pinprick method, liposomally encapsulated Tetracaine® (0.5%) has been shown to be more effective than Tetracaine® in an inert base in producing significant skin

Table 1
Topical Anesthetics

Anesthetics	Ingredients	Vehicle	Application time	Occlusion required	FDA approved	Advantages	Disadvantages	Maximum dose or area
Betacaine-LA®	Lidocaine: Prilocaine: Dibucaine[a]	Vaseline ointment	60–90	No	No	Anecdotal reports of rapid onset	More clinical and safety trials needed	300 cm² (A)
LMX®	4% Lidocaine	Liposomal	60	No	Yes	Liposomal delivery, long duration of action	Post-application residue	100 cm² (C); 600 cm² (A) and (C > 10 kg)
LMX® 5	5% Lidocaine	Liposomal	30	No	Yes	Rapid onset of action	More clinical trials needed	100 cm² (C); 600 cm² (A) and (C > 10 kg)
EMLA Cream	2.5% Lidocaine: 2.5% Prilocaine	Oil-in-water	60	Yes	Yes	Proven efficacy and safety profile	Long application, occlusion required	20 g/200 cm² (A) and (C > 7 y/o and 20 kg)
Tetracaine® Gel	4% Tetracaine® gel[a]	Lecithin gel	60–90	Yes	No	Anecdotal reports of rapid onset	More clinical and safety trials needed	
Amethocaine	4% Tetracaine®		40–60	Yes	No	Rapid onset, prolonged effect	Ester anesthetic, avoid mucosal surfaces	50 mg (A)
Topicaine[b]	4% Lidocaine	Micro-emulsion	30–60	Yes	Yes	Rapid onset, cost-effective	More clinical trials needed	20×15 inches (A)
S-Caine	7% Lidocaine: 7% Tetracaine®	Oil-in-water	30–60	No	No	Unique delivery system	Contains an ester anesthetic, clinical trials ongoing	To be determined

Abbreviations: (A), adults; (C), children.
[a]Compounded, proprietary anesthetic.
[b]Over the counter product.
Source: From Ref. 63.

TOPICAINE

Topicaine contains 4% lidocaine in a gel microemulsion drug delivery system. This product was released in 1997 for use prior to electrolysis and is gaining popularity as a topical anesthetic for laser hair removal. The recommended application time by the manufacturer is 30 to 60 minutes under an occlusive dressing. Topicaine is FDA-approved for the temporary relief of pain and itching on normal intact skin and may be obtained without a prescription. The manufacturer is currently evaluating the systemic absorption of lidocaine after Topicaine application. The maximum area of application should not exceed $600 \, cm^2$ in adults and $100 \, cm^2$ in children (Table 1). Localized adverse events reported have been mild and transient, including erythema, blanching, and edema (57).

Topicaine showed a very rapid onset with a long duration of cutaneous anesthesia in a prospective, randomized, double-blinded, controlled study investigating the efficacy of EMLA, LMX® 5, and Topicaine using a 30-minute application time (48). Equal amounts of the above topical anesthetics plus a control were randomly applied to eight testsites under occlusion on the volar forearms of 24 adult volunteers. The degree of anesthesia was assessed with a Q-switched Nd:YAG laser emitting energy at 1,064 nm. Similar testing was performed 15 and 30 minutes after removal of the anesthetics, with patients' responses being recorded on an ordinal scale of zero (no pain) to four (maximal pain). Maximal pain for each subject was determined by testing untreated volar arm skin with a laser stimulus, which was used as an internal control. Under the parameters of this study, effective anesthesia to laser-induced pain stimuli was demonstrated with Topicaine and LMX® 5 after only a 30-minute application period as compared to control ($p = 0.002$). The highest level of anesthetic efficacy was obtained with Topicaine and EMLA 30 minutes after their removal.

S-CAINE PATCH

The S-Caine Local Anesthetic Patch is a new drug delivery system that utilizes controlled heating to reportedly enhance the rate of anesthetic delivery into the dermis. The patch contains a 1:1 eutectic mixture of lidocaine base (an amide anesthetic) and Tetracaine® base (an ester anesthetic) with a disposable, oxygen-activated heating element. The heating element generates a controlled level of heating (39–41°C) over a period of two hours.

Clinical studies have demonstrated that a 30-minute administration of the S-Caine Patch is efficacious in relieving the pain associated with shave biopsies and venipuncture. In a double-blinded, placebo-controlled clinical trial, the S-Caine Patch provided sufficient anesthesia for a shave biopsy in 72% of the active group compared to 16% of the placebo group ($p < 0.001$) (Rodriguez D, Stewart D, unpublished data). In a randomized, double-blinded, placebo-controlled study in pediatric patients, the active S-Caine Patch was significantly better than placebo in providing cutaneous anesthesia for venipunture after a 30-minute application period ($p < 0.001$). Close to 80% of the patients receiving the active patch reported "no pain" associated with the vascular access procedure compared to 40% with placebo (Eichenfield L, et al., unpublished data).

S-CAINE LOCAL ANESTHETIC PEEL

The S-Caine Local Anesthetic Peel contains a formulation of a 1:1 eutectic mixture of 7% lidocaine base and 7% Tetracaine® base, similar to that of the S-Caine Patch (Table 1). The Peel is a cream which, as it dries, becomes a flexible membrane that is easily removed (Figs. 5 and 6). These unique features of the drug reduce the application time, ease the delivery of anesthetic to contoured regions of the body, and eliminate the need for application under occlusion.

Phase II FDA studies have demonstrated that a 30-minute application of the S-Caine Peel is efficacious in relieving the pain caused by various laser procedures. A randomized, double-blinded, placebo-controlled trial with the S-Caine Peel for local anesthesia prior to pulsed-dye laser treatment on the face was recently completed. The results indicated that

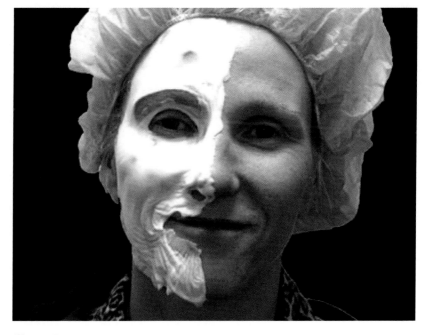

Figure 5
S-Caine Local Anesthetic Peel.

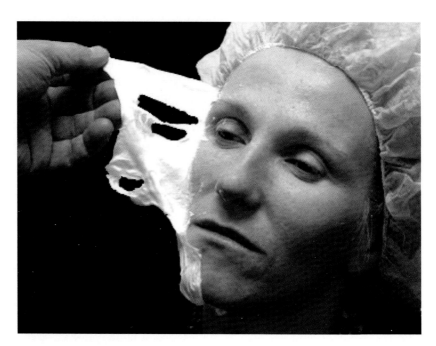

Figure 6
S-Caine Local Anesthetic Peel.

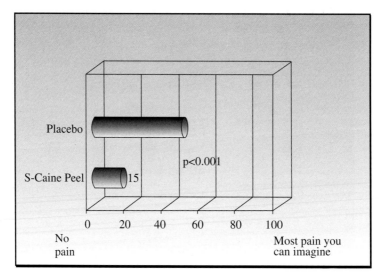

Figure 7
Patients' mean pain evaluations. *Source*: From Ref. 59.

a 20- or 30-minute application of S-Caine Peel was better than placebo in providing local anesthesia prior to pulsed-dye laser treatment of vascular lesions (port wine stains, telangiectases) on the face of adult patients (58). A recent randomized, double-blinded, placebo-controlled trial also demonstrated that a 30-minute application of S-Caine Peel provided effective and safe dermal anesthesia prior to nonablative laser treatment with the 1450 nm diode laser (Fig. 7) (59). The S-Caine Peel was also shown in a randomized, double-blind study of 30 patients to be more effective than EMLA with occlusion when applied 30-minutes prior to full-face single pass CO_2 laser resurfacing (60). Two randomized, double-blinded, placebo-controlled studies showed that a 60-minute application of the S-Caine Peel provided safe and highly effective local anesthesia when used prior to long-pulsed Nd:YAG laser therapy for leg veins (61). In a randomized, double-blinded, placebo-controlled trial, Jih et al. also demonstrated that the S-Caine Peel was safe and effective when applied 60 minutes prior to laser therapy of leg veins using a 1,064 nm long-pulsed Nd:YAG laser (62). The S-Caine Peel is currently in FDA phase III clinical trials and is being studied for local anesthesia prior to laser and surgical procedures after various application times.

COST COMPARISON

A cost comparison revealed that Tetracaine® and Topicaine are the least expensive of the topical anesthetics (Fig. 8). EMLA is also available in a generic preparation at a lower price.

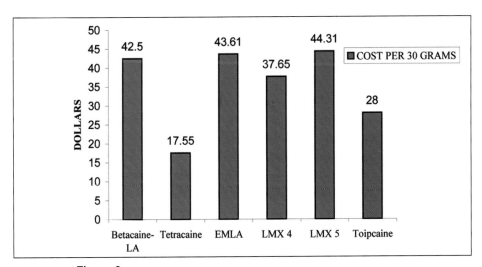

Figure 8
A cost comparison of commonly available topical anesthetic preparations.

CONCLUSION

Topical anesthetics remain a powerful, new advancement for pain relief prior to cutaneous procedures. While there has been a recent release of several new topical anesthetic agents claiming increased efficacy and faster onset, EMLA remains the most widely used topical anesthetic given its proven efficacy and safety by several clinical trials. As the options for the practitioner continue to grow, as well as the demand for faster onset, comparative efficacy and safety trials continue to be of paramount importance.

REFERENCES

1. Rietschel RL, Fowler JF. Fisher's Contact Dermatitis. 4th ed.. Baltimore: Williams and Wilkins, 1995:236–242.
2. Suhonen R, Kanerva L. Contact allergy and cross-reactions caused by prilocaine. Am J Contact Dermatitis 1997; 8:231–235.
3. Mackie BS, Mackie LE. The PABA story. Australas J Dermatol 1999; 40:51–53.
4. Adriani J, Dalili H. Penetration of local anesthetics through epithelial barriers. Anesth Analg 1971; 50:834–841.
5. Covino BG. Local anesthesia. N Engl J Med 1972; 286(18):975–983.
6. Covino BG. Local anesthetic agents for peripheral nerve blocks. Anaesthesist 1980; 29(7):33–37.
7. Hallen B, Olsson GL, Uppfeldt A. Pain-free venepuncture. Effect of timing of application of local anaesthetic cream. Anaesthesia 1984; 39:969–972.
8. Kurien L, Kollberg H, Uppfeldt A. Venepuncture pain can be reduced. J Trop Med Hyg 1985; 88:397–399.
9. Moller C. A lignocaine-prilocaine cream reduces venipunture pain. Ups J Med Sci 1985; 90:293–298.
10. Maunuksela EL, Korpela R. Double-blind evaluation of a lignocaine-prilocaine cream (EMLA) in children. Br J Anaesth 1986; 58:1242–1245.
11. Cooper CM, Gerrish SP, Hardwick M, Kay R. EMLA cream reduces the pain of venepuncture in children. Eur J Anaesthesiol 1987; 4:441–448.
12. Hopkins CS, Buckley CJ, Bush GH. Pain-free injection in infants. Use of a lignocaine-prilocaine cream to prevent pain at intravenous induction of general anaesthesia in 1-5-year-old children. Anaesthesia 1988; 43:198–201.
13. Watson AR, Szymkin P, Morgan AG. Topical anaesthesia for fistula cannulation in haemodialysis patients. Nephrol Dial Transplant 1988; 3:800–802.
14. Bucalo BD, Mirikitani EJ, Moy RL. Comparison of skin anesthetic effect of liposomal lidocaine, nonliposomal lidocaine, and EMLA using 30-minute application time. Dermatol Surg 1998; 24:537–541.
15. Ohlsen L, Englesson S, Evers II. An anaesthetic lidocaine/prilocaine cream (EMLA) for epicutanteous application tested for cutting split skin grafts. Scand J Plast Reconstr Surg 1985; 19:201–209.
16. Lahteenmaki T, Lillieborg S, Ohlsen L, Olenius M, Strombeck JO. Topical analgesia for the cutting of split-skin grafts: a multicenter comparison of two doses of a lidocaine/prilocaine cream. Plast Reconstr Surg 1988; 82:458–462.
17. Goodacre TLE, Sanders R, Watts DA, Stoker M. Split skin grafting using topical local anaesthesia (EMLA): a comparison with infiltrated anaesthesia. Br J Pl Surg 1988; 41:533–538.
18. Arendt-Nielsen L, Bjerring P. Laser-induced pain for evaluation of local analgesia. Anesth Analg 1988; 67:115–123.
19. Hernandez E, Gonzalez S, Gonzalez E. Evaluation of topical anesthetics by laser-induced sensation. Lasers Surg Med 1998; 23:167–171.
20. Friedman PM, Fogelman JP, Nouri K, Levine VJ, Ashinoff R. Comparative study of the efficacy of four topical anesthetics. Dermatol Surg 1999; 25:950–954.
21. Anderson DM. Dorland's Medical Dictionary. 28th ed. Philadelphia: WB Saunders Company, 1994:588.
22. Brodin A, Nyquist-Mayer A, Wadstein T. Phase diagram and aqueous solubility of the lidocaine-prilocaine binary system. J Pharm Sci 1984; 73:481–484.
23. Watson K. Astra markets cream to remove pain of injections. Pharm J 1986; 237:262.

24. Gupta AK, Sibbald RG. Eutectic lidocaine/prilocaine 5% cream and patch may provide satisfactory analgesia for excisional biopsy or curettage with elctrosurgery of cutaneous lesions. J Am Acad Dermatol 1996; 35:419–423.

25. Sherwood KA. The use of topical anesthesia in removal of port-wine stains in children. J Pediatr 1993; 122:S36–S40.

26. Tan OT, Stafford TJ. EMLA for laser treatment of portwine stains in children. Laser Surg Med 1992; 12:543–548.

27. Ashinoff R, Geronemus RG. Effect of the topical anesthetic EMLA on the efficacy of pulsed dye laser Treatment of port-wine stains. J Dermatol Surg Oncol 1990; 16:1008–1011.

28. Evers H, Von Dardel O, Juhlin L, Ohlsen L, Vinnars E. Dermal effects of compositions based on the eutectic mixture of lignocaine and prilocaine (EMLA). Br J Anaesth 1985; 57:997–1005.

29. McCafferty DF, Woolfson AD. New patch delivery system for percutaneous local anesthesia. Br J Aneasth 1993; 71:370–374.

30. Greenbaum SS, Bernstein EF. Comparison of iontophoresis of lidocaine with a eutectic mixture of lidocaine and prilocaine (EMLA) for topically administered local anesthesia. J Dermatol Surg Oncol 1994; 20:579–583.

31. Bjerring P, Arendt-Nielsen L. Depth and duration of skin analgesia to needle insertion after topical application of EMLA cream. Br J Anaesth 1990; 64:173–177.

32. Holmes HS. Choosing A local anesthetic. Dermatol Clin 1994; 12:817–823.

33. Rylander E, Sjoberg I, Lillieborg S, Stockman O. Local anesthesia of the genital mucosa with a lidocaine/prilocaine cream (EMLA) for laser treatment of condylomata acuminata: a placebo-controlled study. Obstet Gynecol 1990; 75:302–306.

34. Adrinai J, Aepernick R. Clinical effectiveness of drugs used for topical anesthesia. JAMA 1964; 188:711–716.

35. Bjerring P, Andersen PH, Arendt-Nielsen L. Vascular response of human skin after analgesia with EMLA cream. Br J Anaesth 1989; 63:655–660.

36. Black RJ, Dawson AJ, Strang WC. Contact sensitivity to lidocaine and prilocaine. Contact Dermatitis 1990; 23:117–118.

37. van den Hove J, Decroix J, Tennstedt D, Lachapelle JM. Allergic contact dermatitis from prilocaine, one of the local anaesthetics in EMLA cream. Contact Dermatitis 1994; 30:239.

38. Jacobson B, Nilssen A. Methemaglobinemia associated with prilociane-lidocaine cream and trimethoprim-sulphamethoxazole. A case report. Acta Anaesthesiol Scand 1985; 29: 453–455.

39. EMLA package insert. Westborough, MA: Astra USA, Inc., 1998.

40. Taddio A, Stevens B, Craig K, Rastogi P, Shlomit B, Shennan A, Mulligan P, Koren G. Efficacy and safety of lignocaine-prilocaine cream for pain during circumcision. N Engl J Med 1997; 336:1197–1201.

41. Engberg G, Danielson K, Henneberg S, Nilsson A. Plasma concentrations of prilocaine and lidocaine and methaemoglobin formation in infants after epicutaneous application of a 5% lidocaine-prilocaine cream (EMLA). Acta Anaestheiol Scand 1987; 31(7):624–628.

42. Eaglstein FN. Chemical injury to the eye from EMLA cream during erbium laser resurfacing. Derm Surg 1999; 25(7):590–591.

43. McKinlay JR, Hofmeister E, Ross EV, Mac Allister W. EMLA cream-induced eye injury. Arch Dermatol 1999; 135:855–856.

44. Brahma AK, Inkster C. Alkaline chemical ocular injury from EMLA cream. Eye 1995; 9:658–659.

45. Foldvari M, Gesztes A, Mezei M. Dermal drug delivery by liposome encapsulation: clinical and electron microscopic studies. J Microencap 1990; 7:479–489.

46. Mezei M. Liposomes as penetration promoters and localizers of topically applied drugs. In: Hsieh DS, ed. Drug Permeation Enhancement. New York: Marcel Dekker Inc., 1993.
47. Gesztes A, Mezei M. Topical anesthesia of the skin by liposome encapsulated tetracaine. Anesth Analg 1988; 67:1079–1081.
48. Friedman PM, Fogelman JP, Levine VJ, Ashinoff R. Comparative study of three topical anesthetics after 30-minute application time. Lasers Surg Med 2000; 26(suppl 12):19.
49. Koppel RA, Coleman KM, Coleman WP. The efficacy of EMLA versus LMX for pain relief in medium-depth chemical peeling: a clinical and histopathologic evaluation. Derm Surg 2000; 26:61–64.
50. LMX package insert. Ferndale, MI: Ferndale Laboratories, Inc., 1997.
51. Betacaine-LA package insert. Tampa, FL: Medical Center Pharmacy, 1997.
52. McCafferty DF, Woolfson AD, Handley J, Allen G. Effect of percutaneous local anaesthetics on pain reduction during pulse dye laser treatment of portwine stains. Br J Anaesth 1997; 78:286–289.
53. Lawson RA, Smart NG, Gudgeon AC, Morton NS. Evaluation of an amethocaine gel preparation for percutaneous analgesia before venous cannulation in children. Br J Anaesth 1995; 75(3):282–285.
54. Molodecka J, Stenhouse C, Jones JM, Tomlinson A. Comparison of percutaneous anaesthesia for venous cannulation after topical application of either amethocaine or EMLA cream. Br J Anaesth 1994; 72(2):174–176.
55. O'Connor B, Tomlinson AA. Evaluation of the efficacy and safety of amethocaine gel applied topically before venous cannulation in adults. Br J Anaesth 1995; 74(6):706–708.
56. Mazumdar B, Tomlinson AA, Faulder GC. Preliminary study to assay plasma amethocaine concentrations after topical application of a new local anaesthetic cream containing amethocaine. Br J Anaesth 1991; 67(4):432–436.
57. Topicaine package insert. Mountain View, CA: ESBA Laboratories, 1997.
58. Bryan HA, Alster TS. The S-Caine Peel: A novel topical anesthetic for cutaneous laser surgery. Dermatol Surg 2002; 28:999–1003.
59. Doshi SN, Friedman PM, Marquez DK, Goldberg LH. Thirty-minute application of the S-Caine Peel prior to nonablative laser treatment. Dermatol Surg 2003; 29:1008–1011.
60. Alster TS, Lupton JR. Evaluation of a novel topical anesthetic agent for cutaneous laser resurfacing: a randomized comparison study. Dermatol Surg 2002; 28:1004–1006.
61. Chen JZ, Alexiades-Armenakas MR, Bernstein LJ, Jacobson LG, Friedman PM, Geronemus RG. Two randomized, double-blind, placebo-controlled studies evaluating the S-Caine Peel for induction of local anesthesia before long-pulsed Nd:YAG laser therapy for leg veins. Dermatol Surg 2003; 29:1012–1018.
62. Jih MH, Friedman PM, Sadick N, Marquez DK, Kimyai-Asadi A, Goldberg LH. 60-minute application of S-Caine Peel prior to 1,064 nm long-pulsed Nd:YAG laser treatment of leg veins. Lasers Surg Med 2004; 34:446–450.
63. Friedman PM, Mafong EA, Friedman ES, Geronemus RG. Topical anesthetics update. EMLA and beyond. Dermatol Surg 2001; 27: 1019–1026.

2

Advanced Cosmetic Use of Botulinum Toxin Type A

Alastair Carruthers
Division of Dermatology, University of British Columbia, Vancouver, British Columbia, Canada

Jean Carruthers
Department of Ophthalmology, University of British Columbia, Vancouver, British Columbia, Canada

Video 1: BOTOX®

INTRODUCTION

When the cosmetic use of botulinum toxin type A (BTX-A) was first introduced in the early 1990s, it was a novel, almost shocking concept; now, however, the cosmetic application of BTX-A is commonly recognized as the gold standard in upper facial rejuvenation. The huge expansion in the acceptance of its use—and the regulatory approval of BTX-A (BOTOX®, BOTOX Cosmetic®, Allergan Inc., Irvine, California, U.S.), for the treatment of the glabella area, in Canada and the United States—has led to a much wider, more scientifically based clinical experience. This chapter will focus primarily on improved uses and advanced cosmetic applications of BTX-A, specifically the BOTOX® and BOTOX Cosmetic® formulations, unless otherwise indicated, since it is with this product that we have had the most experience. It is important to emphasize that before using any product for an indication, physicians should consult the literature available on that specific formulation.

BOTULINUM NEUROTOXINS

Botulinum neurotoxins (BTXs) derive from the bacterium *Clostridium botulinum* and include seven distinct serotypes, identified as A, B, C_1, D, E, F, and G. All BTX subtypes block neuromuscular transmission by binding to receptor sites on motor nerve terminals and inhibiting the release of acetylcholine, but differ slightly in their mechanism of action and clinical effect (1). When injected intramuscularly at therapeutic doses, BTXs produce temporary chemodenervation of the muscle,

19

resulting in a localized reduction in muscle activity. Recommended doses of injected neurotoxin do not result in systemic clinical effects in patients without other neuromuscular dysfunctions.

At present in North America, there are two commercially available toxins: BOTOX®, BOTOX Cosmetic® (BTX-A) and MYOBLOC™ (BTX-B, Elan Pharmaceuticals, San Diego, California, U.S.). BOTOX Cosmetic® is the only botulinum toxin currently approved for cosmetic use in North America, although Dysport® (BTX-A, Ipsen Limited, Maidenhead, Berkshire, U.K.) is available in Europe, and is under consideration for licensing by the U.S. Food and Drug Administration. Since each preparation differs in terms of the *C. botulinum* strain, potency, and manufacturing, the biological behaviors of each are not interchangeable, and the dosages for each product vary.

Comparative Effects of Botulinum Types A and B

BTX-A has been used for aesthetic purposes for over a decade. Numerous clinical trials have established its safety and efficacy for hyperfunctional facial lines; the largest trial documented its superior efficacy over placebo in the treatment of glabellar rhytides, and led to the approval of BTX-A as the only botulinum toxin indicated for cosmetic use in North America (2).

BTX-B (MYOBLOC™) was approved for use in cervical dystonia in 2000, but has been used off-label to treat facial wrinkles and has been evaluated in several smaller clinical trials. Ramirez et al. (3) evaluated BTX-B in 24 patients with facial wrinkles who received 200 to 400 U of BTX-B in the frontalis, corrugators, and orbicularis oculi. Although all patients experienced a rapid onset of near-complete paresis within 72 hours, the duration of effect was suboptimal (mean, eight weeks), and the injections were slightly more painful. Two open-label trials examined BTX-B of 1800, 2400, and 3000 U in the procerus, corrugator supercilii, and orbicularis oculi, and found BTX-B to be effective in treating glabellar frown lines based on photography, patient satisfaction, and improvements in assessment scores (4,5). Both studies suggest that the duration of response was dose related: the mean duration of effect was 8, 9.6, and 10.4 weeks with 1800, 2400, and 3000 U BTX-B, respectively. Finally, Alster et al. (6) assessed the clinical effects of BTX-B in 20 women with vertical glabellar rhytides who experienced less than optimal results with prior BTX-A treatments. After a single treatment of 2500 U BTX-B in five injection sites (procerus, inferomedial corrugators, and superior middle corrugators) bilaterally, average wrinkle scores were reduced by 42% within 48 to 72 hours after treatment, peaking in clinical effect (reduction in wrinkle scores by 78%) at one month. The effect of treatment waned by two months, and no patients maintained improvement at four months. Average pain ratings of 6.6 (moderate pain) were associated with the injections.

BTX-A and BTX-B were compared in a double-blind study of 18 females, with moderate or severe glabellar rhytides, who received 20 U BTX-A or 1000 U BTX-B in the glabellar region (7). At maximum contraction, BTX-A achieved significantly superior improvement over BTX-B at week eight and less pain on injection. BTX-B also adversely affected tear flow when compared with BTX-A at weeks one and four. Overall, BTX-A achieved greater therapy success with longer-lasting results and fewer side effects. In another study of 10 women, Matarasso (8) compared BTX-A (15 U) and BTX-B (750 U) injected into the lateral fibers of the orbicularis oculi muscle and found that BTX-B was associated with slightly increased discomfort upon injection, a faster onset of action, a sensation of "tightness" in the treated area, and a briefer duration of muscle relaxation (8).

Based on the results of these studies, it appears that there are key differences between BTX-A and BTX-B in their effect on injection into the facial muscles. BTX-B has more rapid onset of action and diffuses more widely. At the relative doses used in the above trials (50–100 U of BTX-B to 1 U of BTX-A), BTX-B has a shorter duration of action than BTX-A. Finally, greater pain and possibly other side effects, such as dry mouth, are associated with BTX-B.

Storage and Reconstitution of Commercially Available Preparations

Each vial of BOTOX Cosmetic® contains 100 mouse units of vacuum-dried *C. botulinum* type A neurotoxin complex. The vacuum-dried product should be stored in a freezer at or below −5°C or in a refrigerator between 2°C and 8°C. BTX-A Freezing BTX-A after reconstitution is neither necessary nor desirable. Manufacturer guidelines recommend that BTX-A be reconstituted with sterile 0.9% saline solution without preservatives, and discarded after four hours (1). However, some physicians report using BTX-A 7 to 10 days after reconstitution without altering its potency (9), and Hexsel et al. (10) found no significant differences in efficacy when BTX-A is used within six weeks of reconstitution. Moreover, recent data suggest that reconstitution with preserved saline does not impair the stability of BTX-A (9,11), and a double-blind, randomized, controlled trial comparing preserved and preservative-free saline in 15 patients found that all patients reported 54% less pain on the side of the face treated with preserved saline (12). The study found no difference in treatment efficacy, and reconstituted BTX-A remained stable for up to five weeks.

The appropriate diluent volume must be selected based on the desired concentration of the injection solution, although evidence indicates that higher doses of BTX-A delivered in smaller volumes keep the effects more localized and allow for the precise placement of the toxin with little diffusion, while smaller doses in larger volumes tend to cause more widespread effects (13). In a study of 80 patients receiving a total dose of 30 U BTX-A at dilutions of 100, 33.3, 20, or 10 U/mL in seven injection sites for glabellar rhytides, patients in the lower dilution groups perceived a greater and longer-lasting improvement (14).

Dysport® is available as a lyophilized vial containing 500 U of BTX-A, as well as sodium chloride, lactose, and human serum albumin. There is somewhat less albumin in the Dysport® vial compared to that contained in the BOTOX® vial; it has been suggested that this may account for part of the difference in effectiveness between the Dysport® and BOTOX® units. In Europe, Dysport® is labeled for transport at ambient temperature and storage at 2°C to 8°C, and the guidelines for reconstitution and use are similar to those of BOTOX® (15). Ipsen has an agreement with Inamed Inc., for marketing of Dysport® in North America, and the two companies are currently working towards regulatory approval.

MYOBLOC™ is available in a liquid formulation containing BTX-B 5000 U/mL and is available in 0.5, 1.0, and 2.0 mL vials containing BTX-B, saline, human serum albumin, and sodium succinate as a buffer to preserve acid pH. The pH is approximately 5.6, accounting for the stinging sensation reported on injection. Since this is a liquid formulation, reconstitution is not required; indeed, further dilution is rather complicated in the vial because of the "overfill" of the vials. The clinician with the intention to add saline to reduce the stinging (with benzyl alcohol) would be advised to do so in the syringe and mix the solution well. The unopened vial, like the BTX-A products, is stable for months or years, but once opened, the lability is similar between the products (16).

Immunogenicity

Botulinum toxins are proteins capable of producing neutralizing antibodies and eliciting an immune response, causing patients to no longer respond to treatment (13). The rate of formation of neutralizing antibodies has not been well studied, and the crucial factors for neutralizing antibody formation have not been well characterized (1). However, the total protein concentration and number of units injected are critical in determining potential immunogenicity, and some studies suggest that BTX-A injections at more frequent intervals or at higher doses may lead to a greater incidence of antibody formation (1). The protein concentration in the current lots of BOTOX® is significantly lower than in previous lots, and has been shown to be less antigenic than the original product. Although one of the greatest concerns with the use of BTX-A is the formation of neutralizing antibodies, the overall risk in using BTX-A at recommended doses for neurologic applications is low (less than 5%), and injecting the lowest effective doses, with the longest feasible intervals between injections, will minimize the potential for immunogenicity (1). Lack of effectiveness of BTX-A secondary to the development of immunologic resistance is exceedingly rare in cosmetic patients, and must be distinguished from a much more common degree of resistance, associated with the need for increased doses and probably not due to immunologic mechanisms.

TREATMENT OF THE UPPER FACE

Treatment of the upper face has yielded the greatest clinical experience with cosmetic BTX-A. Although the first published reports of BTX application in the face appeared in 1990, we know that a number of clinicians experimented during the late 1980s, impressed by its ease of technique and obvious benefits and safety (13).

Glabellar Rhytides

Muscles controlling the frown include the corrugator and orbicularis, which move the brow medially, and the procerus and depressor supercilii, which pull the brow inferiorly. Since the location, size, and use of the muscles vary greatly between individuals, individualizing treatment sites and doses to match each patient's needs will optimize the clinical benefits. Although a variety of different injection techniques and doses are described in the literature (13), recent studies suggest that higher doses may be more effective. In a randomized, dose-ranging study of 80 women injected with 10 to 40 U BTX-A, 30 and 40 U produced significantly greater responses with the longest duration on glabellar lines than did 10 or 20 U BTX-A, and peak responder rates and duration of benefit increased significantly with increasing doses (17). At higher doses, many patients experienced clinical benefits lasting three to four months, but some continued to benefit for as long as six to eight months. In an objective analysis of the dose-ranging study, the authors measured changes in eyebrow and eyelid height and found an additional benefit of lateral- and mid-pupil elevation at 30 and 40 U (Fig. 1) (18).

Men injected with current recommended doses may not receive as great a benefit as women. In a study comparing the efficacy and safety of four doses of BTX-A in the treatment of glabellar lines, men were randomly assigned to receive a total of 20, 40, 60, or 80 U in seven sites (19). Preliminary results show that men injected with 80 U achieved a better response rate than those injected with lower doses, and experienced no change in the rate of adverse events, suggesting that male patients are considerably underdosed. Further investigation will determine optimal doses in men; however, we find it useful to halve the volume of saline used to reconstitute the vial when treating males. This technique reduces the injected volume while simply doubling the injected dose.

Horizontal Rhytides

BTX-A in the forehead lessens undesirable horizontal forehead lines for a period of four to six months (13). Again, treatment must be individualized for each patient and injection sites kept well above the brow to avoid ptosis or a complete lack of expressiveness. Patients with a narrow brow (defined as less than 12 cm between the temporal fusion lines at mid-brow level) should receive fewer injections (four sites, compared to five) and lower doses than patients with broader brows. We previously injected a total of 10 to 20 U in four to five sites horizontally across the mid-brow, 2 to 3 cm above the eyebrows (13), but—as seen in the glabella—more recent data suggest that higher doses may be more effective. In a prospective, randomized, double-blind, parallel-group, dose-ranging study of 48 weeks, 60 women received 16, 32, or 48 U BTX-A

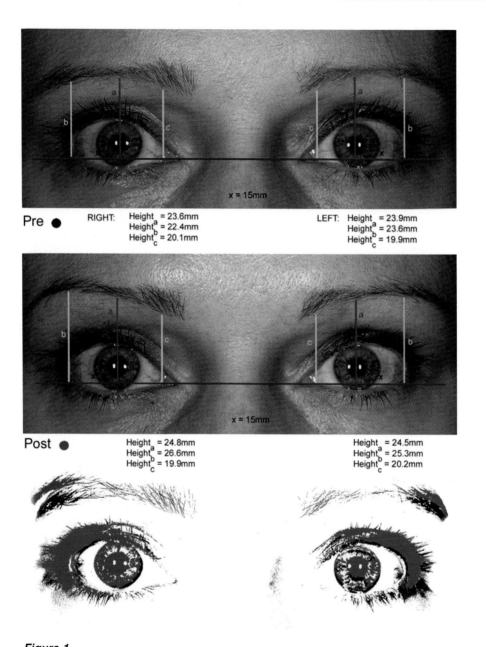

RIGHT:
Height$_a$ = 23.6mm
Height$_b$ = 22.4mm
Height$_c$ = 20.1mm

LEFT:
Height$_a$ = 23.9mm
Height$_b$ = 23.6mm
Height$_c$ = 19.9mm

Pre ●

Post ●

Height$_a$ = 24.8mm
Height$_b$ = 26.6mm
Height$_c$ = 19.9mm

Height$_a$ = 24.5mm
Height$_b$ = 25.3mm
Height$_c$ = 20.2mm

x = 15mm

Figure 1
Individual before (*above*) and after (*below*) 30 U of BOTOX® injected into the glabella area alone. The lower part of the figure is a computer overlay of the two photographs with before (in black) and after (in red). It can be seen that, although the BOTOX® was injected only medial to the pupil majority of the eyebrow elevation is lateral.

in eight sites in the forehead: two in the procerus, four in the frontalis, and two in the lateral orbicularis oculi (half of the doses were injected into the depressors) (20). BTX-A dose of 48 U led to the greatest improvement and duration of response, but adverse effects such as headache, eyelid swelling, and brow ptosis, were more frequent with the higher doses.

Brow Lift

Overactivity of the brow depressors leads to a lowered brow and scowling expression. Medial brow depressors include the corrugator supercilii, procerus, and the medial portion of the orbicularis oculi, while the lateral depressor is the lateral portion of the orbicularis oculi. Treating the glabellar lines often results in an elevation of the brow (13). Huilgol et al. (23) report treating the brow depressors alone to elevate the brow while preserving its natural shape (21). One injection of 7 to 10 U BTX-A in the glabella at the midline (immediately below the line joining the eyebrows), followed by one injection on each side into the supralateral eyebrow (where the orbicularis curves infralaterally, outside the bony orbital rim) resulted in a modest brow elevation (mean, 1 mm) in five out of seven patients. Ahn et al. (22) injected 7 to 10 U into the supralateral orbicularis oculi at three sites below the lateral third of the brow (but superior and lateral to the orbital rim) and produced average midpupillary elevations of 1 mm and lateral brow elevations of 4.8 mm. Huang et al. (23) injected 10 U in four sites along the underside of the lateral half of the brow and 5 U into each corrugator muscle just above and medial to the brow. Brow height at rest increased by 1.9 mm (on the right side) and 3.1 mm (on the left), and the mean increase in brow height on elevation was 2.1 mm on the right side and 2.9 mm on the left.

In a complete analysis of the brow height data from their female glabella dose-ranging study the authors have further explored the benefits and relationship between glabella injection and brow height (24). In this study, injecting a total of 10 U BTX-A into the glabella area produced mild medial brow ptosis, which disappeared after two months. However, injecting a total dose of 20 to 40 U initially produced a significant lateral eyebrow elevation, followed by central and medial eyebrow elevation. This effect peaked at 12 weeks after injection and remained at a significant level at 16 weeks. To our knowledge, this is the first time that an effect of BTX-A caused by injection into skeletal muscle has peaked at 12 weeks rather than the usual four weeks. Since the primary effect is at the lateral side—an area that has not been injected—we presume that this brow lift is due to partial inactivation of the frontalis and not due to the action on the brow depressors, as previously thought. The subsequent central and medial eyebrow elevation could be due to the resetting of the "tone" in the frontalis, causing a gradual lift. Although further investigation is necessary to fully understand the complex, functional interrelationships and, therefore, the control mechanisms involved, we believe that the above data constitute a major advance in our understanding.

Eyebrow Asymmetry and Shaping

Eyebrow asymmetry can be caused by a number of scenarios, including facial nerve trauma following surgical brow lifts, other surgically induced facial paralysis, and habit in those with ipsilateral blepharoptosis and asymmetric nonpathologic facial expression (25). Injection of BTX-A into the frontalis (or overlying) muscle approximately 1 cm above the eyebrow can be an alternative to surgery in patients who desire a more symmetrical appearance.

Injection of BTX-A for glabellar frown lines can cause a mild medial brow ptosis and induce a lateral brow elevation, which gives a more pleasing contour to the eyebrow. Since the lateral, orbital aspect of the orbicularis oculi muscle above the lateral retinaculum serves as an antagonist muscle to the lateral frontalis muscle, adept clinicians can procure the effects of mild brow elevation, creatively improving the shape and position of the eyebrows (25).

CHEMODENERVATION IN THE MID AND LOWER FACE AND NECK

The cosmetic injection of BTX-A in the mid- and lower face and neck has opened up a new avenue of artistry in facial contouring and sculpting. However, previous experience in the indications for its use in the upper face, complete understanding of the resting, dynamic muscular anatomy of the face, and location of the neurovascular bundles are mandatory prior to injection. Incorrect injection can result in catastrophic impairment of function and expression, and the use of electromyographic (EMG) guidance in some patients is recommended (26).

Mid-Face

Crow's Feet

Lateral canthal rhytides are accentuated by contraction of the orbicularis oculi, whose fibers run vertically under the skin at the lateral angles of the eyelids. BTX-A injected subdermally or intradermally relaxes the action of the muscle without completely inactivating the orbicularis oculi, which could interfere with the ability to fully close the eye. Total doses used range from 4 to 5 U per eye to 5 to 15 U per eye over two or three injection sites. We use 12 to 15 U per side, distributed in equal parts over two to four injection sites, and recommend using as few and as superficial injections as possible to minimize bruising (26). Results generally last for three to six months, with few adverse effects noted.

Hypertrophic Orbicularis

Widening the palpebral aperture is part of the new "artistry" of BTX-A in facial contouring and sculpting. In some patients, the act of smiling transiently diminishes the perceived size of the palpebral aperture, especially in

Asian patients, who sometimes desire a more round-eyed, "Western" appearance. Injecting 2 U of BTX-A into the lower pretarsal orbicularis will relax the palpebral aperture at rest and while smiling (26). In a study of 15 women, Flynn et al. (27) injected 2 U subdermally, 3 mm inferior to the lower pretarsal orbicularis, in addition to three injections of 4 U 1.5 cm from the lateral canthus, each 1 cm apart (27). Mean palpebral aperture increase in 86% of patients was 1.8 mm at rest and 2.9 mm at full smile, and results were more dramatic in the Asian eye (Fig. 2). However, be careful to select patients who have had a good preinjection snap test and who have not had lower eyelid ablative resurfacing or infralash blepharoplasties without a coexisting canthopexy to support the normal position of the lower eyelid. Goldman (28) reports a case of a 56-year-old man who developed festooning of the infraocular area two to three days following injections of 10 and 2 U BTX-A in the mid-lateral canthal region and 2 to 3 mm below the ciliary margin mid-pupillary line, respectively.

Nasalis

Frequent contraction of the upper nasalis, which runs from the bony dorsum of the nose inferiorly, contributes to the development of fanning, radial rhytides obliquely across the radix of the nose called as "bunny lines." Treatment allows the underlying mimetic musculature to relax, softening the lines. BTX-A is injected anterior to the nasofacial groove on the lateral wall of the nose and well above the angular vein, and massaged gently afterward to help diffuse the toxin. Injecting in the nasofacial groove is avaided as it can affect the levator labii superioris and levator labii superioris aleque nasi. The lower nasalis fibers drape over the lateral nasal ala and hence can lead to repeated nasal flare, in which the nostrils dilate involuntarily in social situations and give patients the embarrassing appearance of a racehorse. Injection into the lower nasalis fibers will weaken this involuntary action.

(A)   **(B)**

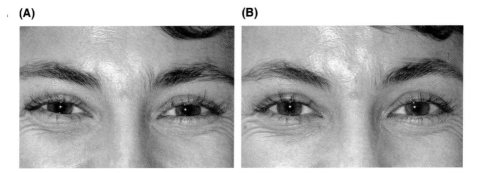

Figure 2
This individual has had 2 U of BOTOX® injected into the orbicularis oculi in the central lower eyelid. (**A**) Before injection; (**B**) after injection, showing widening of the palpebral aperture on maximum smile.

Nasolabial Folds

The nasolabial folds are the curved lines running from the upper border of the lateral nasal ala to just lateral to the lateral angle of the mouth. Weakening the lip elevator muscles, and zygomaticus and risorius muscles, tempting though it may be, will flatten the mid-face and elongate the upper lip, which may not be a desirable outcome for all patients. In patients who have a naturally shorter upper lip, however, injection of 1 U BTX-A into each lip elevator complex in the nasofacial groove will collapse the upper extent of the nasolabial fold, but also elongate the upper lip. As the effect is long lasting ($\pm$ 6 months), patients should be selected carefully and the aesthetic result of the procedure should be fully explained.

Perioral Lip Rhytides

The orbicularis oris is the sphincter muscle that encircles the mouth, lying between the skin and mucous membranes of the lips and extending upward to the nose and downward to the region between the lower lip and chin. Sometimes called the "kissing" muscle, it causes the lips to close and pucker. Overactive orbicularis oris causes vertical perioral rhytides (which are referred to as "smoker's" or "lipstick" lines but often have numerous causes, such as heredity, photodamage, playing musical instruments that require embouchure, and whistling) that radiate outward from the vermilion border. Very small amounts of BTX-A (1–2 U per lip quadrant) are usually sufficient to result in localized microparesis of the orbicularis oris, especially when used adjunctively with a soft-tissue augmenting agent, and can greatly improve the appearance of the lip without creating a paresis that might interfere with elocution and suction. We usually increase the dilution in this area, injecting a total of 6 U BTX-A (reconstituted in 0.24 mL) in a total of eight injection sites, for 0.75 U in 0.03 mL per injection. Carefully measuring the injection sites to balance on either side of the columella or the lateral nasal ala will help alleviate difficulty with postinjection lip proprioception experienced with some patients. Patients who play wind instruments or patients who are professional singers/speakers may not be ideal candidates.

Mid-Facial Asymmetry

Chemodenervation may be useful in patients with mid-facial asymmetry due to innervational or muscular causes. In hemifacial spasm, for example, repeated clonic and tonic facial movements draw the facial midline toward the hyperfunctional side. Relaxation of the hyperfunctional zygomaticus, risorius, and masseter will allow the face to be centered at rest. Likewise, hypofunctional asymmetry, such as that following VII nerve paresis, requires 1 to 2 U injection in the normofunctional side of the zygomaticus, risorius, and orbicularis, and 5 to 10 U in the masseter. In patients who experience asymmetry of jaw movement, 10 to 15 U BTX-A injected intraorally into the internal pterygoid can relax the jaw and relieve discomfort when chewing and speaking.

Lower Face

Depressor Anguli Oris

The depressor anguli oris (DAO) is an important cosmetic muscle, extending inferiorly from the modiolus to the inferior margin of the mandible on the lateral aspect of the chin. Contraction of the DAO causes a downward turn to the corner of the mouth and a negative appearance. Initially, we injected this muscle directly; however, the DAO overlies the depressor labii inferioris, and many patients suffered intolerable, usually asymmetrical, paresis. We now inject the DAO at the level of the mandible but at its posterior margin, close to the anterior margin of the masseter. While the masseter can be easily felt when the teeth are clenched, many patients have difficulty in contracting the DAO voluntarily, although they use it involuntarily all day. A dose of 3 to 5 U usually significantly weakens this muscle, as this is the aim of treatment and not paralysis (Fig. 3).

Melomental Folds

Melomental folds are deep skin folds that extend from the depressed corner of the mouth to the lateral mentum and have traditionally been treated with soft-tissue augmentation alone. However, the combination of soft-tissue augmentation and BTX-A injection into the DAO will lengthen the duration of the augmentation and prevent the repeated molding and contortion of the soft-tissue augmenting agent.

(A)　　　　　　　　　　　　　　　　**(B)**

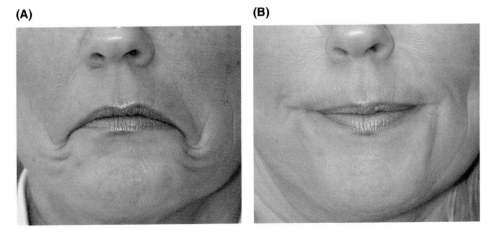

Figure 3
(**A**) shows an individual prior to BTX treatment, forcibly depressing the corners by contracting depressor anguli oris; (**B**) shows an attempt to reproduce this action after injection of 4 U into each depressor anguli oris.

Mental Crease

Softening of the mental crease can be achieved by injecting the mentalis, just anterior to the point of the chin. We initially injected a single dose of 8 to 10 U centrally; however, after observing our patients, it was clear that there are two cutaneous depressions owing to two separate muscles, one on each side of the midline. We now inject 3 to 5 U into each side of the midline under the point of the chin, just anterior to the bony mentum. It is important not to inject at the level of the mental crease, as this will also weaken the lower lip depressors and orbicularis oris, and cause serious adverse effects which can persist for six months or more, depending on the dose. Again, as in the perioral area, weakening rather than paralysis is the aim of treatment. Performing injections as described above will soften many irregularities in this area; especially those created by trauma or surgery, such as chin implant irregularities.

Peau d'Orange Chin

A "peau d'orange" appearance in the chin occurs from a loss of subcutaneous fat and dermal collagen, and is seen when the mentalis and depressor labii muscles are used in speech that requires cocontraction of the orbicularis oris. This was previously treated by soft-tissue augmentation and laser resurfacing. Now, a combination of soft-tissue augmentation and BTX-A injection of the mentalis, or BTX-A injections alone (in those who do not require augmentation) will soften this appearance of the chin.

"Mouth Frown"

Mouth frown—created by permanent downward angulation of the lateral corners of the mouth—is caused by the action of the DAO and the upward motion of the mentalis. We have discussed the injection of the DAO and mentalis separately above, because we initially approached those muscles as separate and distinct areas. However, it is important to look at all muscles *functionally*, as well as *anatomically*, both here and elsewhere. The action of BTX on a single muscle is usually associated with a secondary effect on adjacent muscles, which may produce positive or negative effects. We have found that attempts to weaken the DAO or mentalis alone, while appropriate in some individuals, is ineffective or associated with unacceptable side effects in others. However, if a lower dose of BTX is injected into both muscles at the same time—our optimal treatment for this area at present—the weakening effect is synergistic, and is achieved with fewer side effects. Currently, we inject 3 U of BTX-A into each DAO and each side of the mentalis, for a total of 12 U in a female. This produces a subtle effect which is not as dramatic as the effect in the glabella, where paralysis is the aim in most individuals. We recommend that this technique be used only in individuals who have experienced the effects of BTX in other areas. Patients should be counseled thoroughly, using a hand mirror to demonstrate the aim of treatment, and clinicians should take active and passive photographs, and follow-up two weeks after injection to assess and document the response to treatment, including any side effects.

Lower Facial Asymmetry

In patients who have experienced surgical or traumatic injury to the orbicularis oris or risorius muscle, the unopposed action of the partner muscles in the normally innervated side may lead to decentration of the mouth. BTX-A injected in the overdynamic risorius, immediately lateral to the lateral corner of the mouth, and in the mid-pupillary line will recenter the mouth when the face is in repose. Some patients have congenital or acquired weakness of the DAO, resulting in inability to depress the corner of one side of the mouth; chemodenervation of the partner muscle will restore functional and aesthetic balance.

Masseteric Hypertrophy

BTX-A for contouring in the lower face may be a simple alternative method of shaping the mandible—a relatively common aesthetic procedure among Asians—with a short recovery period, although mostly small studies have published results. To et al. (29) injected 200 to 300 U of Dysport® per side in five patients with unilateral and bilateral hypertrophy of the masseter, and found that three patients needed a secondary injection within one year. von Lindern (30) reported a reduction of the thickness of masseter muscles by half in seven patients with unilateral and bilateral hypertrophy of the masseter and temporalis muscles treated with an average of 100 U of Dysport®. Four patients considered the result satisfactory after a single injection. More recently, Park et al. (31) injected 25 to 30 U BTX-A per side in five to six sites evenly at the prominent portions of the mandibular angle in 45 patients, and found a gradual reduction in masseter thickness during the first three months following injection (average change in masseter thickness, 1.5–2.9 mm, equivalent to 17% to 19% of the original muscle thickness), as measured by ultrasound and computerized tomography. Clinical effects lasted six to seven months following injection before the muscle thickness retreated to its initial size; at 10 months, 36 patients expressed satisfaction with the results. Main local side effects included mastication difficulty, muscle pain, and verbal difficulty during speech, although these effects were relatively transient, lasting from one to four weeks.

Chemodenervation of the Neck

Chemodenervation with BTX-A can be useful in the aging neck, reducing the appearance of necklace lines and platysmal bands.

Necklace Lines

Horizontal necklace lines of skin indentation occur in slightly chubbier necks because of subcutaneous muscular apaneurotic system attachments in the neck. The simplest way to treat these lines is to "dance" along the lines, injecting 1 to 2 U at each site in the deep intradermal plane. Injection is deep dermal, rather than subcutaneous, because there are deeper venous perforators that can bleed, especially lateral in the neck, and the underlying muscles of deglutition are cholinergic and could potentially be affected. Massaging the neck gently after injection can usually prevent bruising. No more than 10 to 20 U is injected per treatment session.

Platysmal Bands

Over time, the cervical skin loses its elasticity, more submental fat becomes visible, and the platysma separates anteriorly, becoming two diverging platysmal bands, the anterior borders of which often tighten and become visible when patients animate their neck as when speaking, exercising, or playing a musical instrument. Kane (32) describes good results of BTX-A for platysmal bands in 44 patients, but cautions that the gold standard for most aging necks remains traditional rhytidectomy surgery. In addition, BTX-A may make platysmal bands appear worse in patients with accompanying jowl formation and bone resorption; it is therefore essential to carefully select patients with obvious platysmal bands, good cervical skin elasticity, and minimal fat descent. Chemodenervation can also be a useful adjunct to traditional facelift surgery (whereby residual postoperative banding that becomes apparent can simply be treated with BTX-A) or as a "rehearsal" for patients not yet ready to undergo traditional rhytidectomy surgery.

The vertically oriented platysmal bands are external to muscles of deglutition and neck flexion. We previously reported one patient treated with 60 U in the neck who developed profound dysphagia, necessitating a nasogastric tube until she could swallow again (26). As additional injections can always be given in subsequent treatments, no more than 30 to 40 U is injected per cervical treatment and caution is exercised.

ADJUNCTIVE THERAPY

BTX-A in conjunction with surgery, soft-tissue augmentation, and laser resurfacing can produce a more polished or refined result and prolongs the effects of other cosmetic procedures. Sometimes there is no replacement for surgery, skin resurfacing, soft-tissue augmentation, or proper skin care; however, neuromodulation has been reported to enhance and increase the duration of other cosmetic procedure results (25).

Surgical Procedures

Since the constant action of facial muscles can interfere with or reverse the results of cosmetic surgery, weakening the muscles with BTX-A before surgery may make it easier to manipulate tissues, allowing for greater surgical correction or better concealment of the surgical incisions. In addition, some experts report that BTX-A during or after the procedure prevented or slowed the return of the wrinkles by reducing the action of the responsible muscles (13).

A variety of BTX-A surgical applications have been reported in the literature. Studies indicate that preoperative relaxation of the muscular brow depressor complex with BTX-A one week prior to brow lift surgery may allow for a greater brow elevation, while postoperative BTX-A may help prolong the benefits of surgery by relaxing the muscles that are working to reestablish the depressed brow (13). Concurrent treatment, BTX-A with periorbital rhytidectomy, has been reported to improve and increase the longevity of the surgical results. Pretreatment of the crow's feet with BTX-A allows the muscles to relax, leading to a more accurate estimation of the amount of skin to be resected during surgery and better placement of the incision (13); excellent improvements in crow's feet by infiltrating a triangular area of the lateral orbicularis oculi have been reported, while the muscle was exposed during blepharoplasty (33). During lower eyelid ectropion and "roundeye" repair, the use of BTX-A transiently weakens the lateral fibers of the orbicularis, which can pull on the medial side of the temporal incision and lead to dehiscence after surgery (13).

Soft-Tissue Augmentation

As previously discussed, BTX-A is used routinely as adjunctive therapy in soft-tissue augmentation to achieve more effective, longer-lasting results, especially in the mid- and lower face. Fagien and Brandt (25) found that BTX-A in patients undergoing soft-tissue augmentation in certain facial areas, (i.e., deep glabellar furrows or lip augmentation) eliminated or reduced the muscular activity responsible for the wrinkles and increased the longevity of the filling agent, such as dermal filler or fat. In a prospective, randomized study of 38 patients with moderate-to-severe glabellar rhytides, BTX-A plus nonanimal stabilized hyaluronic acid (NASHA) led to a better response both at rest and on maximum frown than NASHA (Restylane®, Medicis Aesthetics, Scottsdale, Arizona, U.S.) alone (34). In addition, combination therapy led to a longer duration of response: the median time for return to preinjection furrow status occurred at 18 weeks in the NASHA alone or BTX-A alone groups, compared to 32 weeks in patients treated with BTX-A plus NASHA.

Laser Resurfacing

The adjunctive use of BTX-A with laser resurfacing leads to superior and longer-lasting outcomes and aids the healing of newly resurfaced skin long enough to effect more permanent eradication of wrinkles (13,25), and regular postoperative injections, given every 6 to 12 months, prolong the effects of resurfacing (35). West and Alster (36) found an enhanced and longer-lasting improvement of forehead, glabellar, and canthal rhytides when BTX-A injections were given postoperatively in conjunction with CO_2 laser resurfacing, compared to patients who received laser resurfacing alone. Lowe et al. (37) compared the safety and efficacy of ablative laser resurfacing combined with BTX-A, with that of a placebo for the treatment of crow's feet. BTX-A in conjunction with ablative resurfacing resulted in significantly higher treatment success rates compared with laser alone.

COMPLICATIONS

The complications associated with the aesthetic use of BTX-A are few and anecdotal, and there have been no reported long-term adverse effects or health hazards following its use for any cosmetic indication (38). Most complications are relatively uncommon and are related to poor injection techniques.

Upper Face Complications

Generally, proper injection techniques and patient selection can avoid the most worrisome complications in the upper face—namely brow and lid ptosis and asymmetrical changes to the appearance of the eyebrows.

Brow Ptosis

Brow ptosis, which occurs when the injected toxin affects the frontalis during glabellar or brow treatment, is one of the most undesirable adverse events and is related to poor injection technique. In general, a higher concentration allows for more accurate placement, greater duration of effect, and fewer side effects, since lower concentrations encourage the spread of toxin; there is an area of denervation associated with each point of injection due to toxin spread of about 1 to 1.5 cm (diameter, 2 to 3 cm). All patients are advised to remain upright for two hours and to exercise the treated muscles as much as possible for the first four hours (38). Patients must be advised strictly to avoid rubbing or massaging the injected area for two hours following the treatment.

Brow ptosis can be annoying, lasting for up to three months creating a very negative appearance, and is avoided by proper selection of patients (BTX-A works best in younger patients, aged 20–45 years) and preinjection of the brow depressors if necessary (i.e., in patients with low-set brows, mild brow ptosis, and patients over the age of 50 years) (38). It is important to remember that the brow shape can be changed, and lack of expressivity may be caused by injection of the frontalis lateral to the mid-pupillary line. BTX-A is injected above the lowest fold produced when the patient elevates his or her frontalis and limit the treatment of forehead lines is limited to the portion 3 cm or more above the brow. Injecting the glabella and the whole forehead in one session is more likely to produce brow ptosis (38). Mild brow ptosis responds to apraclonidine (Iopidine® 0.5%), alpha-adrenergic agonist ophthalmic eye drops that stimulate Muller's muscle, which can be helpful for the distressed patient.

Cocked Eyebrow or "Mr. Spock" Eyebrow

A quizzical or "cockeyed" appearance can occur in the brow when the lateral fibers of the frontalis muscle have not been injected appropriately, and the untreated lateral fibers of frontalis pull upward on the brow. To rectify, a small amount of BTX is injected into the fibers of the lateral forehead that are pulling upward; overcompensation can lead to an unsightly hooded brow that partially covers the eye (38).

Upper Eyelid Ptosis

Upper eyelid ptosis, most commonly seen after the treatment of the glabellar complex, occurs when the toxin diffuses through the orbital septum, affecting the upper eyelid levator muscle. Ptosis can appear in as early as 48 hours or as late as 14 days after injection, and can persist from 2 to 12 weeks (38). Again, eyelid ptosis has been linked to poor injection technique; injection of large volumes is avoided, accurately place injections are accurately placed no closer than 1 cm above the central bony orbital rim, and patients are advised to remain upright and not to manipulate the injected area for several hours after injection. BTX-A is not injected at or under the mid-brow (38). Eyelid ptosis can be treated by using apraclonidine, which elevates the lid by 1 to 2 mm and compensates the loss of levator palpebrae superioris (Fig. 4). One or two drops three times a day can be continued until the ptosis resolves. However, it is important to note that allergic contact dermatitis can occur with the use of apraclonidine.

Periorbital Complications

Bruising, diplopia, ectropion, or a drooping lateral lower eyelid and an asymmetrical smile (caused by the spread of toxin to the zygomaticus major) are all reported complications of BTX-A in the periorbital area. It is to be injected laterally at least 1 cm outside the bony orbit or 1.5 cm lateral to the lateral canthus; not close to the inferior margin of the zygoma. Ecchymoses can be reduced by injecting superficially in a

(A)   **(B)**

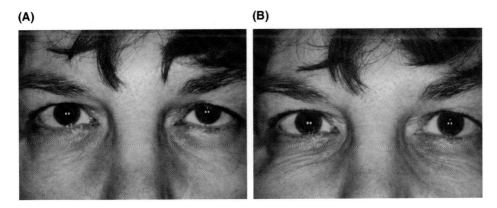

Figure 4
(**A**) shows an individual with mild, left-sided eyelid ptosis following BTX injection. (**B**) shows an image taken 20 minutes later, after two drops of 0.5% apraclonidine were applied to the left eye.

wheal or a series of continuous blebs, avoiding blood vessels by placing each injection at the advancing border of the previous injection.

Injecting the infraorbital orbicularis can produce significant benefit in younger individuals, but the reverse may occasionally be true, especially in older individuals. Patients who are not good candidates are those who exhibit a significant degree of scleral show pretreatment, who have had significant surgery under the eye, who have a great deal of redundant skin beneath the eye, or who have a slow snap test of the lower eyelid, indicating increased lid laxity (38). The vast majority of individuals treated in this area are female, and clinically significant dry eyes are a major problem in this group. Questioning patients about dry eye symptoms (such as whether they experience dry eyes during air travel) may identify individuals who will experience an exacerbation of these symptoms with weakening of the infraorbital orbicularis oculi. If in doubt, a Schirmer's test should be performed.

Lower Face and Cervical Complications

Studies of the lower face report complications such as effects on muscle function and facial expression, usually due to overenthusiastic use of BTX-A in large doses (38). Starting with low doses and injecting more superficially rather than deeply, limits the potential for complications (such as drooling and asymmetry), and injections should be symmetrical to ensure uniform postinjection movement. Injections are avoided in singers, musicians, or other patients who use their perioral muscles with intensity. When injecting the DAO, areas too close to the mouth, injection into the mental fold, and interaction with the orbicularis oris are avoided, as these all of which can result in a flaccid cheek, incompetent mouth, or asymmetric smile. Large doses (greater than 100 U) of BTX-A in the platysma have resulted in reports of dysphagia and weakness of the neck flexors.

CONCLUSION

With wider acceptance and clinical experience, chemodenervation is being applied to increasingly more difficult and complex indications. Treatment of the upper face with BTX-A is no longer considered novel, and once a thorough understanding of the resting and dynamic musculature of the face has been achieved, clinicians are able to branch out into the aesthetic artistry of facial contouring and sculpting. Moreover, the adjunctive use of BTX-A has taken its place in many cosmetic protocols, enhancing or prolonging the effects of other procedures and achieving more aesthetically pleasing results.

REFERENCES

1. Product monograph. BOTOX Cosmetic™ (botulinum toxin type A for injection) purified neurotoxin complex. Markham, Ontario: Allergan Inc., 2001.
2. Carruthers JA, Lowe NJ, Menter MA, Gibson J, Nordquist M, Mordaunt J, Walker P, Eadie N. A multicentre, double-blind, randomized, placebo-controlled study of the efficacy and safety of botulinum toxin type A in the treatment of glabellar lines. J Am Acad Dermatol 2002; 46:840–849.
3. Ramirez AL, Reeck J, Maas CS. Botulinum toxin type B (Myobloc) in the management of hyperkinetic facial lines. Otolaryngol Head Neck Surg 2002; 126:459–467.
4. Sadick NS. Botulinum toxin type B (Myobloc) for glabellar wrinkles: a prospective open-label response study. Dermatol Surg 2003; 29(5):519–522.
5. Sadick NS. Prospective open-label study of botulinum toxin type B (Myobloc) at doses of 2400 and 3000 units for the treatment of glabellar wrinkles. Dermatol Surg. In press 2003.
6. Alster TS, Lupton JR. Botulinum toxin type B for dynamic glabellar rhytides refractory to botulinum toxin type A. Dermatol Surg. In press 2003.
7. Lowe N, Lask G, Yamauchi P. Efficacy and safety of botulinum toxins A and B for the reduction of glabellar rhytids in female subjects. Presented at the American Academy of Dermatology 2002 Winter Meeting. New Orleans, LA, Feb 22–27, 2002.
8. Matarasso SL. Comparison of botulinum toxin types A and B: a bilateral and double-blind randomized evaluation in the treatment of canthal rhytides. Dermatol Surg 2003; 29:7–13.
9. Klein AW. Dilution and storage of botulinum toxin. Dermatol Surg 1998; 24:1179–1180.
10. Hexsel DM, Trindade de Almeida A, Rutowitsch M, Alencar de Castro I, Silveira VLB, Gobatto DO, Zechmeister M, Zechmeister D. Multicenter, double-blind study of the efficacy of injections with botulinum toxin type A reconstituted in 6 consecutive weeks. Dermatol Surg. In press 2003.
11. Huang W, Foster JA, Rogachefsky AS. Pharmacology of botulinum toxin. J Am Acad Dermatol 2000; 43:249–259.
12. Alam M, Dover JS, Arndt KA. Pain associated with injection of botulinum A exotoxin reconstituted using isotonic sodium chloride with and without preservative: a double-blind, randomized controlled trial. Arch Dermatol 2002; 138:510–514.
13. Carruthers A, Carruthers J. Botulinum toxin type A: history and current cosmetic use in the upper face. Semin Cutan Med Surg 2001; 20:71–84.
14. Carruthers A, Carruthers J. Dose dilution and duration of effect of botulinum toxin type A (BTX-A) for the treatment of glabellar rhytids. Presented at the American Academy of Dermatology 2002 Winter Meeting. New Orleans, LA, Feb 22–27, 2002.
15. Package insert. Dysport®: Clostridium botulinum type A toxin-haemagglutinin complex. Maidenhead, Berkshire, UK: Ipsen Limited.
16. Package insert. MYOBLOC™ (botulinum toxin type B) injectable solution. San Francisco, CA: Elan Pharmaceuticals, Inc.
17. Carruthers A, Carruthers J, Said S. Dose-ranging study of botulinum toxin type A in the treatment of glabellar lines. Presented at the 20th World Congress of Dermatology. Paris, France, July 1–5, 2002.
18. Carruthers A, Carruthers J. Botulinum toxin type A (BTX-A) in the treatment of glabellar rhytids: an objective analysis of treatment response. Presented at the American Academy of Dermatology 2002 Winter Meeting. New Orleans, LA, Feb 22–27, 2002.
19. Carruthers A, Carruthers J. Botulinum toxin type A for treating glabellar lines in men: a dose-ranging study. Presented at the 20th World Congress of Dermatology. Paris, France, July 1–5, 2002.
20. Carruthers A, Carruthers J, Cohen J. Dose dependence, duration of response and efficacy and safety of botulinum toxin type A for the treatment of horizontal forehead rhytids.

Presented at the American Academy of Dermatology 2002 Winter Meeting. New Orleans, LA, Feb 22–27, 2002.

21. Huilgol SC, Carruthers A, Carruthers JDA. Raising eyebrows with botulinum toxin. Dermatol Surg 2000; 25:373–376.

22. Ahn MS, Catten M, Maas CS. Temporal brow lift using botulinum toxin A. Plast Reconstruct Surg 2000; 105:1129–1135.

23. Huang W, Rogachefsky AS, Foster JA. Brow lift with botulinum toxin. Dermatol Surg 2000; 26:55–60.

24. Carruthers A, Carruthers J. Glabella BTX-A injection and eyebrow height: a further photographic analysis. Presented at the Annual Meeting of the American Academy of Dermatology. San Francisco, CA, March 21–26, 2003.

25. Fagien S, Brandt FS. Primary and adjunctive use of botulinum toxin type A (Botox) in facial aesthetic surgery: beyond the glabella. Clin Plast Surg 2001; 28:127–148.

26. Carruthers J, Carruthers A. BOTOX use in the mid and lower face and neck. Semin Cutan Med Surg 2001; 20:85–92.

27. Flynn TC, Carruthers JA, Carruthers JA. Botulinum-A toxin treatment of the lower eyelid improves infraorbital rhytides and widens the eye. Dermatol Surg 2001; 27:703–708.

28. Goldman MP. Festoon formation after infraorbital botulinum A toxin: A case report. Dermatol Surg 2003; 29(5):560–561.

29. To EW, Ahuja AT, Ho WS, King WW, Wong WK, Pang PC, Hui AC. A prospective study of the effect of botulinum toxin A on masseteric muscle hypertrophy with ultrasonographic and electromyographic measurement. Br J Plast Surg 2001; 54:197–200.

30. von Lindern JJ, Niederhagen B, Appel T, Berge S, Reich RH. Type A botulinum toxin for the treatment of hypertrophy of the masseter and temporal muscle: an alternative treatment. Plast Reconstr Surg 2001; 107:327–332.

31. Park MY, Ahn KY, Jung DS. Botulinum toxin type A treatment for contouring of the lower face. Dermatol Surg 2003; 29(5):477–483.

32. Kane MA. Nonsurgical treatment of platysmal bands with injection of botulinum toxin A. Plast Reconstr Surg 1999; 103:656–663.

33. Guerrissi JO. Intraoperative injection of botulinum toxin A into orbicularis oculi muscle for the treatment of crow's feet. Plast Reconstr Surg 2000; 105:2219–2228.

34. Carruthers J, Carruthers A. A prospective, randomized, parallel group study analyzing the effect of BTX-A (BOTOX®) and nonanimal sourced hyaluronic acid (NASHA, Restylane®) in combination compared with NASHA (Restylane®) alone in severe glabellar rhytides in adult female subjects: Treatment of severe glabellar rhytides with a hyaluronic acid derivative compared with the derivative and BTX-A. Dermatol Surg 2003; 29(5):802–809.

35. Carruthers J, Carruthers A, Zelichowska A. The power of combined therapies: Botox and ablative facial laser resurfacing. Am J Cos Surg 2000; 17:129–131.

36. West TB, Alster TS. Effect of botulinum toxin type A on movement-associated rhytides following CO_2 laser resurfacing. Dermatol Surg 1999; 25:259–261.

37. Lowe N, Lask G, Yamauchi P, Moore D, Patnaik R. Botulinum toxin type A (BTX-A) and ablative laser resurfacing (Erbium: YAG): a comparison of efficacy and safety of combination therapy vs. ablative laser resurfacing alone for the treatment of crow's feet. Presented at the American Academy of Dermatology 2002 Summer Meeting. New York, NY, July 31–August 4, 2002.

38. Klein AW. Complications and adverse reactions with the use of botulinum toxin. Dermatol Surg 2003; 29(5):549–555.

3

Soft-Tissue Augmentation: Skin Fillers

Jaggi Rao and Janna Bentley
University of Alberta, Edmonton, Alberta, Canada

Mitchel P. Goldman
Department of Dermatology/Medicine, University of California, San Diego, California, U.S.A. and La Jolla Spa MD, La Jolla, California, U.S.A.

Video 2: Skin Fillers

INTRODUCTION

In today's society, individuals are living longer and healthier lives, and as such, the demand for preservation of a more youthful visage has caused a significant growth in the fields of facial rejuvenation and soft-tissue augmentation. It has been estimated that there has been a greater than three-fold increase in total cosmetic procedures from 1992 to 2002 (1). Baby boomers (ages 40–58) account for the largest generational group globally, estimated at 80 million in 2004 (2).

In the past, a youthful appearance was sought through invasive surgical face-lifting techniques. However, there has been a shift in the perception of what constitutes a youthful appearance. Physicians and their patients have moved away from the tight, "pulled back" two-dimensional looks achieved via facelifts and other surgical procedures. The new movement has been toward more conservative approaches that deal with the underlying loss of soft tissue to achieve a plumper, less wrinkled, more three-dimensional appearance. This shift in the perception of the "youthful visage," combined with patient demand for minimally invasive procedures, has led to a major expansion in the field of soft-tissue augmentation.

As we age, our skin is assaulted by the forces of gravity, sun damage, and chronic facial animation, all leading to significant wrinkling, textural distortion, and poor elasticity. There is also loss of dermal thickness and subcutaneous fat, and skeletal and muscular atrophy. The aged face has prominent rhytides in the glabella, forehead, nasolabial folds, and perioral areas. Aging of the lips results in diminished labial volume, circumoral radial grooves, and a "down-turning" at each labial commissure. Subtle enhancement of the lips and filling of the deeper rhytides and

39

folds can produce very significant cosmetic improvement. In addition to stand-alone therapy, the use of exogenous filling agents has expanded to complement other rejuvenative technologies such as botulinum toxin, laser treatment, and intense pulsed light therapy.

Background

The practice of soft-tissue implantation has a long, well-described history since its employment over a century ago. Today, it is a crucial tool in the armamentarium of facial rejuvenation. In 2002, the use of injectable fillers was ranked third in the top five nonsurgical cosmetic procedures, by the American Society for Aesthetic Plastic Surgery (2). Over the last several years, the search for an ideal filling agent has led to a plethora of new agents. There are approximately 40 agents currently being used worldwide. These agents consist of many different biologic and alloplastic materials that can be injected with ease into the dermis and subcutis, and with minimal side effects.

Soft-tissue fillers are indicated for the treatment of cutaneous and subcutaneous defects and deficiencies, revision of depressed scars, improvement in facial contouring, and reduction in facial rhytides and skin folds. Ideally, injectable fillers should be inexpensive, biocompatible, nontoxic, noncarcinogenic, nonimmunogenic, nonallergenic, and non-migratory with long-lasting effects (3).

Although a filling material that satisfies all of the above criteria is yet to be found, there are numerous compounds that fall just short of doing so and are safely and easily administered in the office setting. The most popular of the agents used in the United States are bovine collagen, humanized collagen, and hyaluronic acid (HA) derivatives. The choice of filling substance depends on the type and depth of the target to be treated as well as various patient factors. Health care providers must be judicious, always informing patients of the risks and benefits of treatment and advocating appropriate test doses if necessary to avoid or minimize potential adverse events. Moreover, it is important for injectors to be aware of the various agents available, including their indications and shortcomings, to offer the best available treatment to their patients. Table 1 presents a list of injectable filler products used worldwide at the time of writing.

Classification

Filling agents can be classified according to their longevity in vivo. A histologic comparison study of 10 different soft-tissue fillers for biocompatibility and durability is summarized in Table 2. Temporary fillers can be expected to exert their effects for less than one year. Table 3 lists the temporary fillers available at the time of writing, summarizing key advantages, disadvantages, and regulatory status of each. By definition, permanent fillers maintain their desired effect for greater than one year. Table 4

(*Text continues p. 45.*)

Table 1
Exogenous Soft-Tissue Fillers

Achyal®	Endoplast-50®	Permacol®
AlloDerm®	Evolution®	Plasmagel®
Artecoll®/Artefill®	Fascian®	PMS-350®
Aquamid®	Fibrel®	Profill®
Autologen®	Fibroquel®	Resoplast®
Biocell Ultravital®	Gore-Tex®	Restylane®
Bioplastique®	Human placental collagen	Restylane–Fine Lines®
Captique®	Hylaform® Gel (Hylan B®)	Reviderm Intra®
Recombinant human	Hylan Rofilan® Gel	Sculptra®
collagen: CosmoDerm®,	Isolagen®	Silicone: AdatoSil-5000®,
CosmoPlast®	Juvederm®	Silikon® 1000
Cymetra®	Koken®	Subcision®
Dermal grafting	Atelocollagen®	Zyderm I®
Dermalive®	Meta-Crill®	Zyderm II®
Dermalogen®	Newfill®	Zyplast®
	Perlane®	

Table 2
Histological Comparison of the Biocompatibility and Durability of 10 Commercially
Available Soft-Tissue Fillers

Injectable	Result (in months after procedure)
Zyplast®	Phagocytosed at 6 mo
Restylane®	Phagocytosed at 9 mo
Artecoll®	Encapsulated with connective tissue, macrophages, and sporadic giant cells
PMS-350 (Silicone oil)	Clinically inconspicuous, but dissipated into tissue causing chronic foreign body reaction
Sculptra®	Mild inflammatory response; disappeared clinically at 4 mo
Reviderm Intra® (dextran microspheres)	Pronounced foreign body reaction; disappeared at 6 mo
Dermalive® (HA and acrylic hydrogel)	Induced lowest cellular reaction but disappeared clinically at 6 mo
Aquamid®	Well tolerated and remained palpable, although to lessening degree, over entire testing period; histologically kept in place by fine fibrous capsules
Evolution® (polyvinylhydroxide microspheres suspended in acrylamide)	Well tolerated; slowly diminished over 9 mo
Radiance FN®	Negligible foreign body reaction, but absorbed by skin at 12 mo

Source: From Ref. 63.

Table 3
Temporary Soft-Tissue Fillers

Injectable	Description	Advantages	Disadvantages	Regulatory status
Bovine-based collagen				
Koken Atelocollagen®	Japanese based; no lidocaine in admixture		Skin testing required	Non-FDA approved
Resoplast®			Skin testing required	Non-FDA approved
Zyderm®/Zyplast®	Zyderm® used for more superficial rhytides; Zyplast® best for deeper defects	Well known in the United States; last 3 to 18 mo, with touch-ups at 2 to 3 mo	Skin testing required; rare reports of cyst/abscess formation	FDA approved
Porcine-based collagen				
Permacol®	Acellular cross-linked porcine collagen and elastin fibers	Less immunogenic than bovine collagen	Skin testing required	Non-FDA approved
Human tissue–derived collagen				
Autologen®	Prepared from patient's own skin	No skin testing required; can be refrigerated up to 6 mo	Bruising; costly; time intense; more painful compared to bovine alternatives; multiple treatments needed	No longer available
CosmoDerm®/CosmoPlast®	Human dermal collagen allograft	No skin testing required	Shorter duration of effect; bruising	FDA approved
Cymetra® (Micronized Alloderm)	Micronized human dermal allograft, derived cadaverically	No skin testing required	Bruising; multiple treatments needed; more discomfort	FDA approved

Dermalogen®	Prepared from cadaveric tissue screened for contaminants	No skin testing required (controversial); longer-term filling with multiple injections	More painful compared to bovine alternatives; multiple treatments needed	Manufacturing stopped
Fascian®	Cadaveric donor of thigh connective tissue	Causes stimulation of native collagen; no skin testing required	Bruising; lumpy result on superficial injection	FDA approved
Human-derived product				
Isolagen®	Cultured autologous fibroblasts from patient's own 3 mm punch biopsy	No skin testing required	Costly; less data available	Non-FDA approved
HA based				
Hylaform®/Hylan B® Gel	Extracted from rooster combs	May last longer than bovine counterparts	Possible allergic reaction if avian allergies	FDA approved for filling moderate to severe perinasal or oral wrinkles
Perlane®	Non-animal derived; from streptococcal bacteria fermentation	Useful for deeper defects and lip augmentations, isovolemic degradation	Redness, swelling, itching at site of injection	FDA approval pending
Restylane®	Non-animal derived; from streptococcal bacteria fermentation	Isovolemic degradation, malleable, lasts longer than collagen	Redness, swelling, itching at site of injection	FDA approved for filling moderate to severe perinasal or oral wrinkles
Juvederm®	Non-animal derived; from streptococcal bacteria fermentation	Useful for finer defects, isovolemic degradation	Redness, swelling, itching at site of injection	Non-FDA approved

Abbreviation: FDA, Food and Drug Administration.

Table 4
Permanent Soft-Tissue Fillers

Injectable	Description	Advantages	Disadvantages	Regulatory status
PMMA Artecoll® /Artefill®	25% PMMA microspheres suspended in 75% bovine collagen	Manufacturer claims microspheres not degraded; native collagen forms around product; low incidence of granuloma formation (<0.01%)	Bovine allergy testing required; not to used in areas of thin skin; difficult to remove; may migrate; higher viscosity, thus more technique dependent	Non-FDA approved
Hydroxyapatite Radiesse FN® (Bioform)	Derived from CaHA, found in teeth and bone	Low risk for allergic reaction; native collagen forms around product	May clump; migration possible; if injected next to bone, may get new bone formation/ calcification	FDA approval only for urinary incontinence and vocal cord paralysis
Poly-L-lactic acid Sculptra®	Microspheres of synthetic polylactic acid	Facial volume successfully restored in people with HIV facial lipoatrophy	Granulomas reported; may appear lumpy; erythema; bruising	FDA approval for facial reconstruction in patients with facial lipoatrophy
Polyacrylamide Aquamid®	2.5% polyacrylamide polymer with 97.5% water	Theoretical lower risk of lumpy result due to less provocation of inflammatory response	Minimal data published; monomeric form teratogenic and neurotoxic	Non-FDA approved
Silicone AdatoSil 5000®	Polymer of dimethylpoly-siloxane	Induces fibrous capsule formation causing soft-tissue augmentation	Granulomatous reactions reported; may cause skin necrosis, hardening of the skin; migration and ulceration with large doses reported	FDA approved for ophthalmologic devices
Silikon 1000®	As above	As above	As above	As above

lists the currently available permanent fillers and also compares their main features and regulatory status.

This chapter focuses on the more common biologic and alloplastic agents developed for soft-tissue augmentation. The nature of these agents, their indications and contraindications for usage, as well as their adverse effects are presented in the following sections in groups, according to their duration of effect.

TEMPORARY FILLERS

Bovine-Based Collagen

Bovine collagen was the first soft-tissue filler approved by the Food and Drug Administration (FDA) for facial augmentation in 1981 and is among the most popular substances used for soft-tissue augmentation in the United States. Bovine collagen was first extracted from fresh calf-skin in 1959 by Gross and Kirk at Harvard Medical School (4). It was not discovered until the mid 1960s that the selective removal of the non-helical amino and carboxyl terminal peptides significantly reduced immunogenicity.

The first human trial of injectable bovine collagen filler was conducted by Knapp and Kaplan at Stanford University jointly in the departments of dermatology and plastic surgery in 1977, where investigators reported 50% to 85% improvement in cosmetics of scars, wrinkles, and subcutaneous atrophy lasting 3 to 18 months (5). In a subsequent clinical trial, over 5000 patients were treated with injectable bovine collagen which established excellent clinical correction of rhytides, acne scars, and lip defects. This study also established that 3% of the population had a positive test-dose response, indicating an allergy to bovine collagen (6).

It should be noted that not all scars are correctable with collagen. A stretch test should be performed prior to using these products and other fillers in general, to determine the likelihood of success. Scars that do not flatten out on stretching will not respond because of the underlying stromal tethering (7).

Bovine collagen is manufactured by INAMED Aesthetics (Santa Barbara, California, U.S.) in the form of Zyderm® I, Zyderm® II, and Zyplast® (ZC-1, ZC-2, and ZP). The bovine stock is harvested from a closed American herd, and therefore contamination with bovine spongiform encephalopathy virus or prions is not a concern and has never been noted in over 25 years of use. Zyderm® was FDA approved in 1981 after over six years of clinical trials. This was the first ever xenogenic compound approved by the FDA for soft-tissue augmentation.

Zyderm®/Zyplast®

Zyderm® collagen implantables differ only in the percentage and cross-linking of collagen they contain. Zyderm® I (ZC-1) contains 3.5% bovine collagen (which is 95% type I collagen) and Zyderm® II (ZC-2) contains 6.5% bovine collagen. Both are suspended in phosphate-buffered solution with 0.3% lidocaine. Zyplast® collagen contains 3.5% bovine collagen processed with 0.0075% glutaraldehyde, to cause cross-linking of collagen, which is protective against proteolytic breakdown and is less immunogenic (8). Zyplast® is therefore favored for deeper subcutaneous defects over ZC-1 and ZC-2.

Contraindications to injection with bovine collagen include a history of bovine collagen hypersensitivity (positive test-dose reaction), autoimmune disease, lidocaine hypersensitivity, and anaphylactoid reactions. Relative contraindications include immunosuppressive medications, active inflammatory disease, and active infection (9).

Adverse events are characterized as hypersensitive and non-hypersensitive. The former include erythema and edema of the injection site and, rarely, mild systemic responses. Hypersensitivity reactions have been shown to be associated with anti-Zyderm® antibodies (10). The formation of cysts and small abscesses has rarely been reported at injection sites. Patients who develop this type of complication have a high presence of antibovine antibodies (11). Non-hypersensitive adverse reactions include edema, purpura, local tissue necrosis, and infection, as well as herpes simplex exacerbation (11). Necrosis in the area of injection rarely occurs with treatment of the glabellar region (12). Symptoms include early blanching of the treatment site and pain. If these occur, injection should be discontinued immediately and topical nitroglycerin paste should be applied. There are also isolated case reports of bovine collagen injection causing loss of vision, likely secondary to a vascular occlusion event involving the retinal artery (13). There is no evidence that bovine collagen has a causative role in the induction of autoimmune diseases in humans (14).

Bovine collagen should be available in preloaded syringes and is stored at 4°C, thus preventing cross-linking and premature transformation to a solid gel. Transformation to a solid gel is optimal when it occurs once the product has reached the body temperature.

Skin testing is necessary prior to treatment with bovine collagen; it accurately determines potential allergenicity. The test-dose syringes are preloaded with 0.3 cc of material and are given in the tuberculin skin test style with administration of the material intradermally in the volar aspect of the forearm. Evaluation of the site should be undertaken at 48 to 72 hours post-injection and then again at four weeks. A positive skin test will show signs of erythema, induration, tenderness, or edema at the site of injection and is a contraindication to treatment in the 3% of the population that develop it. Delayed hypersensitivity reactions may also occur, and therefore, we and most other authors advocate a second skin test prior to treatment using the contralateral forearm two to four weeks after the first test dose (15). It is recommended that a single repeat test be done on patients who have been successfully treated for more than two years, prior to administration at another treatment center (14).

Zyderm® (I and II) is injected intradermally via a 30- or 32-gauge needle into the superficial papillary dermis and mid-dermis, while Zyplast® is administered in the deep reticular dermis. Injection of Zyplast® into the superficial dermis has been shown to have undesirable sequelae such as beading and nodule formation (7). Injection technique is the most important factor influencing the outcome of the treatment. Many experienced injectors feel that ZC-1 is the most versatile form of bovine collagen as it is the most forgiving and has less association with beading and overcorrection (14).

Implants usually last three to six months depending on the area injected; however, most experienced users report that touch-ups are generally required at two to three months. Specific indications for Zyderm® include horizontal forehead lines, glabellar lines, crow's feet, nasolabial folds, circumoral and marionette lines, and shallow acne scarring (16). Zyplast® is best for deeper defects such as the nasolabial folds and deep acne scarring. Overcorrection with ZC-1 and ZC-2 by 50% is necessary because of resorption of water in the mixture in the first 24 hours.

Resoplast®

Resoplast® (non-FDA approved) is produced by Rofil Medical International (Breda, Holland) and is another form of bovine collagen. As with the American Zyderm® collagen, a closed herd of healthy animals in Germany is used to derive the calfskins for this product. An effort is made to reduce antigenicity by using formaldehyde for processing the collagen, and neither hormones nor antibiotics are part of the cattle diet. It is available in 3.5% and 6.5% concentrations monomolecular collagen in solution. Skin testing is required. Indications and injection techniques are similar to that of Zyderm® and Zyplast®. The company claims less than a 0.5% risk of allergic reaction, and the intradermal implants last three to six months. Lidocaine is not added to the preloaded syringes, and thus, concurrent use of topical anesthetic or nerve blocks is recommended.

Koken Atelocollagen®

Koken Atelocollagen® (non-FDA approved) is a Japan-based bovine collagen material from Australia-bred calves, and is produced by Koken Corporation Ltd. (Tokyo, Japan). There is widespread use in Asia of this particular compound. On synthesizing Koken Atelocollagen®, the telopeptides found on raw collagen are removed, thus diminishing its antigenicity. It is available as a 2% solution of monomolecular, nonfibrillar collagen. Koken Atelocollagen® is maintained in a buffered solution but does not contain lidocaine. Koken Atelocollagen® is distributed in preloaded cartridges and is injected via 30-gauge needles. Techniques of injection and indications are similar to those of Zyderm®.

Porcine Collagen

Permacol®

> Permacol® (Tissue Science Laboratories, Aldershot, U.K.) is a non-FDA approved form of purified, sterile, acellular cross-linked porcine collagen and elastin fibers. Essentially, it is an acellular dermal matrix. It is thought to be less immunogenic than bovine collagen; and no hypersensitivity reactions have been reported in a recent case series (17). However, the material is still in phase III clinical trials, and further testing is necessary to establish safety and efficacy. There is currently no published experience with this form of soft-tissue filler to date in the United States.

Human Tissue–Derived Collagen

Autologen®

> Autologen® (Collagenesis, Beverly, Massachusetts, U.S.A.) is an autologous injectable collagen consisting of intact human collagen fibrils derived from the patient's own tissue. It requires extensive harvesting and processing from excisional procedures such as abdonmenoplasty or rhytidectomy (18). Two square inches of skin are excised and are sent to the manufacturer. These are processed to create 1 cc syringes of the patient's own material which can be refrigerated for up to six months (3). Autologen® is available in a 5% solution which is injected through a 30-gauge needle into the dermis. No skin test is necessary, and there is no lidocaine present in the suspension. However, a concurrent topical anesthetic or nerve block is recommended. Clinical results report efficacy similar to that of bovine collagen implants (19). Injection with Autologen® is more painful than injection with bovine collagen (19), and the full clinical duration of the implant has yet to be delineated. Autologen® is currently not available in the United States.

CosmoDerm®/*CosmoPlast*®

> CosmoDerm® and CosmoPlast® are distributed by INAMED Aesthetics (Santa Barbara, California, U.S.A.) and both are purified human-based collagen. They are prepared in a phosphate-buffered physiological saline containing 0.3% lidocaine, and CosmoPlast® is further cross-linked with glutaraldehyde to increase its durability. Because these products are human based, skin testing is not required prior to use. CosmoDerm® is used exactly like Zyderm®-1. An overcorrection of 200% is recommended, except for perioral and periorbital lines. CosmoPlast® should be placed in the mid-to-deep dermis, and is used for correcting deeper rhytides, lip augmentation, and smoothing facial scars. Unlike CosmoDerm®, CosmoPlast® should be used to correct the treated area to 100%, without overcorrection. Long-term studies on safety profiles and quality of the cosmetic result have demonstrated these products to be excellent (20). The authors of this chapter have also utilized CosmoPlast® for tissue augmentation of the dorsal hands with success (Fig. 1).

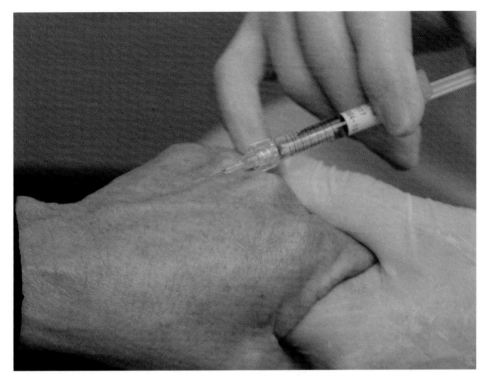

Figure 1
The use of injectable filler for tissue augmentation of the dorsal hands.

Cymetra®

Cymetra® is distributed by LifeCell Corporation (Branchburg, New Jersey, U.S.A.). It is a micronized form of Alloderm. Alloderm is an acellular human dermal allograft prepared in sheets and harvested from tissue banks under sterile conditions. Alloderm is used as a temporary graft in patients with burns or other soft-tissue defects. Cymetra® is injected via dissected dermal tunnels (physical subscision). Prior to injection, the filler is reconstituted using 1 cc of xylocaine. It is implanted via a 26-gauge needle into the subcutis, and the treatment area is gently massaged post-injection. Adverse effects of Cymetra® include transient purpura, erythema, and edema; temporary loss of vision has also been reported. No skin testing is necessary, and the product is FDA approved for the purpose of tissue augmentation.

Dermalogen®

Dermalogen® (Collagenesis Inc., Beverly, Massachusetts, U.S.A.) is a sus pension of injectable human tissue collagen matrix from donor tissue (3). It is very similar to Autologen® except that instead of using the patient's own tissue, the collagen compound is harvested from cadaveric tissue which is screened for viral and bacterial contaminants (21). Collagenesis states that skin testing with Dermalogen® is not necessary and thus, does not supply test syringes. However, a case report describing hypersensitivity and foreign body reaction has been reported (22). Lidocaine is not present in the compound, creating a need for topical anesthetic or nerve block. Dermalogen® is a suspension of collagen fibrils in neutral buffer and is injected similarly to Autologen® via a 30-gauge needle into the superficial dermis. It is manufactured in 3.5% and 2.8% concentrations. Experienced injectors state that the 3.5% concentration is extremely difficult to inject. Dermalogen® should be considered as an option only in those with documented or suspected bovine collagen allergy.

A recent case report of a foreign body, granulomatous reaction to Dermalogen® in a patient desiring lip augmentation was published (22). Dermalogen® was chosen due to concern over the possibility of a past allergic reaction to bovine collagen. A skin test was performed, and at 72 hours there was no reaction; however, at one month post-treatment she developed erythema and induration at the site of implantation. Histologically this was diagnosed to be a foreign body reaction. At two months, the adverse response had resolved without intervention. The patient agreed to have a second test spot of Dermalogen® at a later date, and no early or late adverse reaction occurred.

Even though Collagenesis does not recommend skin testing, this recent case report and experienced injectors' opinion indicate that it would be prudent to perform the regular skin testing with examination of the test site at 48 to 72 hours, and again at four weeks (23).

Fascian®

Fascian® (Medical Aesthetics International, Redmond, Washington, U.S.A.) is a form of particulated fascia lata derived from screened human cadaver specimens. It has been established via clinical trials that particulate fascia lata, when injected intradermally, stimulates native collagen formation in acne scars (24). Fascian® is FDA approved for soft-tissue augmentation. There are three available particle sizes for injection: <2 mm, <0.5 mm, and <0.25 mm. It is reconstituted with 3 cc of 0.3% lidocaine prior to usage, and it is injected via a 16- or 18-gauge needle into the subcutis. Skin testing is not necessary. Due to particle size and product viscosity, some advocate administration via a fat transfer assist syringe device, allowing for more precise control of the microinjection and lessening chances of hematoma formation and tissue damage (25). The product is injected subdermally or intramuscularly for soft-tissue augmentation.

In a study with particulate fascia lata, 81 patients were followed for up to nine months post-injection (26). During this time, no allergic or infectious adverse events occurred, and duration of the soft-tissue augmentation was at least three to four months.

Human Tissue–Derived Noncollagen Product

Isolagen®

Isolagen® is manufactured by Isolagen® Inc. (Exton, Pennsylvania, U.S.A.). It consists of cultured autologous fibroblasts that are isolated and harvested from several 3 mm punch biopsies of the patient's post-auricular skin. These biopsies are sent to the manufacturer, and in six to eight weeks, injections are initiated. Injections of Isolagen® are aimed at the superficial or mid-dermis, and some investigators have performed as many as four injections over a three to six month period (27).

Injections with Isolagen® reportedly have minimal inflammatory or other adverse reactions (27). The product, however, is expensive, and further trials are needed to establish efficacy and practicality. Isolagen® has also been used prior to treatment with biostimulatory lasers such as CoolTouch® (Rosemont, California, U.S.) with excellent results. Isolagen® is presently approved in Australia and England and is awaiting FDA approval in the United States.

HA Compounds

HA-derived fillers were recently developed for the correction of soft-tissue defects and facial contouring via intradermal injection into the dermis. HA is a glycosaminoglycan polysaccharide composed of alternating residues of the monosaccharides D-glucuronic acid and N-acetyl-D-glucosamine forming a linear polysaccharide chain (1). This compound exists as part of the normal constituent of the dermis and provides the elastoviscous matrix within which connective tissue structures are located (1). HA has the ability to attract water and keep the skin firm and moisturized. Glycosaminoglycans, which are abundant in fetal skin, decrease in production with age, leading to fine lines and folds by adulthood (28).

Although HA fillers are nonpermanent, demand is high as patient tolerability is good, and they demonstrate several advantages over other temporary soft-tissue fillers (1). First, HA derivatives confer less risk of immunogenicity because, unlike collagen, HA is chemically identical across all species, eliminating the need for preliminary allergy testing (28). Lowe et al. (29) showed a much lower incidence of allergy (three out of 709, 0.42%) than that reported for collagen (3–4%). HA gels also possess a unique isovolemic pattern of degradation. That is, the HA molecule binds more water as the implant is being degraded within the skin. Hence, its original volume is maintained even with decreasing concentration of the implant. Clinically, this translates into a longer-lasting augmentation effect.

Hyaluronidase has been used by some to correct problems that arise from excessive administration of HA-based products. However from the authors' experience, this is unnecessary. Instead, simple needle puncture (22G) and expression of excess HA or the use of an infrared laser (CoolTouch) or radiofrequency are preferable to break down improperly placed or excessive amounts of HA filler.

Hylaform® Gel, Hylaform–Fine Lines®, and Hylaform Plus® (Hylan B)

Hylaform® Viscoelastic Gel or Hylan B® Gel (Biomatrix, Inc., Ridgefield, New Jersey, U.S.A.) is a sterile, nonpyrogenic, viscoelastic, insoluble, clear, colorless, gel implant derived from rooster combs composed of cross-linked molecules of hyaluronan. Hylaform® is obtained by a chemical cross-linking process using vinyl sulfone in which the hydroxyl groups of the polysaccharide react with each other to form an infinite network through sulfonyl-bis-ethyl-cross-links (28).

The cross-linking agent used is highly soluble in water, which makes it easy to clean the residual chemicals and avian proteins from the gel. The cross-linked hyaluronan forms a gel-like substance, which is then pushed through a sieve, breaking the gel into smaller particles. The smallest particles are packaged into the low-density dermal filler known as Hylaform–Fine Lines®. The medium-sized particles become the product Hylaform®, and the large particles form the high-density product known as Hylaform Plus®. The cross-linking agent and any of the few proteins that remain after processing are largely washed out of the soft, minimally cross-linked matrix.

This gel is well suited for use in dermal augmentation because of its insolubility and resistance to degradation and migration. The high water content mimics the natural hydrating functions of the precursor, HA. The U.S. FDA does not stipulate the requirement for prior skin testing even though this is an avian-derived product. Hylaform® is available in 5.5 mg/mL preloaded 1.0 cc syringes, and is used for lip augmentation and treatment of nasolabial folds.

Adverse reactions are reportedly less than 2%; these include erythema, edema, and purpura at the injection site. One study in guinea pigs showed that tolerability and longevity of this compound were better than that of bovine collagen (30). The authors of this chapter have made direct clinical comparison between Hylaform® and Restylane® for treatment of the nasolabial folds and have found the products to have comparable patient tolerability and overall efficacy (Fig. 2).

Restylane®, Restylane–Fine Lines®, and Perlane®

Restylane®, Restylane–Fine Lines®, and Perlane® (Medicis, Scottsdale, Arizona, U.S.A.) are HA-based soft-tissue fillers derived from *Streptococcus equi* bacterial cultures through fermentation in the presence of sugar. The product is then alcohol precipitated, filtered, and dried. It is cross-linked using a butanediol diglycidyl ether (BDDE) and then heat sterilized.

This highly cross-linked material forms a gel that is stiffer and harder than Hylaform®. The stiffness of the product makes it much more

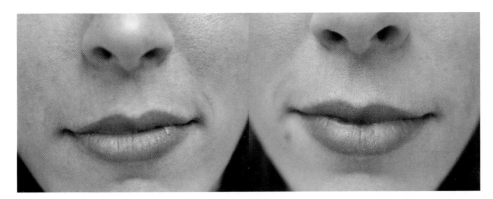

Figure 2
Before and 12 weeks after treatment of Restylane® to the right nasolabial fold
and Hylaform® to the left nasolabial fold.

difficult to wash out the cross-linking chemicals and residual bacterial
proteins. The residual amount of the BDDE cross-linking substance that
remains in the product is thought to lead to the inflammatory reactions
reported with the use of Restylane® and Perlane®. The stiff, gel-like
substance that results after washing and heating the modified HA is then
broken into smaller pieces in a similar fashion as is Hylaform®. The
smallest pieces become Restylane–Fine Lines®, the medium size particles
become Restylane®, and the largest are packaged as Perlane®.

These products have no animal protein components and are
termed "non-animal stabilized hyaluronic acid" (NASHA) derivatives.
Restylane® has been approved in Europe and Canada for the past several
years and used widely in the treatment of rhytides and scars, and in lip
augmentation. It was recently approved for use in the United States (in
December 2003). Restylane® contains 20 mg/mL of partially cross-linked
HA in preloaded 0.4, 0.7, and 1.0 mL syringes. It is injected via a 30-gauge
needle usually under local anesthetic.

Restylane–Fine Lines® is a new, less viscous form of injectable HA
preloaded for use with a 32-gauge needle. It is indicated for finer rhytides
and injected into the superficial dermis.

Perlane® is a more robust form of NASHA and prepackaged in
0.7 mL syringes for injection into the deep dermis/subcutis via a 27-gauge
needle. It is generally used for deeper rhytides and lip augmentations
(Fig. 3).

The non-animal origin of HA gel should, in theory, eliminate the
potential for antigenic stimulation. Safety trials in several animal species
found that a stabilized form of HA does not elicit humoral or cell-
mediated immune reactions (28). Initially, hypersensitivity reactions were
more common with Restylane® and Perlane® due to impurities in the
bacterial fermentation process. However, as more purified HA raw material has been available since 1999, hypersensitivity to the injections has

Polyacrylamide

Aquamid®

Aquamid® (Contura International, Copenhagen, Denmark) is part of a new generation of tissue fillers, composed almost entirely of water. "In Line Cross-Linking Technology" is a new patented method of polymer production that results in a gel that contains 2.5% polyacrylamide (PAAG) and 97.5% water (48). It has been used in Europe for more than 10 years in industry and biomedical research. Cosmetically, it has been used for breast and soft-tissue augmentation. As a polymer, PAAG is considered to be extremely safe and touted as nontoxic, nonteratogenic, and nonbiodegradable (48). It should be noted, however, that the monomeric form of this molecule has been shown to be neurotoxic and teratogenic, but the polymer does not degrade significantly into this dangerous form (49,50).

A pilot study to examine Aquamid's effectiveness as a tissue filler was performed in Sweden for indications such as lip augmentation, cheekbone enlargement, and correction of deep nasolabial folds and glabellar and chin defects. Aesthetic results were reported as positive, with almost 100% patient satisfaction at nine months of follow-up (48).

As Aquamid® is so new, there are little long-term data on safety profiles and duration of effect. However, one recent case report describes a delayed inflammatory reaction in a patient one month after receiving injections for zygomatic facial augmentation (51). The patient developed urticarial plaques near the injection sites within a few days following the initial injections. These resolved, and 10 days later she was treated in the same area with further injections of Aquamid®. The plaques returned, and a draining noninfectious nodule formed in an injected site. Soon after, nodules began to form on both cheeks. Intralesional triamcinalone helped to improve these lesions.

Silicone

AdatoSil 5000®/Silikon® 1000

Silicone is not currently FDA approved for soft-tissue augmentation in the United States, and is indeed illegal in some states such as Nevada. This is as a result of the severity of the side effects reported, misuse of the product, and lack of long-term studies investigating the safety profile with proper injection. However, silicone has been used for over 40 years for soft-tissue augmentation in the United States, Asia, and Europe. More recently two products AdatoSil 5000® and Silikon® 1000 (Alcon Laboratories, Inc., Fort Worth, Texas, U.S.A.) have been FDA approved for usage in ophthalmologic devices. Silicone is a polymer of dimethylpolysiloxane available in liquid or solid form and is the most permanent (that is, longest lasting) injectable available. In soft-tissue augmentation, silicone is injected using microdroplet technique into the subdermal space via a 30-gauge needle. After being injected, the silicone induces fibrous capsule formation surrounding the particles, resulting in augmentation of the soft tissue (52). Numerous injections every four to eight weeks and layering are required with silicone, and undercorrection is recommended. For greater accuracy of microdroplet placement, a recent publication advocated the use of a Becton, Dickinson 3/10 cc insulin syringe swaged with a 28-gauge, 0.5-inch Micro-Fine IV needle to administer Silikon® 1000 (Fig. 7) (53).

(A)

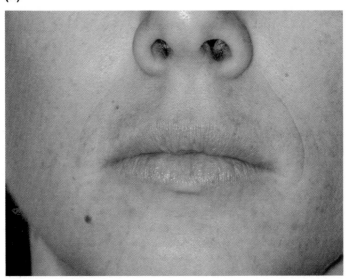

(B)

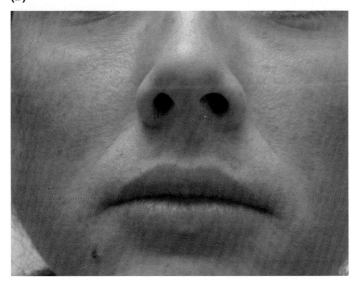

Figure 7
Before (**A**) and after (**B**) silicone treatment of the lips.

Almost all case reports of an adverse reaction do not involve the use of medically pure silicone given in a microdroplet technique. In most foreign countries, silicone is obtained as a nonpurified industrial chemical. A recent case report describes a Hispanic woman who received silicone for lip augmentation in Columbia (54). Approximately six months after the procedure, she developed fevers, chills, and myalgias, along with painfully swollen lips. Her lips underwent ulceration and desquamation, and she developed submandibular lymphadenopathy. She was successfully treated with the immunomodulator Aldara (imiquimod 5%). The microdroplet technique was not used.

In addition to granuloma formation, general inflammation, discoloration, ulceration, local lymph node involvement, and material migration have been reported (52). One dermatologist reports having seen a patient who was experiencing silicone nodule formation (biopsy proven) 36 years following treatment of acne pits (55). Unfortunately, the resultant side effects such as nodularity and cellulitis are notoriously difficult to treat, often involving surgical excision.

Currently, studies are underway to evaluate the use of liquid silicone for HIV-associated facial lipoatrophy. One case report of an HIV-positive man with facial lipoatrophy treated with liquid injectable silicone showed promising results (56).

Box 1
Administration Guidelines

---

1. The treatment area must be assessed for its amenability to correction prior to beginning any tissue augmentation or filling. For example, in correction of scars, a stretch test should be performed to evaluate their candidacy. Scars that do not flatten out on stretching will not respond because of the underlying stromal tethering.

2. Ensure the patient has realistic expectations of the probable result.

3. Regardless of the presence of lidocaine in the various filler admixtures, the concurrent use of a topical anesthetic applied approximately 30 minutes prior to injection or administration of a nerve block may be appropriate for the area of treatment.

4. Herpes prophylaxis in the form of oral antiviral medication is recommended in those patients with a history of cold sores if the lips are to be injected.

5. Generally, a 30-gauge, 0.5-inch needle is a good choice for administration, although variations in caliber and needle length may be appropriate with different products and desired depths.

6. The noninjection hand should be used to stabilize and pull the area of augmentation taut between the thumb and forefinger.

7. Ensure the needle is not blocked by applying slight pressure to squeeze a little bit of product out of its tip.

(*Continued*)

Box 1
Administration Guidelines (*Continued*)

8. There are two main methods used to insert the tissue filler into the appropriate layer of dermis: tunneling and serial puncturing.

   (a) Tunneling:
   - Prior to injection, measure the length of the needle to plan the entry site.
   - Insert the needle at a shallow angle with bevel up, until the hub is flush with the skin.
   - Tilt the needle parallel to skin surface so that skin is tented up over area of augmentation.
   - Smoothly inject the filler as the needle is withdrawn, with each subsequent injection at the advancing edge of previous.
   - Allow the product to flow into the tissue, mindful of variance in flow depending on anatomic site and depth and particular filler viscosity.

   (b) Serial puncturing:
   - In this technique, multiple injections along the length of the area for treatment are made, creating beads of filler.

9. Certain fillers require slight overcorrection of defects, such as ZC-1 and ZC-2, while others require undercorrection as further augmentation may occur over several weeks as the body's natural response to the product compounds the filling material itself.

10. Immediate massage of the treated area to smooth out unevenness and to mold the filler to achieve the desired effect are required following both the techniques mentioned above. It is important to note that pain and possible purpura formation may result from this action. Some advocate the use of external devices, such as a teaspoon, to assist with massage (57). Care must be taken not to overmassage as product effects may be lost.

11. If immediate correction is required, digital pressure can be employed to force the product back out of the dermis through the original entry site. An external instrument, such as a teaspoon, can be used in a hoe-like manner to assist in the extraction of the product (57). A needle and a syringe can also be used to withdraw excess product.

12. Use of ice packs is useful to reduce swelling and pain following the procedure.

13. It is recommended that patients are mindful of the treatment and try to decrease facial movements for the first few days following the procedure to prevent dislodging or contortion of the product.

COMPLICATIONS OF EXOGENOUS SOFT-TISSUE AUGMENTATION

Product Placement

In general, if filler is placed too deeply, the effect is lost quickly. Conversely, if the filler is too superficial, the patient may experience erythema and

(A)   (B)

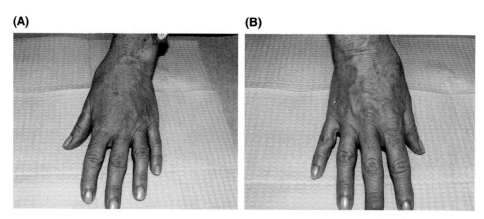

Figure 3
Improved aesthetic results in left hand (**A**) compared to right (**B**) with centrifuged fat at the five month follow-up.

Others, however, argue that centrifugation is an unnecessary step causing undue trauma to harvested cells and raise concern that the centrifuge can be a reservoir for Pseudomonas or other pathogens (Finder K, personal communication, 2001) (24). In one study, centrifugation

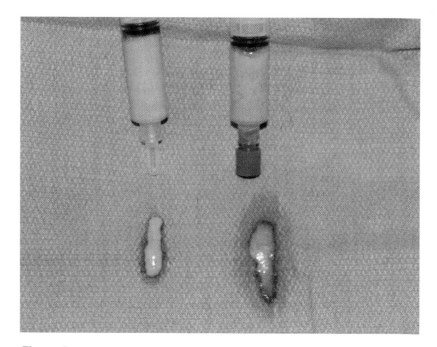

Figure 4
Fat as it appears injected through the syringe: after centrifugation on left, noncentrifugation at right.

at 1000 or 5000 rpm for 15 minutes was shown to disrupt cell morphology (33). Given the results of the study, however, the author now routinely utilizes fat centrifuged for three minutes at 3600 rpm in nearly all cases. Fulton (34) uses centrifuged fat for facial correction, but prefers noncentrifuged fat for larger volume transfer into breasts, biceps, or buttocks. In these situations when larger quantities are transferred, Fulton notes increased lumpiness with centrifuged fat.

INJECTION TECHNIQUES

Illouz (5), Fournier (6), and Coleman (10) advocate injecting small droplets of fat, rather than a large bolus of fat, reasoning that a blood supply is more readily established. In 1994, Carpaneda and Ribeiro (35) demonstrated that smaller injected volumes, less than 3 mm in diameter, had greater graft viability than larger volumes. Even at two months, viable fat cells were noted only in the peripheral zone of larger grafts having diameters of 3.5 mm or greater. Small volume transfer versus overcorrection appears to be favored in the current literature (11,15,16,36,37).

For injection, both blunt-tipped cannulae and needles have been advocated. Some studies have suggested that diameter size be 18 gauge or larger with similar size orifices for transfer between syringes (31,38). In Shiffman's study (23), injection with smaller diameter 20- and 22-gauge needles caused damage to the fat cells with histologic changes in cellular and nuclear morphology. Blunt-tipped cannula reduces risk of bleeding and the rare risk of intravascular injection. However, it is argued that they may be harder to pass through tissue and cause trauma or bleeding in the recipient site. Retrograde filling is always recommended with low injection pressures to avoid a bolus of fat and inadvertent intravascular injection. Transfer of fat to 1 cc syringes is recommended by Coleman and Donofrio (10,32). Low injection pressure is required and larger syringes appear to produce larger particles of fat (Fig. 5). Transfer adapters are available and allow transfer without exposure to air. Prolonged air exposure has been demonstrated to negatively impact fat-cell viability (39).

Various injection strategies have been utilized in the past decade. Fat has been typically transferred only into the subcutaneous space, most often directly under the rhytide or defect site. Two newer approaches have also been recommended for restructuring the aging face: injection into multiple tissue planes (Lipostructure^TM) (10) and intramuscular (IM) injection [fat autograft muscle injection (FAMI)] (40). The author now predominately utilizes the FAMI technique. A more detailed account of this procedure will be presented and demonstrated on the video.

Fat Augmentation into the Subcutaneous Space

Whether blunt-tipped cannulae or needles is utilized, the most common placement of the transplanted fat is in small quantities in different layers

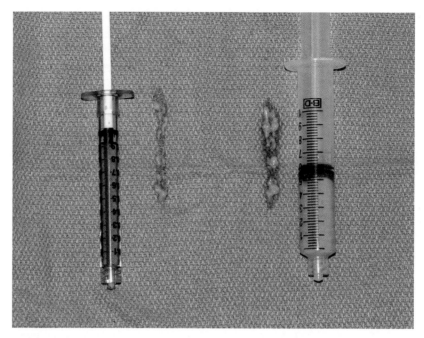

Figure 5
Appearance of small pearls of fat injected through a 1 cc syringe compared to larger particles of fat when the same pressure is applied through a 10 cc syringe.

of the subcutaneous space (11,14,17). The suggested degree of overcorrection has decreased through the years from 50% (1,4) to 30% (14,16), to now minimal to no overcorrection (37,41). Part of the rationale for smaller volumes is not only for improved graft survival, but also for reducing downtime for patients. Postoperative edema is generally proportional to the amount transferred (24,25) Anesthesia is achieved in most cases with regional nerve blocks, supplemented as needed with local anesthesia. Some patients may require additional sedation with oral, IM or Intravenous (IV) medication, depending on individual needs and the extent of the procedure. The cannula is then inserted and advanced to the most distal site. The plunger is withdrawn to exclude intravascular injection. Fat is then injected as the cannula is withdrawn and microdroplets of fat are placed at regular intervals. Recommended syringe size for transfer varies from 10 cc (23,25) to 3 cc (14,16,17) to 1 cc (10,32,42,54). Typical sites for augmentation of the face are shown in Box 2. Other facial and nonfacial indications for fat augmentation are outlined in Box 3.

Lipostructure™

Coleman's method called Lipostructure™ entails an intricate layering of small parcels of fat within multiple tissue planes (10). Not only is the subcutaneous space a recipient site, but also in certain regions fat is

> **Box 2**
> Typical Areas for Fat Augmentation of the Face
>
> 1. Nasolabial fold
> 2. Marionette fold
> 3. Lips
> 4. Glabellar line
> 5. Medial cheeks
> 6. Malar region

placed immediately adjacent to bone or fascia, or within muscle. Only minute parcels of fat are deposited, so that the transplanted droplets are "within 1.5 mm of living vascularized tissue" (10). A full-face correction requires hundreds of passes with a 17- or 18-gauge blunt-tipped cannula attached to a 1 cc syringe. Each pass ideally creates a new tunnel, so the fat "parcels" are adjacent to blood vessels. Typically, less than 0.1 cc of fat is deposited for per pass of the syringe. Quantities injected for the full-face correction often exceed 100 cc. Fat preparation involves gently aspirating the fat, no washing, and brief centrifugation for 30 seconds.

Coleman's method is innovative in that, for the aging face, the entire face is treated not solely under furrows or defects. Coleman's technique can reportedly replace the need for face lifting procedures. A three-dimensional enhancement of youthful facial contours is the goal. Indeed, dramatic before and after results have been published and long-term results have been documented with photography (10). A significant drawback of the Coleman's method is the marked edema seen for weeks to months postoperation. The patient must weigh the benefits of dramatic panfacial correction versus the extended recovery period away from their usual routine.

Modified Lipostructure™

Donofrio (32) has modified Coleman's procedure with a method of "fat rebalancing" also involving the entire face, but with results achieved in

> **Box 3**
> Other Facial and Nonfacial Indications for Fat Augmentation
>
> 1. Acne scars
> 2. Linear morphea
> 3. Other scarring diseases
> 4. Dorsum of hands
> 5. Congenital defects
> 6. Liposuction defects
> 7. Defects from injected materials
> 8. Buttock enhancement
> 9. Breast enhancement
> 10. Cellulite

several (about 6–12) small procedures over a one- to two-year period. Donofrio's (43) analysis of the aging face indicates that fat not only atrophies, but also hypertrophies in some areas. The entire face is treated with smaller total quantities of fat (approximately 20–30 cc), which reduces the downtime for patients from 1 to 10 days depending on the extent of the procedure. Fat is processed atraumatically and injected with blunt-tipped cannulas, using the intricate, repetition pass and layered method recommended by Coleman. Although the first procedure involves fresh fat, subsequent procedures are performed with frozen fat. Like others, simultaneous microliposuction of jowls and other areas is also performed at the first procedure for esthetic rebalancing (37).

Fat Autograft Muscle Injection

A new method for facial volume restoration with autologous fat has been termed as "FAMI" by its developer—French plastic surgeon and anatomist—Roger Amar (40). With this method, fat is injected within or immediately adjacent to the muscles of facial expression, following the patient's natural anatomy. The technique parallels the blood supply and only one to three passes with the syringe are made per area, minimizing trauma and downtime to 5 to 10 days. Additionally, because fat is placed within highly vascularized tissues, the survival of the graft may be optimized. Amar's idea for the FAMI technique was inspired by a study in 1996 in which GuerroSantos et al. (44) demonstrated five-year-survival of fat in rat muscle. The study further found that the muscle thickness continued to increase for six months following fat grafting.

Other evidence supports the notion that fat cells survive optimally near muscle. Nguyen et al. (45) reported in 1990 that muscle was the ideal recipient site when autologous fat was injected into rats. After nine months, fat injected into the subcutaneous plane was completely absorbed and the only site in which autologous fat remained was that injected in the muscle. Fat injection into muscles has also been helpful in other fields of medicine. In otolaryngology, fat has been injected into the vocal cords , resulting in improved muscle function (46–48). In urology, fat has been injected to augment the sphincter tone of the bladder neck muscle (49). Long-term improvement in the function of the rectal sphincter has also been achieved with fat grafting (50). Further, several histologic studies support the improved viability of fat grafts when fat is placed next to well-vascularized tissue (1,4,35). Muscle is also the preferred recipient site among many experienced cosmetic surgeons (37,51). Ultimately, in the FAMI technique, fat implantation hypertrophies the muscles of facial expression, duplicating the contour and support of these muscles in youth.

Indications

Like others (10,42,52), Amar believes much of the aging process is due to panfacial volume loss rather than just gravitational sagging.

Ideal candidates are those with superficial musculoaponeurotic system (SMAS) integrity but pan facial volume loss. These patients are usually 30 to 50 years of age (Fig. 6). The FAMI procedure is also ideal for post-rhytidectomy patients. These patients, in particular, want to avoid a pulled or stretched appearance with second or third lifting procedures. Localized volume loss in areas such as the lips, tear trough deformity, nasolabial folds, chin, and perioral areas is also an indication for FAMI. This technique, like Lipostructure™ and its modifications, is not used to directly fill holes or valleys, but rather to restore the volume surrounding these defects. In restoring the natural projections of the face, FAMI transforms these defects to the smooth, attractive contours of youth. The goals of this technique are shown in Table 1.

FAMI does not replace rhytidectomy in patients with excess SMAS laxity demonstrating exaggerated nasolabial folds or ptosis of the cheek and neck. Patients with significant photoaging would more likely benefit from chemical peeling or laser resurfacing procedures. Alternatives are reviewed with the patient at the time of the consultation. Patients are also asked to bring a photograph, taken 10 to 20 years before, in order to analyze the volumes present in youth (Fig. 7).

Amar's preferred donor site for this procedure is the medial knee or the outer thigh. After a sterile prep and drape, Klein's tumescent solution

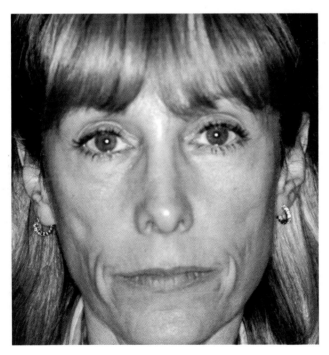

Figure 6
Ideal candidate for FAMI with total facial volume loss.

Table 1
Goals of the FAMI Technique

- Restore youthful projections of the aging face
- Restore continuity of cosmetic units and jawline
- Support free margins of the face
- Restore aesthetic proportions

is infiltrated into the fat surrounding the donor site, but Amar avoids injecting of solution directly into the donor tissue to minimize contact between adipocytes and lidocaine. However, adequate anesthesia may be difficult to achieve unless Klein's solution is infiltrated throughout the area. Harvesting is performed with a blunt-tipped harvesting cannula attached to a 10 cc syringe with low vacuum pressure. Syringes are filled, capped, and set upright to allow fluid separation before the infranatant fat is discarded. The fat is then centrifuged in sterile canisters for three minutes at 3600 rpm. The infranatant fluid and supranatant oily fractions are removed and the fat is transferred to 1 cc syringes with an adapter.

Injection into the muscle requires detailed knowledge of the origin, insertion, and plane of each muscle to be injected (Table 2) (53). Familiarity with the bony landmarks and contours of the skull is also essential (54). The fat is injected in a retrograde fashion along the length of the muscle, usually starting distally from the origin on the bone to the insertion of that muscle. However, sometimes the opposite approach is required owing to the depth of the muscle origin. Usual entry sites are shown in Figure 8. Specific injection cannulae have been developed for specific muscle groups, which enable smooth passes conforming to the contours of the skull (Figs. 9–11). The muscle bundle is filled with one

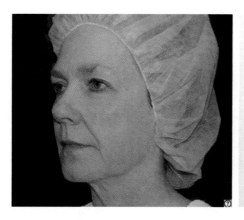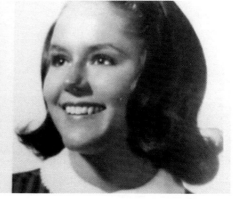

Figure 7
Patient presenting for procedure and as she appeared in a photograph 20 years prior.

Table 2
The Three Planes of the Facial Muscles

Superficial plane:
1. Frontalis
2. Procerus
3. Orbuclaris oculii
4. Zygomaticus minor
5. Depressor anguli oris
Middle plane:
1. Levator labii and alaque nasi
2. Levator labii superioris
3. Orbicularis oris
4. Zygomaticus major
5. Risorius
6. Platysma
7. Depressor labii inferioris
Deep plane:
1. Corrugator
2. Buccinator
3. Levator anguli oris
4. Mentalis

Source: From Refs. 7, 10, 13.

---

to three passes of the cannula, and generally 1 to 3 cc of fat is injected per muscle. Anesthesia is achieved with regional nerve blocks, supplemented with oral or IM sedation. Less frequently, for a full-face procedure in an anxious patient, IV sedation is administered by an anesthesiologist.

Total volumes injected with the FAMI procedure vary with the extent of the treatment area. As little as 3 to 5 cc might be placed into the lateral chin area into the depressor labii inferioris or anguli oris. As much as 60 to 70 cc may be placed for a full-face procedure. In a preliminary report, 20 to 30 cc was used on an average for partial face correction (55). With this amount, patients will have minimal bruising and swelling for five to seven days (Fig. 12). The placement of fat in FAMI procedure is at a deeper plane than in the subcutaneous methods, and one can place more fat without excessive swelling. It is also less traumatic than repetitive pass methods, and even when larger quantities are placed, patients may return to work in 5 to 10 days, depending on quantities injected.

The postoperative course is rather uneventful. Other than the edema, there is generally very little discomfort or bruising. The edema may be alarming to the patient unless forewarned. Our patients are told they will look too full and "monkey-like" for one week. After the period of initial edema, there is gradual loss of swelling, stabilizing at two to three months. Complications have been limited to temporary, palpable lumpiness, which is not generally visible. A notable feature of FAMI is the symmetry of results; even the edema resolves symmetrically.

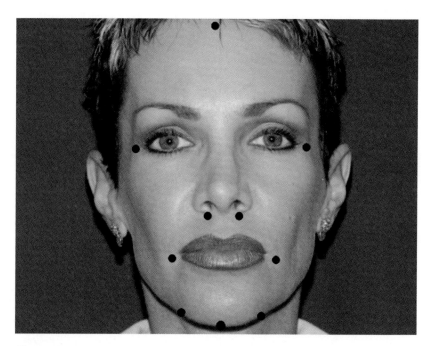

Figure 8
Usual entry sites for FAMI (fat autograft muscle injections) technique.

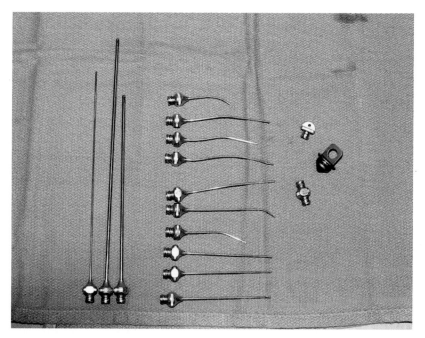

Figure 9
Injection cannula utilized for the FAMI technique.

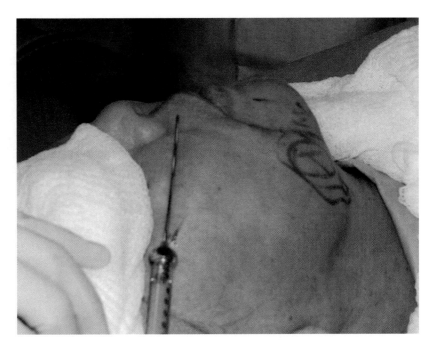

Figure 10
Curved shape of #4 cannula for the zygomaticus minor.

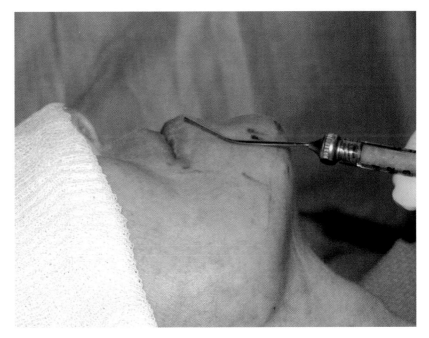

Figure 11
Angled shape of #7 cannula for injection of the depressor labii inferioris.

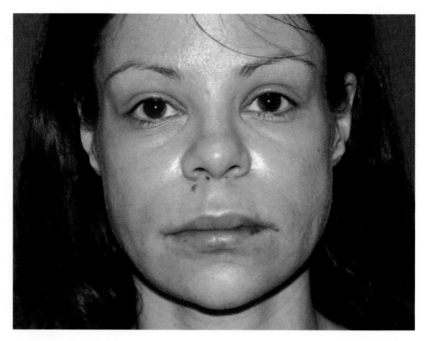

Figure 12
Postoperative patient at five days. Note minimal bruising but significant swelling. A total of 26 cc was placed in the lower face.

Patient satisfaction has been uniformly reported to be good to excellent (Figs. 13 and 14) (55). Amar reports three- to five-year survival (Fig. 15) (56).

COMPLICATIONS OF FAT AUGMENTATION PROCEDURES

Fortunately, the complication rate is low with all fat augmentation techniques. By far, the most serious reported complication is blindness following fat injections to the glabellar lines (57,58). These reports are rare and have involved sharp instrumentation. Avoidance of sharp instruments is recommended in this area, as well as initial withdrawal of the plunger to assure one is not intravascular. Retrograde fill and very low injection pressures will further minimize this risk. Overcorrection is another potential problem, particularly in the infraorbital region resulting in visible, superficial lumps (42). Fat survival in this region is particularly good, perhaps owing to the relative immobility and the vascular bed of the orbicularis oculi muscle. Overcorrection is also visible due to the thinness of the skin. Very small quantities should be placed, if at all, in this area with care to avoid superficial placement (42). Small fatty cysts may also rarely develop in any area. These can be treated with low-dose steroid injection or excision (14,16,42) Additionally, infection is another potential complication. Anecdotal reports have included bacterial

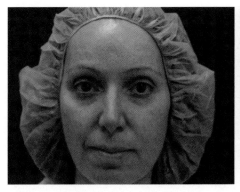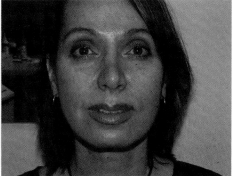

Figure 13
Before and eight months after FAMI procedure.

infection with Pseudomonas, Mycobacterium, and other microbes
(14,42). Often, the centrifuge or instrumentation have been the source.
Fat augmentation should be considered a sterile procedure, including
the use of sterile centrifuge sleeves. Most patients are given prophylactic
antibiotics. Patients with concomitant infections, particularly sinus or
dental, need to be treated adequately before undergoing this procedure
(42). Expected sequelae with this procedure are temporary and include
mild bruising and swelling, and some palpable "lumps."

LONGEVITY OF FAT AUGMENTATION PROCEDURES

Reported long-term results vary from "disappointing" to many years (7–
9,11,16,21,25,37). Eremia and Newman (38) found that the longevity was
related to the recipient site. Good to excellent results were seen at five to

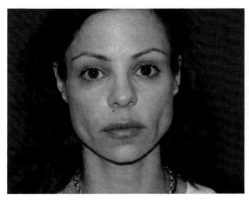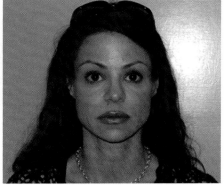

Figure 14
Before and eight months after FAMI procedure.

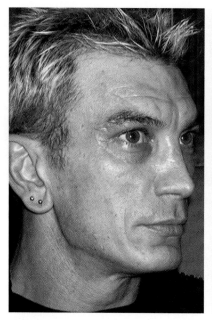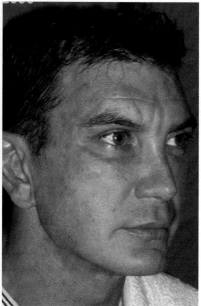

Figure 15
Before and two years after procedure. *Source:* Courtesy of RE Amar, MD.

eight months for the nasolabial and melolabial folds. Fat injections were less effective for the lip and glabellar areas. Indeed, the lips have been least responsive to long-term correction in other reports (16). Others have noted the best survival to be areas of relative immobility such as the fixed scars of linear morphea (25), the forehead (11), the infraorbital area (16), or the backs of the hands (59,60).

Objective measures of long-term results have consisted largely of photography and observation. Newer methods have been utilized in a few studies. Utilizing magnetic resonance imaging of fat transplants, Horl et al. (61) demonstrated 49% volume loss at three months, 55% loss at six months, and negligible decrease in volume between 9 and 12 months. Sadick and Hudgins (62) utilized a marker of site-specific fatty acid composition to document donor fat cell survival in the transplanted site. However, in six patients, undergoing autologous fat transplantation, this marker persisted in only one patient at one year. In the other five patients, either the donor fat did not survive at one year or as Sadick hypothesized the recipient factors triggered conversion to the fatty acid composition of the recipient site. A readily available, practical means of documenting fat cell survival is needed.

TOUCH-UP PROCEDURES

Many who advocate small volume fat transfer recommend touch-up procedures (16,21,32). The rationale for repeated procedures is that small volumes survive best and cause the least downtime for patients. However, small volumes may not be enough to achieve the correction that a patient may need. A typical protocol would have one larger procedure followed by touch-up procedures at three to four month intervals for one year. Variations from this protocol include regular monthly touch-ups for one to two years (32) to repeating the entire procedure every few years as needed (10). Fournier (21) has advocated periodic injections every few years to keep pace with the aging process.

Some surgeons utilize only fresh fat for touch-up procedures, while others regularly utilize frozen fat. The use of frozen fat is controversial. It has been argued that freezing of fat affects its viability, while others contend frozen fat gives satisfactory to even superior results (63–65). Shoshani et al. (66), compared frozen fat versus fresh fat injected into nude mice. Assessments by clinical observation, weight and volume measurement, and histologic parameters demonstrated successful take at 15 weeks in both groups with no statistically significant difference in volume at 15 weeks. Further objective long-term studies will help to address this question.

SUMMARY

Fat augmentation is an effective and popular method of restoring needed volume to facial and body defects utilizing a variety of techniques. There seems to be a consensus regarding gentle handling of the fat and utilizing small volumes during placement. Limited data suggests centrifugation contributes to long-term results. Although fat is nearly the ideal filling substance, there are still many unanswered questions regarding the optimal technique for obtaining the long-lasting results. These questions have been difficult to answer owing to a lack of readily available, effective means of measuring outcome. Scientific research is emerging to address these issues. New concepts of full-face correction utilizing Lipostructure[TM], facial rebalancing, and the FAMI technique offer exciting artistic approaches to the aging face. This is a dynamic field offering the surgeon a creative gratifying procedure and the patient a gratifying natural result.

REFERENCES

1. Niechajev I, Sevuk O. Long term results of fat transplantation: clinical and histological studies. Plast Reconstr Surg 1994; 94:496–506.
2. Neuber F. Fat transplantation. Chir Kongr Verhandl Dsch Gesellch Chir 1893; 20:66.
3. Newman J, Ftaiha Z. The biographical history of fat transplant surgery. Am J Cosmetic Surg 1987; 4:85.
4. Peer LA. Transplantation of tissues. Vol. 2. Baltimore: Williams & Wilkins, 1995:195–230.
5. Illouz YG. The fat cell "graft", a new technique to fill depressions. Plast Reconstr Surg 1986; 78:122–123.
6. Fournier PF. Facial recontouring with fat grafting. Dermatol Clinics 1990; 8(suppl 3):523–537.
7. Kaminer MS, Omura NE. Autologous fat transplantation. Arch Dermatol 2001; 137:812–814.
8. Chajchir A, Benzaquen I, Wexler E. Suction curettage lipectomy. Aesthetic Plast Surg 1983; 7:195–202.
9. Fredricks S. Transplantation of purified autologous fat: A three year follow-up is disappointing [discussion]. Plast Reconstr Surg 1991; 87:228.
10. Coleman SR. Facial recontouring with lipostructure. Clinics in Plast Surg 1997; 24(suppl 2):347–367.
11. Pinski KS. Fat transplantation and autologous collagen: A decade of experience. Am J Cosmet Surg 1999; 16(suppl 3):217–224.
12. Asken S. Autologous fat transplantation: micro and macro techniques. Am J Cosm Surg 1987; 4:111.
13. Chajchir A, Benzaquen I. Fat-grafting injection for soft-tissue augmentation. Plast Reconstr Surg 1989; 85:921–934.
14. Hernádez-Pérez E, Lozano-Guarin C. Fat grafting: techniques and uses in different anatomic areas. Am J Cosmet Surg 1999; 16(suppl 3):197–204.
15. Sommer B, Sattler G. Current concepts of fat graft survival: histology of aspirated adipose tissue and review of the literature. Dermatol Surg 2000; 26(suppl 12):1159–1166.
16. Fulton JE, Suarez M, Silverton K, Barnes T. Small volume fat transfer. Dermatol Surg 1998; 24:857–865.
17. Perez MI. Autologous fat transplantation: Past and current practice. Cosmet Dermatol June 1999; 7–13.
18. Hudson DA, Lambert EV, Bloch CE. Site selection for auto-transplantation: some observations. Aesth Plast Surg. 1990; 14:195.
19. Moore JH, Kolaczynski JW, Morales LM, Considine RV, Pietrzkowski Z, Noto PF, Caro JF. Viability of fat obtained by syringe suction lipectomy: effects of local anesthesia with lidocaine. Aesth Plast Surg 1995; 19:335–339.
20. Alexander RW, Maring TS, Aghabo T. Autologous fat grafting: a study of residual intracellular adipocyte lidocaine concentrations after serial rinsing with normal saline. Am J Cosmetic Surg 1999; 16(suppl 2):123–126.
21. Fournier PF. Fat grafting: my technique. Dermatol Surg 2000; 26(suppl 12):1117–1128.
22. Fagrell D, Eneström S, Berggren, Kniola B. Fat cylinder transplantation: an experiemental comparative study of three different kinds of fat transplants. Plast Reconstr Surg 1996; 98:90–98.
23. Shiffman MA, Mirrafati S. Fat transfer techniques: the effect of harvest and transfer methods on adipocyte viability and review of the literature. Dermatol Surg 2001; 27(suppl 9):819–826.
24. Coleman WP. III. Fat transplantation. Dermatol Clinics 1999; 17(suppl 4):891–898.
25. Markey AC, Glogau RG. Autologous fat grafting: comparison of techniques. Dermatol Surg 2000; 26(suppl 2):1135–1144.

26. Jones JK, Lyles ME. The viability of human adipocytes after closed-syringe liposuction harvest. Am J Cosmetic Surg 1997; 14(suppl 3):275–279.

27. Lewis CM. Correction of deep gluteal depression by autologous fat grafting. Aesth Plast Surg 1992; 16:247–250.

28. Johnson G. Body contouring by microinjection of autogenous fat. Am J Cosm Surg 1987; 16:248–262.

29. Griffin EI. Results of fat transfer survey: criteria and interpretation. American Academy of Dermatology, Mar 21, 1999.

30. Butterwick KJ. Hand Study. Lipoaugmentation for the aging hands: a comparison of the longevity and aesthetic results of centrifuged vs. non-centrifuged fat. Dermatol Surg 2002. (In Press).

31. Shiffman MA. Effect of various methods of fat harvesting and reinjection. Am J Cosmet Surg 2000; 17(suppl 2):91–97.

32. Donofrio LM. Structural autologous lipoaugmentation: a pan-facial technique. Dermatol Surg 2000; 26:1129–1134.

33. Chajchir A, Benzaquen I, Moretti E. Comparative experimental study of autologous adipose tissue processed by different techniques. Aesthetic Plast Surg 1993; 17:113–115.

34. Fulton JE Jr. Breast contouring by autologous fat transfer. Am J Cosmet Surg 1992; 19:273–279.

35. Carpaneda CA, Ribeiro MT. Study of the histological alterations and viability of the adipose graft in humans. Aesth Plast Surg 1993; 17:43.

36. Ersek RA, Change P, Salisbury MA. Lipo layering of autologous fat: An improved technique with promising results. Plast Reconstr Surg 1998; 101(suppl 3):820–826.

37. Guerrerosantos J. Long-term outcome of autologous fat transplantation in aesthetic facial recontouring: sixteen years of experience with 1936 cases. Clin Plast Surg 2000; 27:515–543.

38. Eremia S, Newman N. Long-term follow-up after autologous fat grafting: analysis of results from 116 patients followed at least 12 months after receiving the last of a minimum of two treatments. Dermatol Surg 2000; 26(suppl 12):1148–1158.

39. Agris J. Autologous fat transplantation: a 3-year study. Am J Cosmet Surg 1987; 4:95–102.

40. Amar RE. Microinfiltration adipocytaire (MIA) au niveau de la face, ou restructuration tissulaire par greffe de tissue adipeux. Ann Chir Plast Esthét 1999; 44(suppl 6):593–608.

41. Pinski KS, Roenigk HH. Autologous fat transplantation: long-term follow-up. J Dermatol Surg Oncol 1992; 18:179–184.

42. Berman M. Rejuvenation of the upper eyelid complex with autologous fat transplantation. Dermatol Surg 2000; 26:1113–1116.

43. Donofrio LM. Fat distribution: a morphologic study of the aging face. Dematol Surg 2000; 26:1107–1112.

44. GuerreroSantos J, Gonzalez-Mendoza A, Masmela Y, Gonzalez MA, Deos M, Diaz P. Long-term survival of free fat grafts in muscle: an experimental study in rats. Aesthetic Plast Surg 1996; 20:403–408.

45. Nguyen A, Pasyk KA, Bouvier TN, Hassett CA, Argents LC. Discussion: comparative study of survival of autologous adipose tissue taken and transplanted by different techniques. Plast Reconstr Surg 1990; 85(suppl 3):378–386.

46. Zaretsky LS, Shindo ML, deTar M, Rice DH. Autologous fat injection for vocal fold paralysis: long-term histologic evaluation. Ann Otol Rhinol Laryngol 1995; 104(suppl 1):1–4.

47. Mikaelian DO, Lowry LD, Sataloff RT. Lipoinjection for unilateral vocal cord paralysis. Laryngoscope 1991; 101:465–468.

48. Bauer CA, Valentino J, Hoffman HT. Long term results of vocal cord augmentation with autogenous fat. Ann Otol Rhinol Laryngol 1995; 104:871–847.

49. Gonzalez de Garibay AS, Castillo Jimeno JM, Villanueva Perez I, Figuerido Garmendia E, Vigata Lopez MJ, Sebastian Borruel JL. Treatment of urinary stress incontinence using paraurethral injection of autologous fat. Arch Esp Urol 1991; 44:595–600.

50. Shafik A. Perianal injection of autologous fat for treatment of sphincteric incontinence. Dis Colon Rectum 1995; 38:583–587.

51. Fulton JE. Fat transfer: historical perspectives. Am J Cosmet Surg 1999; 16(suppl 3):193–194.

52. Berman M. Opinion: The aging Face: a different perspective on pathology and treatment. Am J Cosmet Surg 1998; 15(suppl 2):167–172.

53. Salasche SJ, Bernstein G, Senkarik M. Muscles of facial expression. Surgical Anatomy of the Skin. Appleton & Lance198869–87.

54. Gray H. The facial muscles. In: Gross CM, ed. Anatomy of the Human Body 107th ed. Philadelphia, PA: Lea & Febiger, 1969:382–390.

55. Butterwick KJ, Lack E. Facial volume restoration with fat autograft muscle injection (F.A.M.I.): preliminary experience with a new technique. Dermatol Surg. (In Press).

56. Amar RE. Fat autograft muscle injection. Presented at AACS Annual Meeting, Feb 2002.

57. Dreizen NG, Framm L. Sudden unilateral visual loss after autologous fat injection into the glabellar area. Am J Ophthalmol 1989; 107(suppl 1):85–87.

58. Teimourian. Blindness following fat injections. Plast Reconstr Surg. 1988; 80:361.

59. Aboudib JHC Jr, deCastro CC, Gradel J. Hand rejuvenescence by fat filling. Ann Plast Surg 1992; 28:559–564.

60. Abrams HL, Lauber JS. Hand rejuvenation: the state of the art. Dermatol Clin 1990; 8:553–561.

61. Horl HW, Feller AM, Biemer E. Technique for liposuction fat reimplantation and long-term volume evaluation by magnetic resonance imaging. Ann Plast Surg 1991; 26:248.

62. Sadick NS, Hudgins LC. Fatty acid analysis of transplanted adipose tissue. Arch Dermatol 2001; 137:723–727.

63. Jackson RF. Frozen Fat–Does it work? Am J Cosmet Surg 1997; 339–343.

64. Takasu K, Takasu S. Long-term frozen fat transplantation. Int J Cosmet Surg 1999; 7:33–38.

65. Saylan Z. Frozen fat: better than fresh fat. Int J Cosmet Surg 1999; 7:39–42.

66. Shoshani O, Ullmann Y, Shupak A, Ramon Y, Gilhar A, Kehat I, Peled IJ. The role of frozen storage in preserving adipose tissue obtained by suction-assisted lipectomy for repeated fat injection procedures. Dermatol Surg 2001; 27:645–647.

5

Liposuction

Gerhard Sattler
*Center for Cosmetic Dermatologic Surgery, Rosenparkklinik,
Darmstadt, Germany*

Video 5: Liposuction of Inner Thighs

INTRODUCTION

Liposuction is the surgical procedure of removing fat cells by using specially designed suction devices. Using stiff hollow cannulas, the subcutaneous fat can be removed through tiny incisions. On minimizing the total number of adipocytes, fat cannot be stored in the treated body areas any longer. Since its first description in 1975, the method has constantly been improved. Today, liposuction should rather be called "liposculpturing," as the precise forming of body areas (body contouring) is possible. It is the most common procedure performed in cosmetic surgery worldwide. Besides the cosmetic indications, liposuction has been established as an effective treatment in noncosmetic indications as well. By setting up internationally accepted guidelines for liposuction, renowned medical societies try to establish high quality standards to achieve predictable operative outcome and minimal surgical risk (1).

HISTORY OF LIPOSUCTION

Georgio and Arpad Fischer from Rome were the first to give a description about removing fat using cannulas inserted through tiny incisions (2), in the year 1975. They invented a machine to suction unprepared fat through hollow needles from patients under general anesthesia. This so-called "cellusuctiotome" was a single piece suction machinery with an attached hollow cannula. The fat was fragmented by a motorized cutting blade. This procedure suffered from high intraoperative risks such as severe blood loss and poor aesthetic results as well as a high rate of postoperative complications (e.g. dents and seromas). Thus, the interventions were often unsatisfactory.

Yves-Gerard Illouz, a surgeon from Paris, learned Fischer's technique, instead of the specially designed complicated suction machine. He started then to use a commercially available suction system (initially used for abortions), thus making the procedure easier for other surgeons. He also introduced the so-called "wet technique." To facilitate aspiration of the adipose tissue and reduce blood loss he administrated a physiologic saline solution mixed with hyaluronidase into the operation site (3). Pierre Fournier from Paris showed how to receive better, and more regular results by using the "crisscross-technique." Furthermore, he is a pioneer in the field of fat and collagen transfer and the inventor of syringe liposuction as which can be used an alternative to suction pumps (4).

In 1983, the American Society of Liposuction Surgery was founded. Dermatology became one of the main specialities, Especially after introduction of the tumescence technique by Jeffrey Klein (discussed below), with dermatologists performing and constantly improving the tumescent liposuction technique. Today, tumescent liposuction is the method of choice due to its high safety profile. In a survey performed by Hanke et al. (5) in 1994, this aspect was dramatically demonstrated: from the 15,336 patients who underwent liposuction in tumescent anesthesia, no severe complications such as blood transfusions or hospitalization were reported.

TUMESCENT LOCAL ANESTHESIA

Jeffrey Klein, a dermatologist and pharmacologist from San Juan Capistrano/California, first described the tumescent technique, a combination of the wet technique and a local anesthetic procedure, is the year 1987. By this technique, large volumes of physiologic saline (tumescere = to swell) were administrated with added lidocaine anesthetic solution. This idea revolutionized the history of liposuction, as tumescent liposuction minimized the operative and anesthetic risks, and turned the operation into an outpatient procedure (6,7).

The formulation used by Klein is shown in Table 1. The concentration of the local anesthetic in this solution was 0.0475%. In the course of time, various research groups modified the composition and recommended different volumes of the Klein's solution. In Europe, lidocaine was replaced by prilocaine, which causes less systemic toxicity, although it does cause formation of methemoglobin (discussed under the topic—New developments).

The tumescent solution is infiltrated subcutaneously into the surgery area. Infiltration should be continued until a "watermelon-like" consistency

Table 1
Klein's Tumescent Solution

Component	Amount
Lidocaine 1%	50,0 mL
Epinephrine 1:1000	1,0 mL
Sodium bicarbonate 8.4%	12,5 mL
Trimacinolone-acetonide	10 mg
physiologic saline (NaCl 0.9%)	1000 mL

of the area to be treated is achieved. The injection can be done manually with syringes if only small areas are to be treated. For liposuction surgery, the use of mechanical roll pump systems is recommended because large volumes of tumescent solution must be installed (up to 6 L). To benefit from the special effects of tumescent technique, it has proved to be useful to allow the solution to take effect for 30 to 60 minutes (discussed under the topic-Current concepts of Liposuction).

Owing to the epinephrine in the tumescent solution, which leads to a vasoconstriction, systemic absorption of the lipophilic local anesthetic is delayed. This means that though large quantities of local anesthetics are used, plasma levels generally stay below $2 \mu g/mL$ (8). Because of the special pharmacogenetics of the tumescent solution, dosages of up to 35 mg/kg lidocaine or 50 mg/kg prilocaine are considered safe when using the tumescent technique (9,10).

Infiltration should be done slowly to allow a painless spread in the tissue—however, slow infiltration leads to delayed systemic absorption. The anesthetic effect is long lasting for 8 to 16 hours, thus giving post-operative analgesia as well.

The tumescent solution acts like an interstitial infusion thus compensating intraoperative fluid losses. The solution stabilizes the subcutaneous connective tissue, which is consequently less traumatized. This also makes the procedure less painful for the patient and physically less strenuous for the surgeon. The patient is able to cooperate even when he is awake; he can shift the position on the operating table when required or even get up during operation to control the result already, achieved result in a standing position.

Further advantages of tumescent liposuction are (10):

- Absence of the need for a general anesthesia
- Significantly reduced blood loss
- Immediate patient mobilization
- Significantly shorter period
- Convalescence
- Long lasting postoperative analgesia

All these advantages make tumescent liposuction an ideal out-patient procedure and, nowadays, the method of choice. New developments during the last decade have furthermore helped to facilitate the procedure and improve aesthetic outcome (discussed under the topic New Developments).

PHYSIOLOGY OF LIPOSUCTION

Liposuction is not a method to reduce overweight or correct general obesity. Liposuction is ideal to remove isolated, disproportional fat deposits, and to achieve a proportional and harmonic body contour. When used this way, it can be called liposculpturing.

During a diet, the volume of the adipocyte cells can be reduced, but their number stays the same. This theory explains why patients keep on putting weight in the same circumscript areas like abdomen or thighs, where a great number of adipocytes exist.

The distribution of fat is determined by genetic aspects such as race and sex. Women tend to put on weight at the lateral thigh ("saddle bag deformity"), the lower abdomen, the hip, and the gluteal region while men develop fat deposits rather in the upper and lower abdomen, the hip, the neck, or the back.

Because of the genetic fixation of fat depositions, even excessive physical training cannot remove fat in determined areas. Raised muscle activity has no influence on the reduction of overlying adipose tissue.

Liposuction is the only method to remove this circumscript fat deposits that are resistant to diet and training. In an area where adipocytes are removed through liposuction, the effect stays permanent, even when the patient is putting on weight in other areas. It reduces the number of adipocytes that can store lipids. An influence on the fat metabolism, which might play a beneficial role in reducing morbidity associated with obesity (diabetes, high blood pressure), is discussed.

EVALUATION OF PATIENTS

The ideal patients are younger than forty years of age and have an elastic skin turgor. They should have normal weight, no anamnestic data for disorders in wound healing, bleeding diathesis or thrombosis, and only circumscript fat deposits.

On the other hand, the advantages of tumescent technique offer the opportunity to widen the therapeutic range to patients up to 80 years of age, as long as they are generally healthy and do not show any risk factors.

Preoperative Investigations

On the first visit, the patient is informed about the operation, potential risks, and the expected outcome. Thorough clinical examination of the general health status as well as the regions to be lipocontoured, and an appropriate medical history is a standard health care procedure. The patient should be evaluated in standing and sitting positions, the skin turgor must be checked, particularly its elasticity, and the presence of dimpling and striae need to be evaluated. Blood tests including those for coagulability factors, electrolytes, liver, and kidney parameters should be conducted. If there are any anamnestic hints for coagulability disorders, bleeding diathesis, or a raised risk of thrombosis in the personal or family history, then all the relevant clotting factors should be investigated.

The only absolute contraindication is a known allergy to the anesthetic in the tumescent solution. Special caution and appropriate supervision are necessary in patients with marked myocardial weakness because of the danger of volume overload, and in patients with a known tendency to develop a high-grade cardiac arrhythmia because of the proarrhythmic effect of local anesthetic drugs. Severe liver or kidney dysfunctions, convulsions, as well as disturbances in coagulation should be ruled out. Drug interactions need to be considered.

When using prilocaine as local anesthetic, a lack of the metabolizing enzyme glucose-6-phosphate-dehydrogenase needs to be ruled out. If this enzyme is found to be reduced, lidocaine can be used instead.

An unrealistic patient's expectation regarding the operative outcome might be a contraindication as well.

To show the patient the results that can be achieved by liposuction surgery, it might be useful to present pre- and postoperative pictures of other patients.

If finally the patient and the surgeon come to the conclusion that a liposuction is indicated, an informant written consent must be obtained.

Planning of the Operation

Nowadays, virtually the whole body can be treated by liposuction.

Very good retraction leading to excellent postoperative outcome can be expected in

- Neck and cheeks
- Male breast
- Upper and lower abdomen
- Waist
- Inner part of the knee
- Lower legs and ankles.

Good retraction with corresponding good results can be expected in

- Upper and lower back
- Upper arms
- The flanks and hips
- Lateral and medial thighs

Areas that are more difficult to treat are the ventral parts of the upper thighs, axillar region, and the inner part of the gluteus. Liposuction of the female breast is also possible but needs a very experienced surgeon.

If the removal of large volumes of fat or the treatment of several areas is planned, serial liposuctions are recommended. Although general obesity cannot be treated with liposuction alone, it might help to treat the most distracting fat deposits by liposuction, thereby creating a new attitude and motivation for changes in lifestyle.

TECHNIQUE OF LIPOSUCTION

Preoperative Preparations

On the actual day of surgery, the areas that will be treated are marked. Pre-existing irregularities that must be respected during liposuction are outlined. Then photographs are taken to document the preoperative status.

In most cases, it is recommendable to give an oral or IV-sedation, e.g., diazepam, before starting the infiltration of the tumescent solution.

Surgical Setting

Sterile conditions and certain hygienic standards must be obeyed. The elimination of microorganisms can be achieved by various sterilization procedures, such as boiling, steaming, autoclaving, or using radiation. Before starting the surgery, the skin is disinfected; skin disinfection should be repeated at regular intervals during surgery. The surgeon should wear sterile gloves and clothing.

The vital signs should be monitored routinely. Every 15 minutes, blood pressure and pulse should be monitored. The use of a pulse oximeter is recommended to control blood oxygenation, especially when using prilocaine as local anesthetic drug (induces formation of methemoglobin). According to the liposuction guidelines of the American Society of Liposuction Surgery (ASLSS) and the American Academy of Cosmetic Surgery (AACS), at least one healthcarer in the operating room must have adequate training in cardiopulmonary resuscitation (1). Oxygen supply should be available.

Tumescent Local Anesthesia

The infiltration should be done slowly. To shorten the infiltration procedure, it can be helpful to perform parallel infilliation using multiple needles at different sites (e.g., using the Stenger-Sattler Distributor, shown in the video).

Tumescent solution is infiltrated until a watermelon-like consistency of the tissue is achieved. Owing to the vasocompression and vasoconstriction occurring in the infiltrated area, a "blanching effect" occurs.

After infiltration, the tumescent solution should be allowed to soak in, for at least 30 minutes to one hour to show any effect. It can be necessary to reinfiltrate and then to achieve the ideal watermelon-like tissue turgor required for correct tumescent liposuction. We suggest using the term "state of tumescence" (Fig. 1).

Additional Sedation and Analgesia

The tumescent anesthesia is sufficient for most patients. In nervous patients, or when treating sensitive areas, it might be useful to give additional sedation or analgesia.

For sedation, the IV-use of benzodiazepines such as midazolam has been in use for some years. Nowadays, short acting hypnotics such as propofol are also administered.

For an additional analgesia if, required, short acting opioids such as remifentanil have showed to be very effective.

When using additional sedation or analgesia, a continuous monitoring of all vital functions is essential; an anesthetist should be on call.

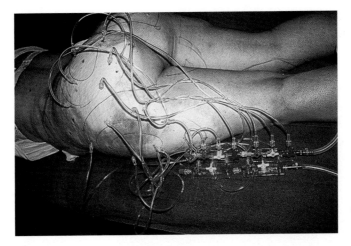

Figure 1
State of tumescence while infiltrating the gluteal region with the Stenger distributor.

General Technique of Liposuction

To begin the actual suction of the adipose tissue, small liposuction cannulas, attached to a suction system via a flexible tube, are inserted through small incisions at the edges of the site of surgery. The incisions should be placed in skin folds or areas covered with hair to hide potential tiny scars.

Liposuction is done in various layers, in a crisscross method. To prevent irregularities, each area has to be treated from different sides and angles, but the main suction direction should be parallel to the longitudinal axes of the body (treating of inner thigh). Only deep layers are treated in other directions. This prevents irregularities and saves the lymphatic vessels. A multipositional approach, with the patient actively changing positions, is generally recommended.

If fat transfer is planned, the fat should be gathered in a sterile container (Fig. 2) (11). Liposuction should not be done too superficially. It depends on the form and size of the cannula how much adipose tissue is left subcutaneously. Small cannulas, as to with diameters ranging from 2 to 4 mm, lead to a smoother more regular result. The result can be controlled intraoperatively by the touch and pinch test. Before finishing surgery, the patient is checked in various positions including the standing position. This can help detect fat deposits that have not yet been treated or any side differences. If necessary, corrections can be done immediately.

At the end of surgery, the patient should stand upright for a short time. Because of gravity, a great amount of the tumescent solution will thus drain automatically. The incisions are then closed with sterile wound strips and the patient is wrapped in absorbent dressings and a compression garment. These compression garments are to be worn for

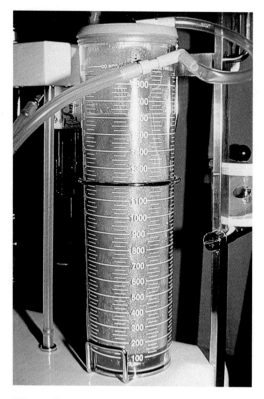

Figure 2
Liposuction aspirate with only fat as supranatant.

one to four weeks, depending on the operation site, the laxity of tissue, and the patient's comfort.

Recommended Volumes of Removal

According to the liposuction guidelines of the ASLSS and the AACS, liposuction surgery using the tumescent technique has been demonstrated to be a safe procedure in the routine removal of volumes of up to 4000 mL of supranatant fat. The maximum volume may go up to 5000 mL of supranatant fat, removed in an ideal patient with no comorbidities. Megaliposuctions, with the removal of more than 6000 mL supranatant fat, should be restricted, experienced surgeons such that it is performed only by involved in clinical research in a hospital setting (1).

Perioperative Medication

Prophylactic antibiotic therapy is recommended. Although the early ambulation of patients prevents venous stasis and the risk of thrombosis, we have established a perioperative anticoagulation scheme, with low molecular heparins, for five days postoperatively to minimize the risk of deep leg vein thrombosis and pulmonary embolism—rare but major complications.

POSTOPERATIVE FINDINGS

Most patients recover within 24 hours after surgery. To prevent postoperative pain, a mild analgetic drug such as paracetamol can be administered. Postoperative swelling and bruising for the next five to seven days may occur. The patient must be informed that tumescent solution will keep draining from the incision sites for one to two days postoperatively. Minor irregularities and soreness are expected sequelae, which usually resolve spontaneously within the first two weeks postoperation.

Normal activities can be performed after two or three days, but greater physical efforts should be avoided for at least five to seven days. Walking and light physical training is recommended from the day after surgery.

Postoperative visits should be scheduled at 2, 8, and 12 weeks after operation, to get a good follow-up. In some cases, "touch ups" are required to optimize the result. They should be done only after complete wound healing has taken place, at the earliest 12 months after the first liposuction.

An important aspect of liposuction is the retraction of the skin. Within four months after surgery, a three-dimensional shrinking and wound healing of the subcutaneous tissue takes place, which retracts the overlying skin as well.

This effect varies in different regions. Best retraction is seen in the neck, the male breast, waist, abdomen, inner knee, ankle, and calf. Good retraction can be found in cheeks, upper arm, hip, lateral thigh, lateral knee, and suprapatellar region, whereas retraction is only moderate on the back, lower abdomen, pubis region, medial and proximal thigh, and in the gluteal region.

To give an overview about possible complications, the incidence of complications after liposuction is shown in a collective report of 4831 patients treated in our clinic, in Table 2.

Nonsatisfactory cosmetic outcome may occur, especially with inadequate operating techniques, as Figures 3–5 demonstrate. These pictures

Table 2
Incidence of Complications After Liposuction in Tumescent Local Anesthesia in a Collective of 4831 Patients

Big asymmetry	0
Superinfected hematoma	0
Seromas	15
Irregularities/dents	2
Persisting scar at incision site	1
Wound infections	2
Pulmonary embolism	0
Blood loss requiring blood transfusion	0
Electrolytic disorders	0
Deep vein thrombosis	5

show patients that presented to our clinic with the question of correcting operations after unsatisfying first liposuction treatment in other clinics.

NONCOSMETICAL INDICATIONS FOR LIPOSUCTION

There are a number of noncosmetic disorders that can effectively be treated with liposuction; some examples are:

- Lipoma
- Reconstruction of the skin and subtissues in flap elevations, subcutaneous debulking, or flap movement
- Gynecomasty or pseudogynecomasty
- Mammahyperplasia
- Buffalo hump in Cushing's syndrome
- Lipolymphedema
- Axillary hyperhidrosis
- Compartmentsyndrom caused by hematoma
- Various pathologic disorders of the fat tissue such as lipodystrophia or *Lipomatosis dolorosa* and others (11)

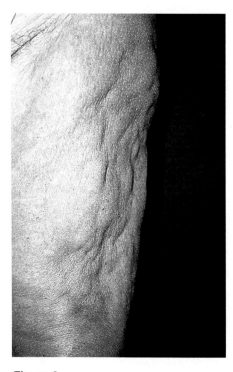

Figure 3
Postoperative result after liposuction in the early (1975) "dry technique" (i.e., without tumescence infiltration).

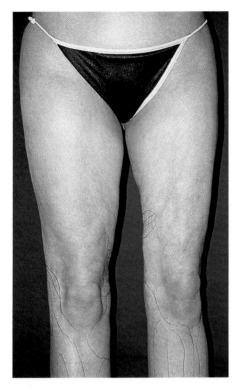

Figure 4
Postoperative result after overcorrection of inner thigh in tumescence technique.

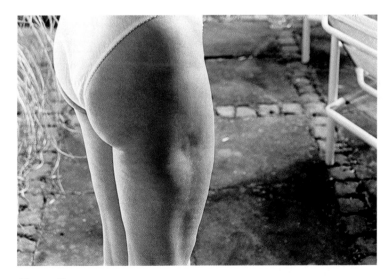

Figure 5
Postoperative result after liposuction of lateral thigh with overcorrection over the trochanter region caused by incorrect positioning of patient on the operating room table during liposuction.

NEW DEVELOPMENTS IN LIPOSUCTION

Important new developments took place during the last decade. New cannulas and liposuction-assistant techniques changed the technical side of the procedure. Improvement and changes in the tumescent solution made the use of greater volumes possible and safer. On the basis of growing clinical experience and findings, the concept of physiodynamics of tumescent liposuction as well as of wound healing developed further, which has consequences in the planning and, technique of liposuction (9).

Current Concept of Physiodynamics and Wound Healing After Tumescent Liposuction

During and after infiltration of the tumescent solution, the distribution takes place in several stages (Fig. 6).

Initially there is a suprafascial hydrodissection along the septa of the fibrous tissue. The solution then starts to gather around the fat lobules in the paralobular space. Allowing a penetration time of 30 to 60 minutes, the solution will lead to an intralobular, infiltration which will, as a result of the interstitional pressure and diffusion forces, finally lead to a homogenization of the adipose tissue. This effect is important to facilitate the suction process and to get regular postoperative results. The softened, prepared fat can be aspirated with small nontraumatic cannulas, thus reducing tissue traumatization and destruction of subcutaneous connective tissue, blood, and lymph vessels. These structures are essential for wound healing and skin retraction, and help create a predictable cosmetic outcome (Fig. 7).

When all the tumescent solution is drained from the surgery site, a process of continuous adherence and shrinking of the subcutaneous wound is initiated, which results in a global three-dimensional wound contraction and finally a horizontal subcutaneous scar. Maximum shrinking is seen normally after four months, but total time of wound healing continues for up to 18 months (Fig. 8).

In the same process, the shrinking of the connective tissue fibers leads to a skin retraction. A liposuction using tumescent technique, with correct suction process at all layers of the subcutaneous tissue, causes an "interstitial skin reduction flap."

The whole process of healing is significantly determined by the operation technique.

Current Concept of Planning and Carrying Out Tumescent Liposuction

To achieve an ideal healing process with corresponding ideal results, the use of a standardized operation technique is recommended. Thin, blunt-tipped, atraumatic cannulas or vibrating cannulas (discussed below)

(A)   **(B)**

(C)   **(D)**

(E)   **(F)**

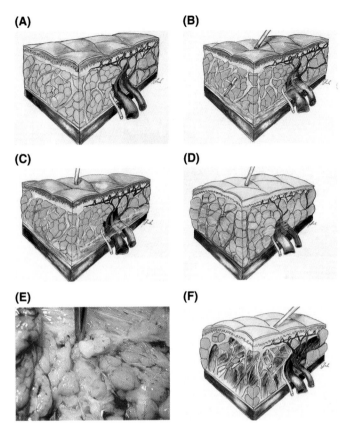

Figure 6
(**A**) Section of skin and subcutaneous adipose tissue before tumescenct local anesthesia. (**B**) First state of distribution of tumescence solution along the fibrous septae causing hydrodissection. (**C**) State of paraseptal and perilobular distribution of tumescence solution. (**D**) State of homogenization of the subcutaneous tissue. (**E**) Intraoperative site of the state shown in (**D**) (homogenization of adipose tissue). (**F**) Result after removal of adipose tissue with remaining connective tissue.

should be preferred to save the subcutaneous fibrous and the connective tissues and vessels.

To achieve the necessary interstitial tissue pressure, "supertumescence" with building up of high tissue turgors should be reached. Infiltration of the tumescent solution should be done slowly; to save time infiltration can be done parallel with multiple needles at different sites (e.g., by using the Stenger–Sattler distributor). The solution must be allowed to soak in for at least 30 minutes.

Suction must be done at all layers of the subcutaneous space. The correct use of tumescent local anesthesia in combination with atraumatic cannulas reduces friction as far as possible. After 20% to 30% of the tumescent

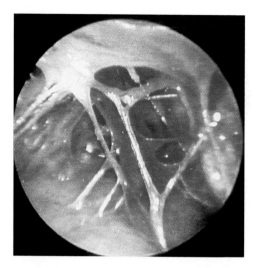

Figure 7
Endoscopic picture after complete liposuction of the lateral lower leg demonstrating of persisting fibrous tissue without adipocytes.

fluid is removed, manual tissue stabilization (discussed below) performed by an assistant compensates the developing laxity of the skin turgor.

Postoperatively, a thorough drainage of tumescent solution must be achieved by leaving the incision sites open and wearing compression garments.

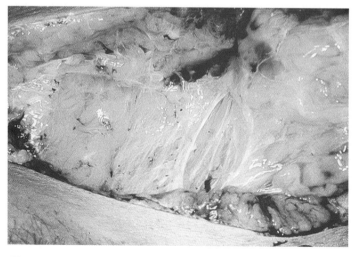

Figure 8
Formation of a subcutaneous scar 12 months after liposuction. Photograph taken during abdominoplasty.

Technical Developments

To obtain an atraumatic suction technique, technical developments led to an improvement of cannulas and liposuction-assisting devices.

Manual Liposuction, 24-Hole Cannulas

If correct tumescent local anesthesia is performed, then suction can be done with thin, blunt-tipped cannulas. The connective tissue can further be spared when cannulas with multiple suction holes are used (24-hole cannulas). After building up the suction force, a number of holes (10–12,12–16) will be occluded by fibrous tissue. The remaining holes stay effective in liposuctioning, so the cannula cannot build up a higher suction force due to occlusion of the holes. As the suction force decreases, the holes that were previously blocked will reopen.

When using two- or three-hole cannulas, it easily happens that all holes are occluded simultaneously. In this case, the suction force increases rapidly thus reinforcing the occlusion. Liposuction can be continued only after cleaning of the cannula or destruction of the blocking tissue.

The developed suction force in a 24-hole cannula is just strong enough to remove the fat cells but too weak to suck in and destroy fibrous tissue or vessels. In this way, blockage of the cannula and destruction of the connective tissue is prevented and the treatment is subtler.

Ultrasound-Assisted Liposuction (UAL)

To facilitate fat aspiration in difficult areas such as the male breast or back or in secondary sites, a number of new suction devices were developed starting in the late1980s.

In 1987, Scuderi and DeVita (12) and Zocchi (13) first described a method of homogenizing the fat with ultrasound waves. The suction cannulas were attached to an ultrasound generator and ultrasound waves sent into the tissue supposedly destroy the adipocytes.

There are some severe disadvantages when using this technique. The cannulas must have a comparatively larger volume. A large number of seromas and skin burns and persisting hypo- or hyperaesthesias as a result of destruction of the myelin sheath of peripheral nerves were reported (14). There was even speculation about a potential carcinogenic risk. Therefore, the American Society of Dermatologic Surgery rates ultrasound assisted liposuction as an experimental method with no extended clinical use (15,16).

Powered Liposuction/Vibrating Cannulas

In 1995, Charles Gross (17), an ENT surgeon at the University of Virginia, described a new technique he used in liposuction of the neck called "lipo-shaving." An engine-powered cannula with an integrated rotating blade was used to destroy adipocytes under direct visual or endoscopic control.

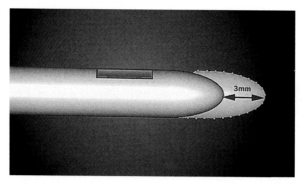

Figure 9
Demonstration of vibrating cannula technique.

This idea started the invention of a new generation of cannulas, first with rotating blades but later with oscillating blades.

The latest development is cannulas without blades but with a vibrating grip that leads to vibration of the cannula when passing through the tissue (Fig. 9). One rationale behind the use of vibrating cannulas is the different inertness of various materials whereas, the cannula passes fibrous tissue without damaging it, the homogenized fat can be aspirated. The other aspect that aids this effect is the difference in velocity of the vibration and the presence of the suction force. If the vibration speed is higher than the speed of the airflow of the suction, the suction can only withdraw the liberated, homogenized fat. The cannula will escape and spare the tissue structures that have tight attachments.

Vibrating cannulas facilitate the treatment of fibrous or pretreated areas. Because they pass easily through the tissue and do not tangle with the fibers, they make the procedure more comfortable for the patient and the surgeon.

Severe complications have not been reported.

Further improvements of the cannulas and grips are expected, which will lead to a wide spread usage of this suction device as it shows greater benefits in achieving good operative outcome (18).

Table 3
Sattler's Tumescent Solution with Reduced Prilocaine

Prilocaine 1%	40.0 mL
Epinephrine 1:1000	1.0 mL
Sodium bicarbonate 8.4%	6.0 mL
Triamcinolon-acetonide 10 mg	1.0 mL
Physiologic saline (NaCl 0.9%)	1000.0 mL
	1048.0 mL solution 0.038%

Table 4	
Tumescent Solution After Schneider-Affeld and Friedrich	
Prilocaine 2%	10.0 mL
Lidocaine 2%	10.0 mL
Epinephrine 1:1000	0.66 mL
Sodium bicarbonate 8.4%	6.0 mL
Triamcinolon-acetonide 40mg	0.33 mL
Physiologic saline (NaCl 0.9%)	1000.0 mL
	1026,99 mL solution 0.037%

Endoscopic Liposuction

Liposuction is an operation without direct visual control. Endoscopic liposuction can be used to visualize what is happening in the subcutaneous space during liposuction. This method helped to control the technique and quality of liposuction and to give a further understanding of physiodynamic processes in the adipose tissue. It is not routinely used clinical procedure, but has helped in the development of new, useful liposuction devices.

Refinements of the Tumescent Solution

In the course of time, the original Klein tumescent solution was modified by various working groups.

We first replaced lidocaine as local anesthetic with prilocaine because of its lower systemic plasma levels, which is relevant when using large volumes.

As a result of clinical observations, prilocaine could be reduced by 20% from the initial 50 mL/L to 40 mL/L, which resulted in a reduced local anesthetic concentration of 0.038% (Table 3).

Table 5		
Volumes of Tumescent Solution: Comparison of 1992 and 1997 Recommendations		
	1992	1997
Abdomen	800–1000 mL	5000 mL
Hips (both sides)	400–1000 mL	5000 mL
Waist (both sides)	400–1000 mL	3000 mL
Lateral thigh (both sides)	500–1200 mL	4000 mL
Ventral thigh (both sides)	600–1200 mL	4000 mL
Medial thigh (both sides)	255–700 mL	3000 mL
Knee (both sides)	200–500 mL	2000 mL
Male breast (both sides)	300–800 mL	3000 mL
Neck	100–200 mL	800 mL

In clinical trials, Schneider-Affeld and Friedrich combined lidocaine and prilocaine to decrease the side effects of a single agent. Their solution is shown in Table 4.

As a consequence of reduction of the local anesthetic concentration and the growing knowledge of delayed absorption, the quantities of tumescent solution used in one session could be raised. The possibility to use more quantities of tumescent solution widens the therapeutic range. Today, up to 6 liters of tumescent solution are used in one session.

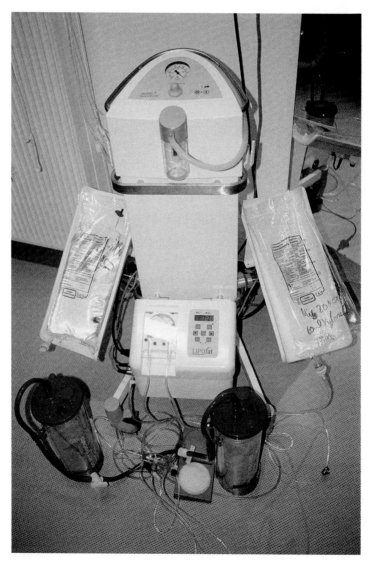

Figure 10
Modern liposuction equipment with infiltrating pump connected to a Stenger distributor, a suction system, and warming devices for tumescence solution.

Clinical experience showed the better effects of super-tumescence when using large volumes; because of the reduction of tissue traumatization, the complication rate is also reduced.

Table 5 gives a comparison of the initially recommended amounts of solution and the amounts used in 1997 and are still used today.

The use of trimacinolone in the solution is discussed, many physicians do not add it any more. The initial rationale for its use, the prevention of postoperative inflammation, is no longer relevant. Meanwhile, other effects like psychovegetative stabilization as well as a regulative effect on the blood circulation play more important roles.

Over the past years, the tumescent technique has evolved from a mainly anesthetic procedure to an essential part of successful liposuction, as it is crucial for the described processes of physiodynamics and wound healing, and determines the course of the surgery and postoperative outcome.

Improved Operating Techniques and Positioning of Patient

Besides technical and pharmacological improvements, clinical experience led to improvements in the operation procedure.

The operative outcome can mainly be improved through active cooperation of the patient who is awake. It helps the suction process if the patient is able to contract the underlying muscles to build a firm base and change positions if necessary.

(A) **(B)**

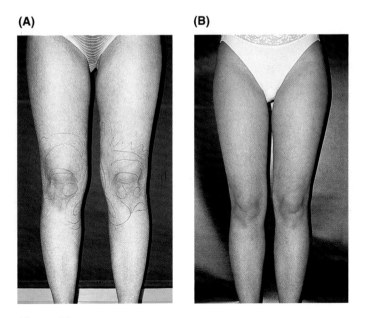

Figure 11
(**A**) Preoperative findings in a 20-year-old patient with lipomatosis of the thighs. (**B**) Postoperative results four months after liposuction via tumescence technique with 24-hole cannulas.

(A)   (B)

(C)   (D)

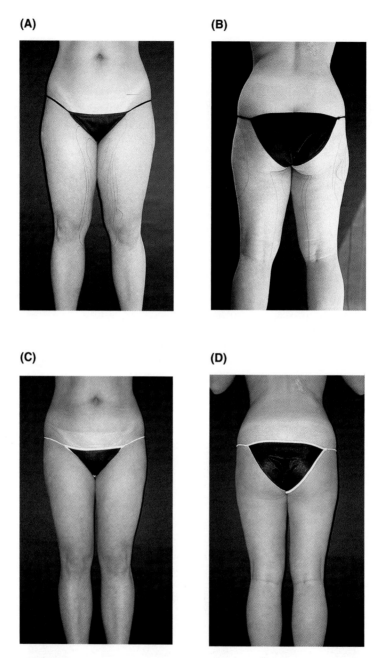

Figure 12
(**A**) and (**B**) Lipomatosis of hip, medial and lateral thighs in a 42-year-old
patient, preoperative findings. (**C**) and (**D**) Postoperative result one year later.

The operative outcome can significantly be improved by a correct positioning of the patient on the operating table and an easy access to the surgery site.

Experience has shown that it is better to treat the medial thighs not with the patient lying on his or her back but on the side with the leg to be treated stretched out on the operating table and the other leg in a 90 degree angle, to stabilize the position. With this positioning, there is a far better access to the fat deposits.

When treating the back or flanks, it is better to position the patient on the side, with the back overstretched. With this improved positioning, the overlying skin as well as the underlying muscles are stretched, which makes the aspiration of subcutaneous fat easier.

Manual assisted skin stabilization technique (MASST). Everyone performing liposuction surgery in tumescent technique has experienced that the stabilizing effect of the tumescent solution on the tissue decreases constantly because it is removed along with the fat by the suctioning process. Thus, liposuctioning gets more difficult as shearing forces on the tissue get stronger. This can be counteracted efficiently when the tissue is bimanually stabilized by stretching it with the help of an assisting person (nurse).

Last but not least, all the minor improvements that give the patient more comfort during the whole procedure should be provided. They include devices to warm sheets, blankets, and the tumescent solution to body temperature as well as a pleasant atmosphere created by music

(A)   **(B)**

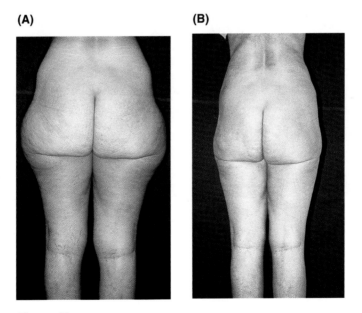

Figure 13
(**A**) Marked saddle bag deformity in 52-year-old patient. (**B**) Result after three liposuction sessions using tumescence anesthesia in yearly intervals, 6 years after the last liposuction.

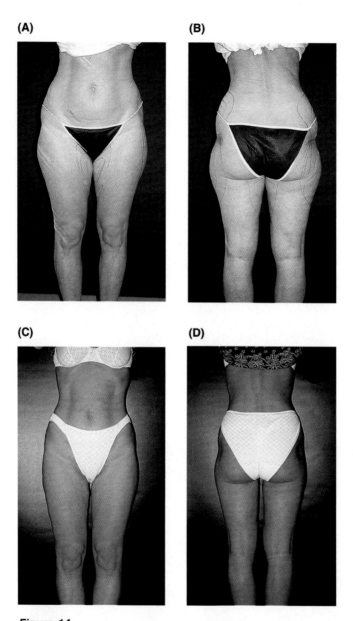

Figure 14
(**A**) and (**B**) Preoperative finding before liposuction of the hip, medial and lateral thigh as well as the knee region with vibrating cannulas. (**C**) Postoperative result after 12 months.

and room furnishing. When planning the surgery suite, it is important to include a bathroom within the easy reach of the patient (Fig. 10).

SUMMARY

The invention of the tumescent technique by Jeffrey Klein revolutionized the history of liposuction.

This technique formed the basis on which numerous developments in the field of liposuction took place within the last 25 years. Today, liposuction in tumescent local anesthesia (a term coined by our group) is the most commonly performed cosmetic procedure worldwide.

Owing to the improved operation techniques as well as refinements in the tumescent solution and the cannulas used, a substantial reduction of risks and side effects could be achieved. Thanks to all these improvements, we have reached a point today where this operation technique can offer a predictable and highly satisfactory cosmetic result with minimal risk.

To show the extent of cosmetic outcomes, we include some pre- and postoperative findings (Figs. 11–14).

Further progress can be expected through the development of more effective but at the same time more subtle cannulas. To find the best tumescent solution, pharmacological studies are planned.

REFERENCES

1. American Society of Liposuction Surgery (ASLSS) and American Academy of Cosmetic Surgery (AACS): Guidelines for Liposuction Surgery, 2001.
2. Fischer A, Fischer G. Revised technique for cellulitis fat reduction in riding breeches deformity. Bull Int Acad Cosmet Surg 1997; 2:40–41.
3. Illouz Y. Bodycontouring by lipolysis: a 5-year experience with over 3000 cases. Plast Reconstr Surg 1983; 72:511–524.
4. Fournier P. Body Sculpturing Through Syringe Liposuction and Autologous Fat Reinjection. Samuel Rolf International, 1987.
5. Hanke CW, Bernstein G, Bullock BS. Safety of tumescent liposuction in 15336 patients— national survey results. Dermatol Surg 1996; 22:459–462.
6. Klein JA. The tumescent technique for liposuction surgery. Am J Cosmet Surg 1987; 4:236–267.
7. Sommer B, Sattler G, Hanke CW. Tumeszenzlokalanästhesie. New York: Springer Berlin Heidelberg, 1999.
8. Sattler G, Rapprich S, Hagedorn M. Tumeszenz-Lokalanästhesie- Untersuchung zur Pharmakokinetik von Prilocain Z Hautkr. 1997; 7:522–525.
9. Sattler G, Sommer B. Tumescent Liposuction in Germany: history and new trends and techniques. Dermatol Surg 1999; 25:221–223.
10. Lillis PJ. Liposuction surgery under local anesthesia. Limited blood loss and minimal lidocaine absorption. J Dermatol Surg Oncol 1988; 14:1145–1148.
11. Sattler G, Hasche E, Rapprich S, Mösler K, Hagedorn M. Neue operative Behandlungs-möglichkeitren bei benignen Fettgewebserkrankungen. Zeitschrift H+G 1997; 8:579–582.
12. Scuderi N, DeVita R. Nuove prospettivo nella liposuzione: La lipoemulsificazione. Giorn Chir Plast Ricostr Este 1987; 1:33.
13. Zocchi ML. Ultrasonic liposculpturing. Aesthet Plast Surg 1992; 16:287–298.
14. Scheflan M, Tazi H. Ultrasonically assisted body contouring. Aestet Surg 1996; 16: 117–122.
15. Topaz M. Possible long-term complications in ultrasound-assisted lipoplasty induced by sonolumiscence, sonochemistry and thermal effect. Aesthet Surg 1998; 18:19–24.
16. ASDS: Statement on ultrasonic liposuction. Dermatol Surg 1998; 24:1035.
17. Gross CW, Becker DG, Lindsey WH, Park SS, Marschall DD. The soft tissue shaving procedure for remove of adipose tissue. Arch Otolaryngol Head Neck Surg 1995; 121: 117–1120.
18. Coleman WP III. Powered liposuction. Dermatol Surg 2000; 26(4):315–318.

6

Laser-Assisted Blepharoplasty

Alina A. M. Fratila
Jungbrunnen-Klinik Dr. Fratila GmbH, Bonn, Germany

Video 6: Blepharoplasty: Lower Eye
Video 7: Skin Resurfacing
Video 8: Blepharoplasty: Upper Eye

INTRODUCTION

Signs of aging in the orbital region are the first to be noticed. Today, aesthetic blepharoplasty is a procedure tailored for the individual. A meticulous ophthalmologic examination of the patient and listening to their concerns and expectations are mandatory for a good result and patient satisfaction. The sayings "more is better" and "one operation fits all" are no longer the general opinion on eyelid surgery. Aesthetic eyelid surgery has a unique position among other aesthetic surgical procedures, and the aesthetic surgeon has the major responsibility of creating a near-perfect surgical outcome. Asymmetries of as little as 1 mm may compromise the ideal result and make the patient unhappy. Using the free beam UltraPulse® CO_2 (UPCO$_2$) laser (Lumenis Inc., Santa Clara, California, U.S.A.) as a superior incisional instrument to perform blepharoplasty, the surgeon may better recognize the supporting structural deficiencies (because of the ability of the "light scalpel" to cut and cauterize simultaneously) thus producing almost perfect postoperative symmetry. The advantages of using the UPCO$_2$ laser are evident: minimal intraoperative bleeding and, thus, superior visualization, shorter operating time, and reduced postoperative bruising and swelling.

HISTORY

Although the initial use and presentation of the laser-assisted blepharoplasty technique was first demonstrated by Sterling Baker in 1983 at the Byron Smith Study Club during the American Academy of Ophthalmology Meeting in Chicago and published in the *Yearbook of Ophthalmology* in 1984, the acceptance of the CO_2 laser beam as a superior incisional tool and the recognition of the accuracy of the laser-assisted technique among ophthalmic plastic surgeons and surgeons performing blepharoplasty in general have been very sluggish (1). There is, of course, the learning curve and the high cost of the UltraPulse® CO_2 laser to be considered as well as but a step into this revolutionary innovation should be considered by all surgeons performing blepharoplasty. As Will Rogers said, "even if you're on the right track, you'll get run over if you just sit there" and Sterling Baker also added, "any physician who proposes to treat a patient with a new modality should have enough respect for both the patient and the technology to obtain appropriate training and to develop effective skills" (2). The French surgeon Bourguet was the first to describe the transconjunctival approach for lower eyelid blepharoplasty (3) in his 1924 publication. In 1983, Baylis published the technique in the *Ophthalmic Plastic and Reconstructive Surgery Journal* (4). In 1987, the dermatologist Laurence David was the first to use CO_2 laser for transconjunctival blepharoplasty (5). The advantages and disadvantages of using the CO_2 laser as an incisional tool in blepharoplasty have been discussed in several articles (6,7), but today, there is no doubt that laser-assisted blepharoplasty of the upper and lower eyelid (transconjunctivally) in combination with $UPCO_2$ laser skin resurfacing of the periorbital skin is the state-of-the-art technique in esthetic eyelid rejuvenation (personal communication, 1996).

SURGICAL ANATOMY OF THE ORBITAL UNIT

The upper and lower eyelids are composed of skin (the anterior lamella), of the orbicularis muscle and the tarsus (the middle lamella or supportive layer), and of the conjunctiva (the posterior lamella). The eyelid skin, very thin and hairless, lies on a thin layer of subcutaneous tissue. Just beneath the skin lies the orbicularis oculi muscle, divided into three regions, the pretarsal and the preseptal regions (the palpebral portion) and the orbital region (Fig. 1). The orbicularis oculi muscle is innervated by the zygomatic branch of the facial nerve. The muscle fibers of the orbital portion originate at the medial canthus and the function of these concentric loops is to close the eyes. The palpebral portion of the orbicularis muscle is formed by semicircular muscle fibers that extend from the medial to the lateral canthus. Beneath the orbicularis muscle lies the orbital septum, a fibrous structure that divides the orbit into an anterior compartment and a posterior compartment (Fig. 2). The orbital septum of the upper eyelid extends from the periosteum of the orbital rim down to the levator aponeurosis approximately 5 mm above the tarsal plate. In the lower eyelid, the orbital septum joins the capsulopalpebral fascia, which is also approximately 5 mm below the tarsal plate. A weakened orbital septum will allow the fat pads to prolapse forward. The preaponeurotic fat is divided into two compartments in the upper eyelid (medial and central) and the precapsulopalpebral fat into three compartments in the lower eyelid (medial, central, and lateral) (Fig. 3). The lacrimal gland is located in the lateral preaponeurotic compartment of the upper eyelid. The medial fat pad, in both upper and lower eyelids, is more pale and fibrous. Between the medial and central fat pads lies the inferior oblique muscle in the lower eyelid and

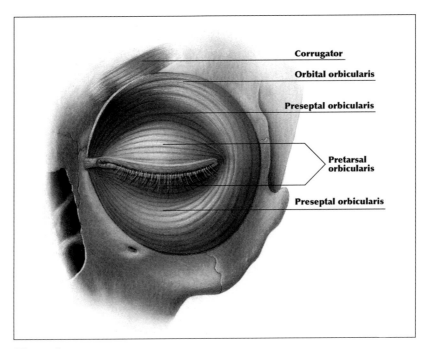

Figure 1
The periorbital muscles.

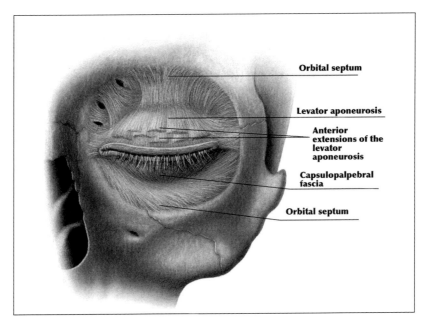

Figure 2
Orbital septum.

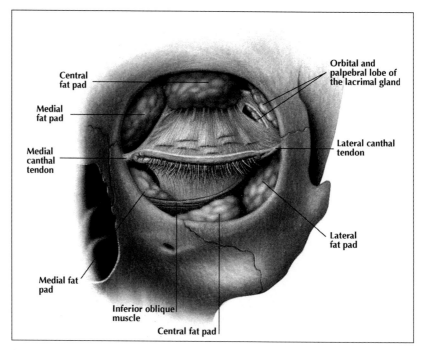

Figure 3
The upper and lower eyelid fat pads.

fibers from Whitnall's ligament in the upper eyelid. The fat pads are well-vascularized and careful dissection, during blepharoplasty, is mandatory to avoid retrobulbar hemorrhage. The upper eyelid is elevated by the levator palpebrae superioris muscle, which arises from the orbital apex and after turning into levator aponeurosis, inserts into the anterior surface of the tarsal plate. Anterior extension of the aponeurotic fibers inserts into the eyelid skin beginning 2 mm above the superior margin of the tarsus, thereby creating the supratarsal crease (Fig. 4). Deep below the levator palpebrae superioris muscle lies Muller's muscle, an extension of the levator muscle that inserts into the superior margin of the tarsal plate. The levator palpebrae superioris muscle is innervated by the oculomotor nerve (cranial nerve III) and the Muller's muscle by the sympathetic fibers from the superior cervical ganglion. The equivalent of the levator aponeurosis in the lower eyelid is the capsulopalpebral fascia extending from the inferior rectus muscle (lower lid retractor) anterosuperiorly to the inferior border of the tarsal plate. The fibrous band surrounding the inferior oblique muscle, Lockwood's ligament, is the equivalent of Whitnall's ligament, and the inferior tarsal (Horner's) muscle the equivalent of Muller's muscle. The tarsal plates are made of dense connective tissue and are approximately 30 mm long. The upper tarsus is centrally 10 mm wide, and the lower tarsus is only 4 to 5 mm wide. In the tarsal plates, the meibomian glands are located. Conjunctiva, the posterior lamella, covers the sclera

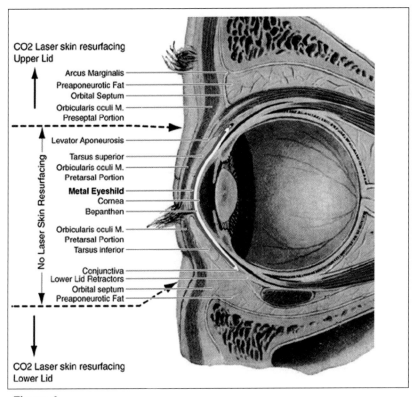

CO2 Laser skin resurfacing
Upper Lid

- Arcus Marginalis
- Preaponeurotic Fat
- Orbital Septum
- Orbicularis oculi M. Preseptal Portion

- Levator Aponeurosis
- Tarsus superior
- Orbicularis oculi M. Pretarsal Portion
- **Metal Eyeshild**
- Cornea
- Bepanthen

- Orbicularis oculi M. Pretarsal Portion
- Tarsus inferior

- Conjunctiva
- Lower Lid Retractors
- Orbital septum
- Preaponeurotic Fat

No Laser Skin Resurfacing

CO2 Laser skin resurfacing
Lower Lid

Figure 4
Cross-sectional diagram of the upper and lower eyelids.

and cornea and reflects back on the upper and lower eyelids' inner surface, which being firmly adherent to the tarsal plates. For further details on the surgical anatomy of the eyelids, the author recommends the following studies (8–12).

INITIAL CONSULTATION

It is important to understand what makes the patient unhappy. The patients have to explain what they would like to improve; if they can point out the exact esthetic concern, the patients are good candidate for aesthetic surgery. Their motivation, personality, and intentions should also be evaluated. For example, do the patients have realistic expectations? Does the patient believe that the cosmetic outcome will improve their relationships and enhance their career? If the patient's answer is yes, the patient may not be a good candidate for the operation. A safe procedure is recommended and the patient is informed about additional procedures that might be appropriate. The patient is made aware of the side effects and complications. Other possible therapeutic procedures, degree of improvement, and healing time are also explained.

The patient has to accept that additional surgery may be necessary and that the result of the treatment is unpredictable. During the first consultation, show the patient before-and-after photographs of other patients and a patient during dressing change. A video demonstration of the laser procedure may be useful. Informational brochures should contain written recommendations about preoperative skin care and postoperative management.

At the first preoperative consultation, the patient's medical history and general health status must be assessed. Did the patient have a previous cosmetic procedure like blepharoplasty, dermabrasion, chemical peeling, or a face-lift? Are they satisfied with the results? If the patient has a previous cosmetic procedure and is dissatisfied with the results for no apparent reason, there is a high probability that they will not be satisfied with an additional surgical procedure. Is there a history of poor healing and keloid formation or hyperpigmentation? The possible psychiatric disturbances have to be found and the patient's acceptance of risks and downtime has to be evaluated. The general medical history should include specific questioning about allergic reactions, itching, sensitive skin, hypertension, diabetes, autoimmune disease, immunodeficiency, hepatitis, bleeding disorders, HIV, and thyroid function. Does the patient smoke (number of cigarettes smoked daily and/or alcoholic drinks with type and amount on a daily basis)? The use of aspirin-containing medications and nonsteroidal anti-inflammatory medications should be discontinued for approximately two weeks preoperatively.

The ophthalmologic history includes visual acuity, use of contact lenses or glasses to improve vision, and previous ophthalmic surgery. Is the superior visual field decreased by the upper eyelids or does the patient have recurrent, severe eyelid- and periorbital edema? Is there any chronic eyelid disorder such as tearing, dryness, frequent blinking, mucous discharge, or crusting of the lid margins? Is there facial muscle weakness, Bell's palsy, or trauma (13)?

RELATIVE CONTRAINDICATIONS

The relative contraindications for blepharoplasty are myxedema, hyperthyroidism, sarcoidosis, Sjögren's syndrome, pemphigoid, myasthenia gravis, and Graves' dysthyroid ophthalmopathy. Conditions such as the presence of malignant lesions, malar or midface hypoplasia (polar bear configuration), proptosis or shallow orbits, exophthalmos, tear trough deformity, lower lid laxity, midface or suborbicularis oculi fat (SOOF), and descent and malar festoons require an alteration in technique (14).

PREOPERATIVE DOCUMENTATION

Preoperative photographs are obligatory. There should be slides and polaroid pictures of the full face, close-up views of eyes—both eyes together and each eye separately, relaxed and smiling, and in upgaze. In addition, close-up lateral views along with right and left oblique views should be performed.

LASER-ASSISTED UPPER EYELID BLEPHAROPLASTY

Aesthetic upper eyelid blepharoplasty has become one of the most widely accepted and frequently performed cosmetic procedures. At first sight, the procedure seems to be simple to perform. This impression of simplicity is deceiving, especially when dermatochalasis and supporting structural deficiencies are simultaneously present.

In 1984, Sterling Baker's experience with the use of the continuous wave (CW) CO_2 laser for incisional blepharoplasty of the upper eyelid in 40 patients was published (1). Dermatochalasis, muscle hypertrophy, fat protrusion, upper eyelid ptosis, and prolapse of the lacrimal gland are the most common deformities associated with upper eyelid blepharoplasty. The bloodless surgical field, when performing $UPCO_2$ laser-assisted upper eyelid blepharoplasty, makes the correction of ptosis, as well as the repositioning of prolapsed lacrimal glands, easier. The quality of the scar after laser blepharoplasty is indistinguishable from that of scalpel incisions. Moreover, the re-creation of the upper eyelid crease, perhaps because of heat fixation, and the bloodless dissection when performing the transpalpebral eyebrow lift are the unique features of laser upper eyelid blepharoplasty. Two to three months after blepharoplasty, there are no noticeable differences between patients operated with the CO_2 laser and those operated with the scalpel, but the immediate postoperative period is much more agreeable, with less swelling and bruising.

Aesthetics of Eyelid–Eyebrow Complex

The shape and configuration of the eyebrows and the eyelid–eyebrow complex (Fig. 5), as well as the fullness of the SOOF, known to other authors to as retroorbicularis oculi fat (ROOF) (15), should always be analyzed before surgery. In males, the eyebrows are normally straight and located slightly above or on the orbital rim. In females, the eyebrows may be in a straight (seen mainly in models), curved, or arched form and are in a higher position relative to the orbital rim. The arched configuration has a peak normally located between the middle and lateral thirds of the eyebrow and is more elevated temporally than nasally. Although guidelines for normal eyebrow positioning are well-described in medical texts, each individual's specific anatomy must be discussed with the patient using, if necessary, old photographs. To achieve satisfactory results, the surgeon has to be sure that the patient understands that an eyebrow ptosis cannot be treated with blepharoplasty and a simultaneous surgical technique for eyebrow elevation may be necessary (Fig. 6A and B). Together, the surgeon and the patient must identify the specific esthetic concerns and the patient must have realistic expectations.

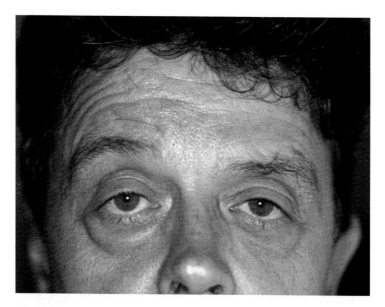

Figure 5
This patient requested upper eyelid blepharoplasty and was not aware of the asymmetry. It is imperative to check for symmetry preoperatively and to bring to the patient's attention the deformity before surgery: eyelid ptosis with right greater than left levator dehiscence and with compensatory eyebrow elevation, lateral canthus lies inferior to the medial canthus, scleral show, prolapse of the infraorbital fat pads more accentuated on the right side.

(A)   **(B)**

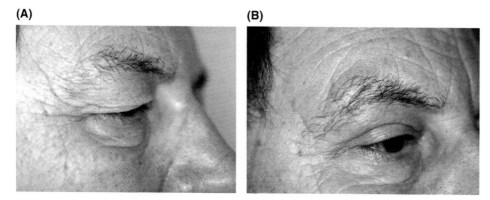

Figure 6
(**A** and **B**) Preoperative view and postoperative result following midforehead brow lift and upper eyelid blepharoplasty. Note the invisible scar on the forehead three months postoperatively hidden in a deep wrinkle. In this case, a direct approach was preferred because the patient was over 70 years old and had a wide forehead with deep wrinkles.

Ptosis may affect the medial or lateral aspect of the eyebrows. Analyzing the male patient photographs at a younger age, may help in deciding if elevation of the eyebrow is necessary. Usually, the distance from the eyelid crease to the inferior border of the eyebrow is twice the distance from the eyelid margin to the eyelid crease, with smaller variations in men as compared with women. If upper eyelid lateral fullness is present, one should discriminate between bony prominence, prolapsed lacrimal gland (Fig. 7D), SOOF hypertrophy, and lateral brow ptosis. If ptosis of the eyebrow is causing the fullness of the eyelid–eyebrow complex, an eyebrow lift should first be performed (15). Whenever possible, preferably, the eyebrow is elevated by first performing an endoscopic forehead lift (Fig. 8A and B), a temporal brow lift, or a midforehead brow lift (Fig. 6), a browplasty (direct brow lift) (Fig. 7), or an open forehead lift (pretrichal).

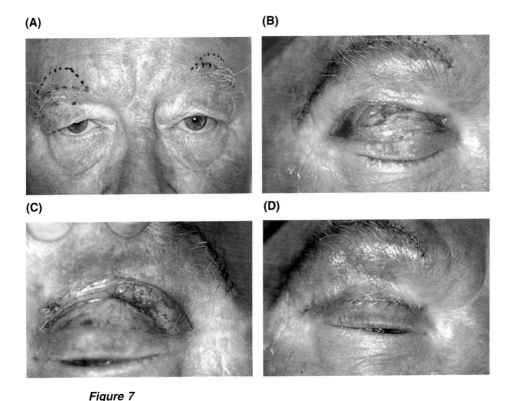

(A) **(B)**

(C) **(D)**

Figure 7
(**A**) Patient with asymmetric brow ptosis, right more than left, marked dermatochalasis both upper and lower eyelid, prolapse of the medial and central fad pads but also of the lacrimal gland, scleral show, and lower lid laxity. (**B**) Intraoperative view after eyebrow lift through direct approach, notice the prolapsed lacrimal gland (right eye). (**C**) Intraoperative view after repositioning of the lacrimal gland within the lacrimal fossa (horizontal mattress suture is placed through the periosteum of the inner aspect of the superior orbital rim—the lacrimal fossa—and the outer pole of the lacrimal gland) and lateral canthopexy (left eye). (**D**) Immediate postoperative result.

(A) **(B)**

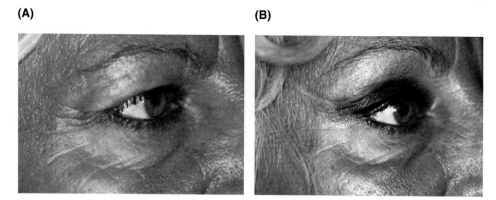

Figure 8
(**A** and **B**) Preoperative view and postoperative result 17 days after endoscopic forehead lift and upper eyelid blepharoplasty.

Upper Eyelid Examination

The preoperative ophthalmological examination must include analysis of
the palpebral aperture. The normal palpebral aperture measures 10 to
12 mm vertically and approximately 30 mm horizontally. Normally, the
upper eyelid covers 1 to 2 mm of the superior, and the lower eyelid just
touches the inferior corneal limbus with no "scleral show" (sclera between
the inferior limbus and the lower eyelid margin is visible) (15). If the superior limbus is visible, a thyroid disease may be present. If there is a scleral
show, lower eyelid laxity or retraction may be a concern. Ptosis is present
when the upper lid droops more than 2 mm over the iris in primary gaze.
Ptosis can be congenital or acquired and may be present asymmetrically.
It can be classified as mild: 1 to 2 mm, moderate: 2 to 3 mm, and severe:
greater than equal to 4 mm (13).

Shape and configuration of the eyelid fold should be analyzed.
Normally, the upper eyelid fold is present 8 to 10 mm above the lid margin
(in males somewhat lower than in females). Asymmetry of the upper-eyelid
crease should be demonstrated to the patient prior to surgery. If the superior
sulcus is relatively deep, conservative removal of the orbital fat is recommended to avoid skeletonization of the eye (Fig. 9C).

Analyze the location of fat pad protrusion—usually medial and
centrolateral in the upper eyelid and lateral, central, and medial in the
lower eyelid. Gentle pressure on the globe through a closed eyelid will
show the location and the size of the individual fat pads.

The patient is referred to an ophthalmologist, prior to the operation, for examination; visual acuity, visual field, presence or absence of
corneal scars or injury, corneal diseases, heterophoria, and strabismus
to exclude an enophthalmos are noted and the status of the ocular media,
macula, and optic nerve is checked. The levator excursion is normally
15 to 18 mm but levator excursion of 10 to 14 mm is acceptable. Tear
production, should also be analyzed.

(A)   **(B)**

(C)

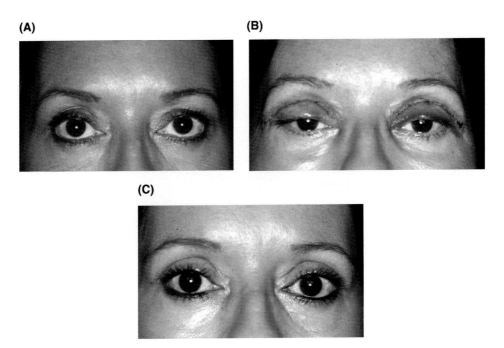

Figure 9
Preoperative view (**A**), one day postoperative (**B**) and four weeks after upper eyelid blepharoplasty and lateral canthopexy (**C**). Note the deep-set upper eyelid crease on the right side with asymmetry of the dermatochalasis and the scleral show preoperatively (**A**). In (**B**) (one day postoperative), note the typical blepharoptosis because of the supratarsal fixation made for a better definition of the upper eyelid crease. Preaponeurotic fat was not removed.

Marking Surgical Incision Lines

It is imperative that the surgical incision lines are marked prior to the local infiltration of anesthetic solutions with a marking material resistant to the surgical preparations. The preaponeurotic fat pads should be marked preoperatively with the patient sitting upright and gazing up. The surgical lid crease in the upper eyelids is marked 9 to 10 mm above the lash line in the pupillary axis. At the medial and lateral aspects, this line should never be closer than 5 mm to the superior punctum or to the lateral canthal angle (Fig. 10). It should extend medially to a line drawn vertically through the superior punctum. The superior incision line is placed no closer than 1 cm from the inferior border of the eyebrow—the transition zone between the thicker skin of the eyebrow and the thinner skin of the eyelid (15). Preferably, the lines are marked with the patient lying down while we do our final check of the marking symmetry in a sitting position.

Anesthesia

Local anesthesia and IV sedation are generally preferred. Inject approximately 2 mL of lidocaine 1% with epinephrine and hyaluronidase

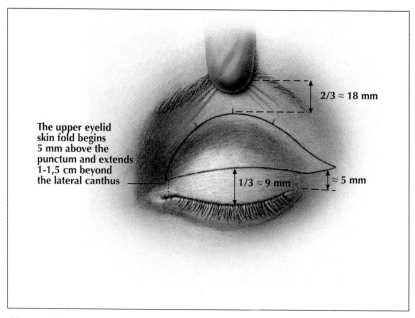

Figure 10
Marking the surgical incision lines on the upper eyelid.

subcutaneously, making a "bleb" at the lateral canthus (Fig. 11). Massage it gently through the entire upper eyelid in both directions. This very much reduces the risk of postoperative ecchymosis by reducing the necessity of multiple injections.

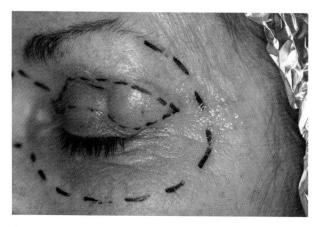

Figure 11
A "bleb" of local anesthesia at the lateral canthus is gently massaged through the entire upper eyelid in both directions.

The globe has to be anesthetized with a topical local anesthesia for it to be able to tolerate the David–Baker retractor or the metal eye shields. The undersurface of the protective shields is lubricated with Methocel® gel.

In the author's experience, the use of general anesthesia is more comfortable for the patient.

Surgical Procedure

Protect the operated eye with the David-Baker retractor (16) while the skin incision is performed with the $UPCO_2$ laser using the 0.2-mm hand piece in UltraPulse® mode at 15 mJ and 4 W. Some surgeons prefer 25 mJ/pulse at a power of 5 W (15) or even CW CO_2 laser at 6 W. Incise the skin flap at a constant speed (usually about 1 cm/sec). If slowed down, the incision will be deeper. One should stay in focus and should not use multiple passes. If the patient requires early suture removal, the skin incision may be performed with a scalpel, but the risk of bleeding is higher. The temporal portion of the incision should extend only through skin to avoid cutting terminal branches of the lacrimal artery, which pass between skin and orbicularis muscle at the level of the lateral orbital rim (15). A skin orbicularis muscle flap, is raised centrally and nasally.

Grasp the skin flap with a forceps at the temporal end of the marked ellipse and perform the excision of the skin flap with the $UPCO_2$ laser using the 0.2-mm beam diameter defocused in CW mode and with a power setting of 6 W. With gentle traction on the flap, once the orbital rim has been crossed, the plane of dissection is deepened to excise a skin-muscle flap (Fig. 12A). Protection of the nose with the Jaeger stainless steel plate is mandatory. The surgical apparatus is kept anterior to the orbital septum at all times.

Defocus the beam and vaporize any bleeding vessels. Always have a cautery unit available in case a vessel gets away.

At this surgical step, the David–Baker retractor is replaced with stainless steel shields to avoid pressure trauma and prolonged edema of the pretarsal skin. This permits better ballottement of the globe and exposure of the preaponeurotic fat pads (Fig. 12B).

The septum is opened superiorly over the fat pad to avoid injury to the levator aponeurosis, using the Rabkin spatula as a backstop (Fig. 12C). The spatula is passed beneath the septum and this is incised across its entire extent (Fig. 12D). First, the middle (Fig. 12E) then medial fat pads (Fig. 12F) are resected using a wet cotton-tipped applicator or the Rabkin spatula as a backstop. Remove only the fat herniating anterior to the orbital rim; avoid removal of excessive fat as this leads to skeletonization or an "A" shape deformity of the eyelid.

If fullness of the lateral brow is because of the descent of the SOOF, sculpt this region with the CO_2 laser defocused beam (Fig. 12G).

To create a more defined lid crease, remove the metal eye shield. This facilitates visualization of the iris ensuring symmetric placement of crease-defining sutures (supratarsal fixation). Place three interrupted

(A)   (B)

(C)   (D)

(E)   (F)

(G)   (H)

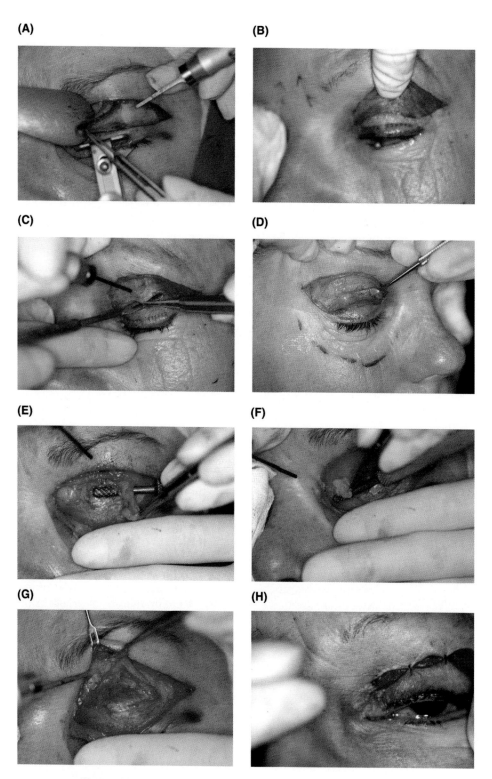

Figure 12
(*Caption on facing page*)

7–0 Prolene sutures through the skin, the levator aponeurosis at the superior tarsal border, and through the skin again on the superior border of the wound (Fig. 12H). These sutures are removed after three days. The most frequent error is an asymmetric placement of the sutures medially, which can create a very apparent difference in lid crease position and depth of the sulcus in the upper eyelids. The goal of aponeurosis fixation sutures is to stretch the pretarsal skin vertically and create a defined superior lid crease (Fig. 9B).

A running subcuticular suture using 7–0 Prolene is recommended and should be removed after 10 days. If the skin incision is performed with a scalpel, remove the suture after 5–7 days.

Postoperative Management

An ophthalmic ointment is applied to the suture three to four times a day and the patient is instructed to use ice compresses for ten minutes every hour for the first two days.

The patient is recommended to avoid airline travel a week after the operation, because changes in atmospheric pressure could precipitate an orbital hemorrhage (15,17). The patient should sleep with the head elevated, avoid heavy bending and exercise for at least one week, and may resume contact lens wear and makeup after two weeks.

LASER-ASSISTED LOWER EYELID BLEPHAROPLASTY

Traditionally lower eyelid blepharoplasty has been performed transcutaneously, with a subciliary approach. Currently, a superior method for rejuvenation of the lower eyelid is the transconjunctival approach to remove the herniated orbital fat pads using the CO_2 laser as a "light scalpel" in combination with periorbital $UPCO_2$ laser skin resurfacing to improve wrinkling of the periorbital skin, including crow's feet, and to give the skin a firmer look (Fig. 13A and B) (18). The surgeon may use either the regular CW CO_2 laser or the $UPCO_2$ laser in CW mode to perform the transconjunctival incision. Based on the author's clinical experience and literature review research, it is believed that transconjunctival incisions performed with the $UPCO_2$ laser in CW mode have a smaller zone of lateral thermal coagulation than those performed with the standard CW CO_2 laser, allowing the incision to heal better. For laser skin resurfacing of the periorbital skin, the author

---

Figure 12
(*Facing page*) (**A**) A skin-muscle flap is raised centrally and nasally. (**B**) David-Baker retractor is replaced with stainless steel shield to avoid pressure trauma and prolonged edema of the pretarsal skin. (**C**) The septum is opened over the Rabkin spatula as a backstop. (**D**) Using Rabkin spatula as a backstop the septum is opened in its entirety. (**E**) The middle fat pad is resected. (**F**) The medial fat pad is resected. (**G**) The SOOF is partly vaporized with the CO_2 laser defocused beam. (**H**) Supratarsal fixation for a better definition of the upper eyelid crease.

(A)   **(B)**

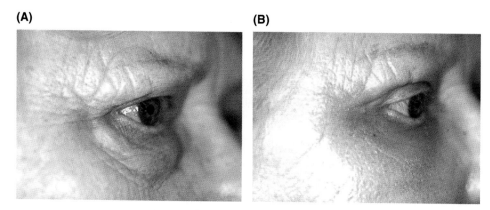

Figure 13
(**A** and **B**) Preoperative view and postoperative result three weeks after upper eyelid blepharoplasty, transconjunctivally lower eyelid blepharoplasty and UPCO$_2$ laser skin resurfacing periorbitally. Note the erythema after laser skin resurfacing, which may persist up to two months but may be covered easily with make-up (e.g., Unifiance Optic Smoothing^{TM} make-up).

only recommends the UPCO$_2$ laser to avoid scarring, hypopigmentation, and other complications related to the CW or superpulse CO$_2$ lasers. The Er:YAG laser may be used for laser skin resurfacing as well, but the tightening effect on the skin is often not enough to achieve a satisfactory cosmetic result.

The indications for operating on the lower eyelid may be either esthetic or functional. The functional indications for lower eyelid blepharoplasty are beyond the purpose of this article.

Because there is no single procedure that produces a satisfactory outcome in every patient, esthetic lower eyelid blepharoplasty demands a precise evaluation to select the most appropriate surgical approach. Today's patients desire rejuvenation without complications such as lower lid retraction or skeletonization of the periorbital region. This has resulted in a renaissance of transconjunctival blepharoplasty. It is the technique of choice when only herniated fat pads need to be removed from the lower eyelid. Because transconjunctival lower eyelid blepharoplasty often requires combining with periorbital laser skin resurfacing to correct skin laxity (dermatochalasis and wrinkling of the lower lid), it is very important for the patient to be informed about additional risks and downtime. Following CO$_2$ laser resurfacing, the skin may be red for weeks and often, male patients may not be willing to accept the use of concealing cosmetics.

Preoperative Examination, Patient Selection, and Procedure Selection

A thorough ophthalmologic examination should be performed before every blepharoplasty, but the surgeon himself has to examine and pay attention to the most important aspects. The lateral canthus should be

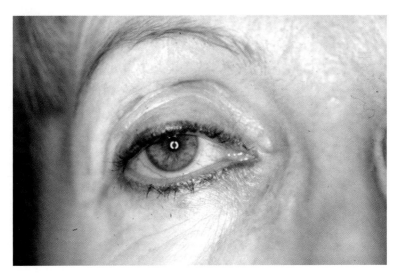

Figure 14
Round eye with scleral show and a sad look; the lateral canthus is lower than the medial one.

at or slightly above the mid-pupillary line (20° angle) i.e., approximately 2 mm higher than the medial canthus (Fig. 9C) (15). If not, a round eye with a sad look will characterize patient's expression (Fig. 14). The inferior eyelid fold lies 3 to 4 mm below the eyelid margin medially and 5 to 6 mm laterally.

When the position of the globe relative to the orbital rim is analysed from a lateral view, we are dealing with a favorable anatomical situation if an imaginary line through the ocular globe, lower lid, and malar eminence is oriented anteriorly. This situation indicates a positive vector relationship. In contrast, a negative vector relationship indicates a higher risk of an unfavorable result with lower eyelid retraction and scleral show when performing additional laser skin resurfacing or chemical peeling for rejuvenating the sun-damaged skin (Fig. 15). The removal of skin from the lower eyelid must be also very conservative. Otherwise, the proptotic appearance of the globe may create an esthetically unacceptable "staring" look. Attention should be turned to orbicularis oculi pars pretarsalis hypertrophy and to whether this is a concern for the patient. Periorbital wrinkles, so-called "crow's feet," are no longer an indication for incisional infraciliary blepharoplasty. Contrarily, pronounced festoons are difficult to deal with and may require wide preparation of the skin down to the orbital rim. The skin should be inspected for surgical scars, epicanthal fold, canthal webs, or pigment lesions.

Lower eyelid laxity should be tested with both the "snap back" test (checking the lower lid horizontal laxity) and the pinch or "pull out" test (checking the canthal tendon laxity). If the lower eyelid remains depressed for more than three seconds after downward traction (Fig. 16C)

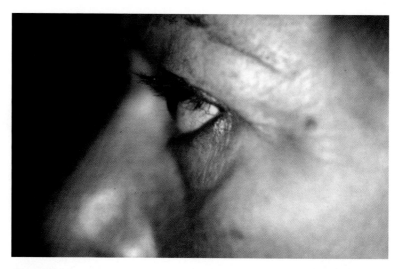

Figure 15
Negative vector relationship. Same patient as in Figure 25 (A and B).

(A)   **(B)**

(C)

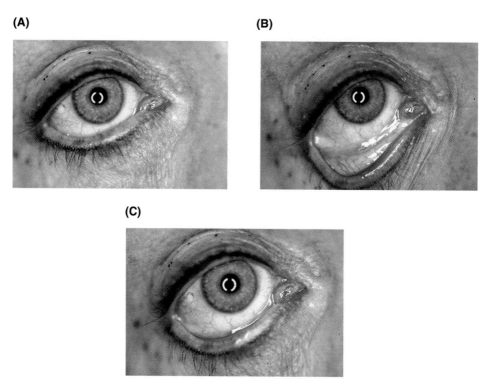

Figure 16
(**A**) Note the position of the lower eyelid after traditionally subciliary approach
performed in another clinic; 2 mm of scleral show is seen in primary gaze, the
lateral angle lies below the medial canthal angle and the rounded eye gives a
very sad look. Snap back test: After downward traction for five seconds (**B**),
the lower eyelid remains depressed more than three seconds (**C**).

or can be distracted (pinched or "pulled out") more than 8 mm, a simultaneous canthoplasty or another lower eyelid tightening procedure must be performed at the time of surgery to avoid lower eyelid retraction with the rounded eye, sad look, and scleral show (Fig. 16A) (18).

Special attention should be paid to the lower eyelid punctal position, entropion, ectropion, tear film abnormalities, recurrent severe eyelid, and periorbital edema in the past (likely because of allergic reaction or lymphedema), or more permanent swelling infraorbitally (pseudoherniation of orbital fat) enhanced by the upward gaze. Has the patient had previous surgery or cicatricial changes in the inferior fornix conjunctiva? Are they complaining about the prominent orbicularis oculi muscle, pars pretarsalis, and the crow's feet, which accentuate when laughing? In accordance with individual situations, several operation techniques may be advisable.

Botulinum Toxin Type A

The indication for treatment with botulinum toxin type A is the occurrence crow's feet when smiling. If wrinkling around the eye persists at rest and/or moderate dermatochalasis is present, botulinum toxin type A is recommended in combination with $UPCO_2$ laser skin resurfacing of the periorbital area (Fig. 17). Usually, subcutaneously injection of 12 units of Botox® (or 36 units of Dysport®) on each side is satisfactory for most individuals. The total dose for each eye is divided into four injection points: 3 U to the lateral sub-brow region, 4 U at the level of the lateral canthus and 2 cm lateral to the lateral canthus, 3 U 1.5 cm inferior and slightly medial to the second point, and 2 U infraorbitally, with avoidance of the pretarsal orbicularis. The main complications owing to injection in this area are bruising, diplopia, drooping of the lateral lower eyelid, ectropion, and an asymmetric smile, if the effect of the toxin is spreading into zygomaticus major (19). Botulinum toxin A maybe injected 2 weeks before laser skin resurfacing or after healing. The idea of using Botulinum toxin A before surgery is that the resurfaced skin will heal at rest and the risk of wrinkle recurrence is low. However, even when snap back test and pull out test are normal, the risk of producing a temporary ectropion immediately postoperatively in this case is higher and thus, the author prefers to inject Botulinum toxin A one month after laser skin resurfacing. This seems to reduce the postoperative edema periorbitally as well, because the natural massage of the muscle activity will better transport the lymph fluid.

Periorbital UltraPulse® CO_2 Laser Skin Resurfacing

It is the physician's method of choice when dermatochalasis or static wrinkling is to be treated. Herniated lower eyelid fat pads may be present (Fig. 18C). Chemical peeling as a medium-depth chemical peeling or deep phenol peeling will achieve the same result, but there are several advantages in using laser skin resurfacing over chemical peeling: an

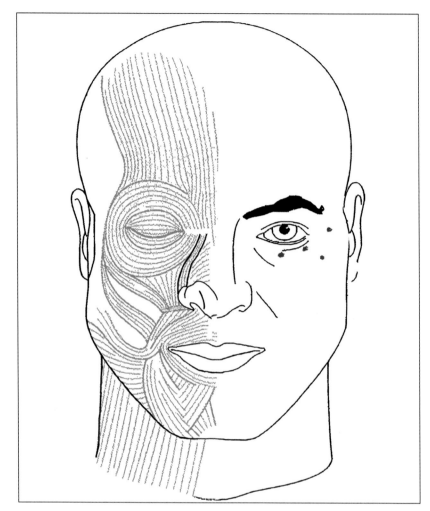

Figure 17
The injection points for botulinum toxin type A periorbitally.

immediate tightening of the skin occurs and surface correction is clearly seen, there is less postoperative swelling, and there are no systemic risks (cardiac, renal) similar to those with deep phenol peeling. The postoperative erythema, which may persist for three weeks up to two months is the only concern after $UPCO_2$ laser skin resurfacing. To avoid persistence of erythema, laser skin resurfacing, periorbitally, with Er:YAG laser was recommended, but in our experience the tightening effect and the cosmetic outcome is not as successful as after $UPCO_2$ laser skin resurfacing. The author prefers to combine $UPCO_2$ laser skin resurfacing of the periorbital area with medium depth chemical peeling of the rest of the face to avoid notable differences between resurfaced area and nonresurfaced facial skin.

(A) **(B)**

(C)

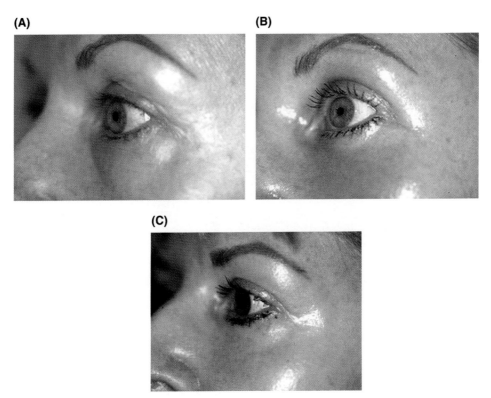

Figure 18
Preoperative view (**A**) with minimal dermatochalasis of the upper eyelid and minimal prolapse of the fat pads medially. Three weeks (**B**) and six years (**C**) after transconjunctival lower eyelid blepharoplasty, UPCO$_2$ laser skin resurfacing periorbitally, and injection of botulinum toxin type A for the crow's feet area.

This combination procedure helps reducing the operation and healing time as well as the cost of the operation, giving an even and better cosmetic outcome simultaneously (Fig. 19C). When we combine chemical peeling and laser skin resurfacing for rejuvenation of the face, first, the chemical peeling is performed excluding the periorbital area (and the perioral area if this supposed to be treated as well) (Fig. 19B). Then laser skin resurfacing follows and thus, a minimal overlap of the two procedures will not have the same side effect as that arising from penetration of chemical solution into the denuded area after the laser skin resurfacing. In our experience, when using the UP5000^{TM} CO$_2$ laser with the computer pattern generator (CPG: UltraScan$^®$ 5000^{TM}) for periorbital skin resurfacing, the parameters given in Table 1 have proved to be safe. Because the skin is thicker in the crow's feet area, the same parameters as for resurfacing of the facial skin can be used. With UltraScan$^®$ 5000$^®$, the spot size is 2.25 mm and therefore, when using the UltraPulse$^®$ Encore^{TM} CO$_2$ laser with the CPG (UltraScan$^®$ Encore^{TM}) the spot size of 1.3 mm has to be taken into

(A)   (B)

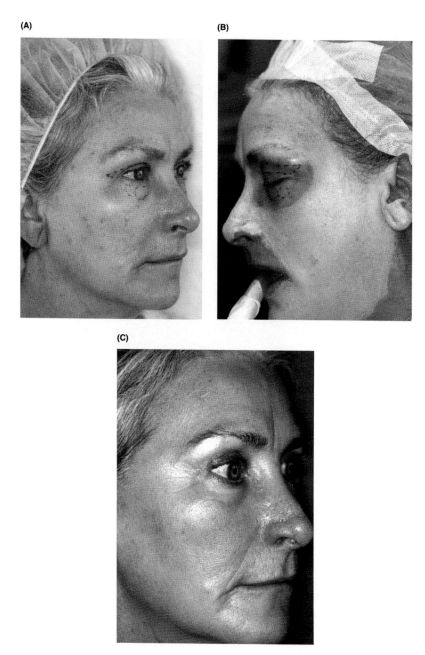

(C)

Figure 19
Preoperative (**A**) and intraoperative (**B**) view, and postoperative result (**C**) five
months after medium depth chemical peeling on the face, upper and transconjunctivally lower eyelid blepharoplasty in combination with $UPCO_2$ laser
skin resurfacing perioral and periorbital.

Table 1
Suggested Parameters Using the UltraScan® 5000™

Region	Passes	Energy (mJ)	Fluence (J/cm^2)	Repetition rate (Hz)	Pattern	Size	Density
Eyelid	1st	250	6.2	200	3	5	5
	2nd	200	5.0	200	3	5	4
Crow's feet	1st	300	7.5	200	3	5	6
	2nd	250	6.2	200	3	5	5
	3rd	200	5.0	200	3	5	4

consideration and thus the energy must be lowered to obtain the same fluence (Table 2). Usually, we do not treat the pretarsal skin because this might increase the postoperative edema (Fig. 4).

After laser skin resurfacing of the periorbital region, we protect the wound with an occlusive dressing, like Silon-TSR® (Bio Med Sciences, Allentown, Pennsylvania, U.S.), for about 1 week (Fig. 20). The dressing makes the wound less susceptible to infections, guarantees a moist environment of the wound, results in no crust formation, reduces discomfort, pain and burning sensation, and shortens the postoperative erythema (20). Changing the dressing is very simple and is performed every second day. Silon-TSR® is transparent and thus the wound can be easily examined, microperforations allow the exudate to run off, is not adhesive to the wound, is simple to change, and is delivered also in "Face-mask" design. The most important benefit of using the Silon-TSR® dressing is shortening of the postoperative erythema and reducing the burning sensation.

After 10 days, the skin is completely healed and a light make-up can be used to cover the erythema. Sun exposure should be avoided for at least three months, and also strenuous activities, increased cranial pressure (vomiting, constipation, etc.) and extreme heat or cold temperatures.

Table 2
Suggested Parameters Using the UltraScan® Encore™

Region	Passes	Energy (mJ)	Fluence (J/cm^2)	Repetition rate (Hz)	Pattern	Size	Density
Eyelid	1st	80	6.0	200	3	5	5
	2nd	70	5.2	200	3	5	4
Crow's feet	1st	100	7.5	200	3	5	6
	2nd	80	6.0	200	3	5	5
	3rd	70	5.2	200	3	5	4

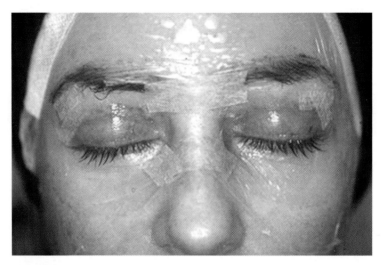

Figure 20
Postoperative view two days after upper and transconjunctivally lower eyelid blepharoplasty in combination with UPCO$_2$ laser skin resurfacing periorbital and forehead. Note the absence of crust formation and the minimal erythema under the occlusive dressing with Silon-TSR®.

Transconjunctival Approach

Herniated lower eyelid fat pads are the indications for performing this operation. If crow's feet, dermatochalasis, or moderate festoons are also a concern, first the CO$_2$ laser–assisted transconjunctival lower eyelid blepharoplasty is performed. A medium depth chemical peel for the facial skin follows (the periorbital skin is excluded) in combination with periorbital UPCO$_2$ laser skin resurfacing in the same operation session. Botulinum toxin type A treatment of the crow's feet area is recommended to avoid recurrence of the periorbital wrinkles. The surgical technique of the CO$_2$ laser–assisted transconjunctival blepharoplasty may be performed even if laxity of the lateral canthal tendon is present. However, a lower eyelid tightening procedure [lateral canthoplasty (21) or lateral tendon to periosteum canthopexy (22)] should be additionally performed. CO$_2$ laser-assisted transconjunctival blepharoplasty requires the use of only a few instruments and is time-saving. With some experience, the operating time may not exceed 15 minutes.

Mark the prolapsed orbital fat pads on the lower eyelid with the patient sitting up with view upgaze.

Topical anesthesia of the conjunctiva using two drops of topical anesthetic in the inferior cul-de-sac is only necessary if the operation is performed under local anesthesia. When both transconjunctival blepharoplasty and laser skin resurfacing are performed, additional IV sedation or even general anesthesia is more comfortable for the patient. Inject 2 mL of lidocaine 2% with epinephrine (1:100,000) transconjunctivally using a 36-gauge needle. We use a mixture of 1:9 mL hyaluronidase–lidocaine because hyaluronidase helps diffuse the local anesthetic throughout the lower eyelid (18,23).

Protect the globe using a Jaeger stainless steel plate with Methocel® gel as a lubricant in the eye to be operated on and a stainless steel shield, also with Methocel® gel, in the opposite eye.

The assistant's fingertips at the lid margin are gently pulling the lower lid downward and the surgeon is holding the Jaeger plate and the laser hand piece. When Jaeger plate is swept back from the orbital rim it produces bulging of fornix of conjunctival recess and the prolapsed fat pads are exposed (Fig. 21A). Be careful not to trap the upper eyelid eyelashes against the cornea, producing erosion on the globe.

Make the transconjunctival incision 6 mm below the eyelid margin, and extend the incision almost from side to side (from the medial caruncle to the lateral canthus).

Use the 0.2-mm focused hand piece of the UPCO$_2$ laser in CW mode with a power of 6 W and perform two to three passes. Use the laser focus guide for the blunt dissection during the procedure.

The first pass transects the conjunctiva and the second one, the lower eyelid retractors. Stay anterior to the orbital rim and avoid the inferior oblique muscle found between the nasal and middle fat pads (18).

With one hand, the assistant is now pulling the lower eyelid away placing a 9-mm DesMarres lid retractor into the incision (Fig. 21B). With the Jaeger plate in the other hand, the assistant is protecting and gently pulling down the globe, to help bulging the prolapsed orbital fat.

With the third pass, the fascia over individual fat pockets is opened. Always have a cautery available in case a big vessel is getting away. Fat pads (lateral, middle, and medial) are transected with the CO$_2$ laser slightly defocused using DesMarres retractor as backstop. Because the

(A)   **(B)**

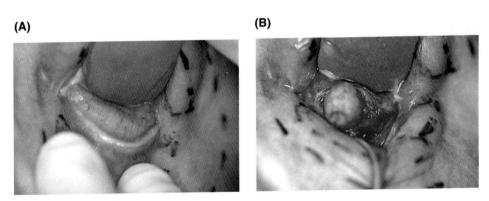

Figure 21
(**A**) Transconjunctival lower eyelid blepharoplasty, intraoperative view: Jaeger plate swept back from the orbital rim produces bulging of fornix of conjunctival recess. (**B**) Fat pads are transected using DesMarres retractor as backstop.

fat found laterally is commonly the most difficult to excise, start sculpting this fat pad first. Excise only the fat that prolapses anteriorly to the orbital rim and avoid larger blood vessels. Remember, what Dr. Sterling Baker likes to say, "The vessel not cut is the one that will not bleed" (18).

Remaining redundant lobules of fat can be vaporized in situ (but this makes visual comparison of the amount of fat resected less accurate).

Suturing of the transconjunctival incision is not necessary. Irrigating the wound with saline at the end of the operation will help to identify small bleeders.

Judge the amount of fat to be resected by visual quantification of fat pads on ballottement of the globe.

At the end of the operation, the lower lids should be gently pulled upward to prevent adhesion of the incision to the orbital rim.

Now, $UPCO_2$ laser skin resurfacing may be performed if necessary (Fig. 13 A and B). If not, the infraorbital area is compressed with suture strips to prevent swelling and hematoma in this area.

Cold packs are applied in the postsurgical care unit and the patient is instructed to keep the head elevated for at least one week postoperatively. Prophylactically, topical antibiotic/steroid eye drops are prescribed for a week. Contact lenses should not be worn for about two weeks (Fig. 22A and B).

Transcutaneous Subciliary Approach

Considerable dermatochalasis and festoons in combination with prolapsed preaponeurotic fat pads lateral, central, and medial, as well as orbicularis oculi hypertrophy require a transcutaneous subciliary approach. Excessive lower eyelid laxity because of inadequate orbicularis muscle tonicity and/or weakening of the lateral canthal ligament should be treated with an additional procedure either to tighten the lateral canthal tendon (for instance canthopexy or canthoplasty) or to reinforce the anterior

(A)   **(B)**

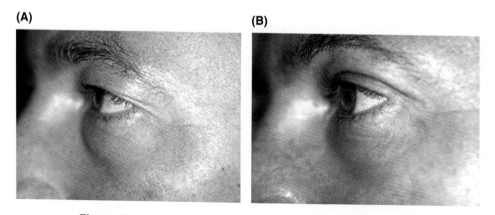

Figure 22
(**A**) Preoperative view and (**B**) postoperative result three months after upper and transconjunctivally lower eyelid blepharoplasty in a male patient.

lamella using Adamson's technique (24–26). According to the author and other physicians, this technique seems to be the method of choice to consolidate the anterior palpebral wall (27).

Use 3 mL of 2% lidocaine with 1:100,000 epinephrine and hyaluronidase. Local anesthesia is injected subcutaneously into the lower eyelid using one or two skin punctures. Avoiding forward and backward motions through the orbicularis muscle, the chance of hematoma formation is minimized. The addition of hyaluronidase into the anesthetic mixture enhances diffusion of the anesthetic solution by increasing tissue permeability.

To allow maximal hemostatic effect of the epinephrine, gentle pressure is applied to the eyelids for about 10 minutes.

Start the skin incision with the scalpel 1 cm lateral and 2 mm inferior to the lateral commissure, if possible, in a natural "crow's foot" and continue with the infraciliary skin incision using Westcott scissors to dissect the skin and the underlying orbicularis muscle. The infraciliary skin incision ends 2 mm beneath the inferior punctum and is facilitated by using traction suture with 4–0 silk to put the lower lid on upward tension.

The author prefers the combined technique of a skin flap with preservation of the orbicularis oculi pars pretarsalis followed by a skin muscle flap dissection in the avascular preseptal plane down to the orbital rim (14).

After incision of the skin, transect the orbicularis muscle beyond the lateral canthal angle using the CO_2 laser beam (for better coagulation). The infraorbital skin–muscle flap is dissected downward using the fully rectified waveform of the Ellman radiosurgical unit (Surgitron Radiolase). The cutting and coagulating capability of this needle, used as a monopolar unit, is excellent while producing minimal lateral heat and tissue damage. It is more precise than the free beam CO_2 laser, for this dissection.

Open the orbital septum making three very small horizontal incisions in the medial, central, and lateral portion of the septum just above the preaponeurotic fat pads which are vaporized in situ or resected using CO_2 laser in CW mode with 6 to 8 W (Fig. 23A). Balloting on the globe will help; the fat pads protrude into the surgical field but anyway, start with the temporal fat pad to facilitate its removal. Avoid traction on the fat pads and so retrobulbar hemorrhage, which may be related to this maneuver. The medial and central fat pads are separated by the inferior oblique muscle, which should not be injured.

Make a small orbicularis muscle flap, which will support the anterior lamella out of the inferolateral portion of the orbicularis, beyond the lateral canthal angle. With help of the CO_2 laser, create a tunnel deep on the periosteum of the superolateral orbital rim. Pass the muscle flap through the tunnel (Fig. 23B). The incision of upper eyelid blepharoplasty can be used, if both procedures are performed simultaneously; if not, perform a small incision in the upper eyelid crease. Anchor the muscle flap using Monocryl 5–0 or even Vicryl 5–0 (Fig. 23C). A nonresorbable suture is not necessary because scar tissue develops very soon in the periorbital area and will stabilize the result (Fig. 24A–D).

(A)   **(B)**

(C)

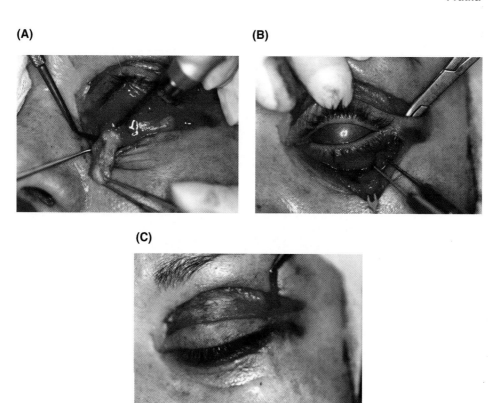

Figure 23
Transcutaneous subciliary approach for lower eyelid blepharoplasty, intra-operative views: (**A**) The fat pads on the lower eyelid are resected through stab incisions using CO_2 laser in CW mode. (**B** and **C**) A small orbicularis muscle flap is passed through a tunnel deep on the periosteum and anchored to the orbital rim.

If only a slight laxity of the anterior lamella is present, it is enough to simply reinforce the skin by means of a suture that anchors the orbicularis muscle to the periosteum directly below the retinaculum (27,28).

After suturing the muscle flap to the periosteum and draping the skin flap over the lower eyelid, resect the excessive skin both infraciliary and at the lateral canthus.

A nonresorbable running suture like Prolene 7–0 is preferably used to close the incision across the lower eyelid, which is removed after three days.

Use a pressure dressing with Suture-Strips on the lower eyelid area to prevent postoperative edema and hematoma (Fig. 24D).

Instead of CO_2 laser–assisted fat pad resection, preservation and repositioning of orbital fat pads may be recommended in patients with prominent orbital rim or tear trough deformity or depression in the nasojugal groove area. This technique described by many authors (22,29–32) may be performed both through transcutaneous and transconjunctival approach,

(A)

(B)

(C)

(D)

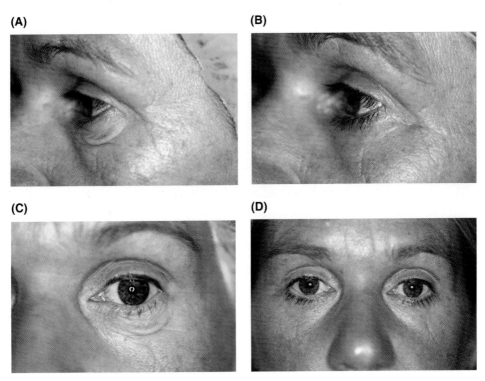

Figure 24
Preoperative views (**A** and **C**) and postoperative result (**B** and **D**) three
months after lower eyelid blepharoplasty, transcutaneous subciliary approach.

converting the double convexity deformity present. The author prefers fat
grafting (microlipoinjection) to the periorbital area using saddlebags fat as
the donor region (33).

A positive side effect after rhytidectomy with SMAS suspension
using a pronounced upward rotation, well-appreciated by the patients,
is filling the depressed area over the inferior orbital rim (Fig. 25A and
B). To avoid wrinkling of the infraorbital area, a canthopexy of the lateral
canthus should be explained to the patient and performed simultaneously.

COMPLICATIONS AND THEIR TREATMENT

Laser-assisted blepharoplasty is a more visual surgical technique with less
tactile feedback to identify anatomic planes, as opposed to the classical
blepharoplasty method using "cold steel" or even radiowave surgery.
However, both techniques accomplish the same goals and lead to the
same complications. Nevertheless, some complications are theoretically
more common for laser surgery (like wound dehiscence) or even typical
of the laser technique (e.g., burns). On the other hand, other complications

(A)   **(B)**

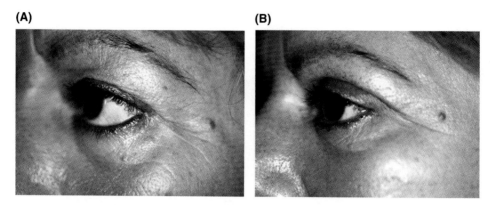

Figure 25
(**A**) Preoperative view and (**B**) postoperative result five weeks after rhytidectomy, upper eyelid blepharoplasty, and lateral canthopexy.

are less frequent in laser-assisted blepharoplasty and, therefore, are well-
received by the patient, e.g., intraoperative bleeding, postoperative hematoma or bruising, and eyelid malposition of the lower eyelid. A remarkable
aspect is the absence of complications such as distorting scars or rounding
of the lateral portion of the lower eyelid after transconjunctival laser-
assisted lower eyelid blepharoplasty.

Complications may occur because of inadequate surgeon and/or
patient education and improper use of the laser itself (17). Complications
may be minor and temporary; others may be major and/or permanent.

Some complications may occur intraoperatively, some postoperatively. Talking about complications is mandatory to focus on their prevention and management. Therefore, a presentation of the most frequent
intra- and postoperative complications seems to be more appropriate.

As with every cosmetic procedure, the surgeon must be aware of
problems occurring with an unenlightened patient or with those having
unrealistic expectations concerning both the risks of surgical techniques
coupled with the required downtime and as well as the intended outcome.
Using clear and concise written material, the patients should be able to
understand if they are good candidates for the procedure, whether there
are patient-related contraindications, the preoperative and postoperative
instructions, as well as the most important surgical steps. A well-educated
patient will recognize side effects or even complications and will report
these to the surgeon or is able to take care of them himself using first aid.

One of the most common causes of postoperative dissatisfaction is an
incomplete excision of the medial fat pad in upper eyelid blepharoplasty *and
of the lateral fat pad* in the transconjunctival lower eyelid blepharoplasty.
We recommend starting with the excision of the lateral fat pad in the lower
eyelid and removing both the anterior portion (very close to the central fat
pad) and the posterior lateral portion of this fat pad, which is tightly adherent to the capsulopalpebral fascia (CPF) (34,35). To avoid *skeletonization
of the eye*, the surgeon should be conservative with the resection of the fat

pads. The medial fat pad in the upper eyelid can be resected quite well without esthetic compromise. One should be prudent and avoid cutting the big vessels in this region, especially the artery. If too much fat is excised in the lower eyelid, a sunken eye may develop.

Postoperatively, the patients may be also very disappointed with an *asymmetrical palpebral aperture or asymmetrical upper eyelid crease.* This side effect is very often seen when inexperienced surgeons perform the operation first on one eye and after several days or even weeks, on the other one (Fig. 26). To avoid this side effect, a meticulous operation and suture technique must be performed and the surgery should be done on both eyes simultaneously. If the side effect still occurs, one of the most common causes could be asymmetrical, postoperative swelling. Therefore, we recommend leaving it untouched until postoperative edema has subsided. A decision must then be made as to whether the lower one of the two creases should be raised or the higher one of the two creases should be lowered. Some oculoplastic surgeons assert it is easier to cut a higher suture and refix skin edges to a lower position on the aponeurosis. However, we have had first hand experience with the opposite. A female patient had been operated on twice by an aesthetic surgeon who routinely performed blepharoplasty, on one eye and on the other one, some weeks later. She had a lower incision on the left upper eyelid (Fig. 27A), no definition of the upper eyelid crease (Fig. 27B) and with the eye closed, no skin excess, that is to say a *pseudodermato-chalasis* with the eyes opened (Fig. 27B). Another skin excision would certainly lead to lagophthalmos. We reoperated the patient, performing a small, 1 mm wide skin excision and elevated a skin-muscle flap down to the orbital septum. The septum orbitalis was opened and a supratarsal fixation, 9 mm from the lid margin, was performed for a better definition

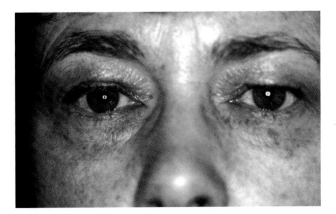

Figure 26
Note the asymmetrical upper eyelid crease after upper eyelid blepharoplasty performed in another clinic: first one eye, and after two weeks the other eye, was operated on.

COMPLICATIONS AFTER BLEPHAROPLASTY

Minor Complications

Dissatisfied Patient

- Aesthetic compromise:
  Palpebral aperture or upper eyelid crease asymmetry
  Inadequate or excessive fat removal
  Unacceptable scarring
    Hypertrophic scar
    Wound dehiscence
    Dog-ear medial or lateral aspect
    Suture tunnel
- Complications related to laser skin resurfacing periorbitally or typical for laser surgery in general:
  Burns
  Loss of eyelashes
  Synechia
  Milia
  Erythema, transitory or persistent
  Hyper- or hypopigmentation, transitory or persistent
- Eyelid malposition:
  Retraction
  Ptosis
  Paresis
  Ectropion (transitory)
  Entropion
  Punctal obstruction
  Lagophthalmos
  Scleral show
- Corneal changes:
  Desiccation
  Keratoconjunctivitis sicca
  Exposure keratitis
  Inability to wear contact lenses
  Tear film abnormalities
  Epiphor
  Erosions, corneal abrasion
  Ulceration
- Minimal visual disturbance
- Chemosis
- Subconjunctival hemorrhage
- Pupillary changes

(Continued)

COMPLICATIONS AFTER BLEPHAROPLASTY (*Continued*)

Major Complications

- Retrobulbar hemorrhage/hematoma
- Blindness
- Glaucoma
- Extraocular muscle disorders
- Diplopia
- Prolapse
- Infection: orbital cellulitis, abscess
- Less frequent complications
- Epicanthal fold
- Cysts formation
- Eyelid numbness

---

of the upper eyelid crease. The pseudodermatochalasis was so corrected and the symmetry of the upper eyelid crease reestablished (Fig. 27C).

Pronounced dermatochalasis of the upper eyelid may demand excessive skin removal in the medial and lateral aspect of the upper lid. First, possible ptosis of the eyebrow must be analyzed, then a repositioning of the ptotic eyebrow has to be considered, explained to the patient, and performed before upper eyelid blepharoplasty. If redundant skin in the medial and lateral aspect of the upper eyelid is still a problem, M-plasty to avoid *dog-ears* may be performed (12). With a normal eyebrow position, only an ellipse shaped excision of the skin laterally, ending at the orbital rim is required. An M-plasty on the lateral aspect of the upper eyelid may leave a complex scar, which cannot be hidden in a natural fold like e.g. a crow's foot. On the medial aspect of the upper eyelid, an M-plasty is a good solution to prevent prolonging the scar over the thick nasal skin, which can be clearly seen. This technique, however, is more appropriate for elderly patients with thin skin. Younger patient with relatively thick skin may complain about the dog-ear resulting from the M-plasty itself. If this aspect is a concern, an elliptical excision of the dog-ear should be performed as soon as possible by prolonging the scar medially, but very conservatively so not to produce an epicanthal fold or leave a visible scar.

Intraoperative Complications

Most of the intraoperative complications are related to improper use of the laser itself, e.g., violation of laser safety, an inadequate surgical technique because of inappropriate surgeon education, orbital hemorrhage and thus failure to identify the anatomic planes properly, and injury to extraocular muscles (17).

The surgeon, his operative staff, and anesthesiologist must be well-educated in laser safety. Special goggles for staff, a proper endotracheal

(A)   **(B)**

(C)

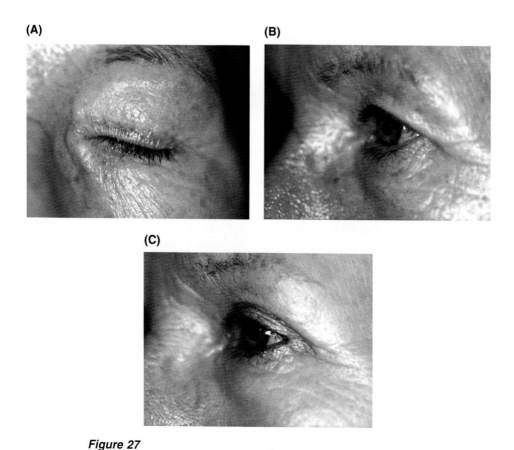

Figure 27
(**A–C**) Note the lower incision on the left upper eyelid (3 to 4 mm from lid
margin) after upper eyelid blepharoplasty (**A**) performed in another clinic: first
one eye and after one week the other eye was operated on. The left eye was
operated twice by the first aesthetic surgeon because the patient complained
on pseudodermatochalasis. Even after the second operation the pseudodermatochalasis persisted (**B**). (**C**) demonstrates the postoperative result after
the author performed a supratarsal fixation for a better definition of the upper
eyelid crease with no skin excision.

tube, stainless steel shields to protect the patient's eyes, a Jaeger stainless
steel plate, and only instruments with nonreflecting surfaces that could
come in contact with the laser beam must be used. The shields, the Jaeger
plate, and the David-Baker retractor (16) must be large enough to cover
the entire globe to prevent *burns* and *ulceration* or *penetration injury* to the
globe. If any of these complications occurs, they have to be recognized on
site and an ophthalmologist should immediately come to examine the
injury. The perforation of the globe may lead to retinal or choroidal
detachment, loss of intraocular contents, and permanent blindness (17).
Avoid direct lasering of the metal eyeshield, although studies have
demonstrated that even repetitive applications of the laser beam to the

external surface of the shield will not substantially increase the temperature on the other side in contact with the globe to be able to produce a thermal denaturation or any injury to the cornea (36). To avoid *corneal abrasion* or erosions, stainless steel shields should be gently cleaned by the staff, and each of these should be sterilized in separate paperbags. All the surfaces of the instruments in contact with the surface of the globe should be polished and always checked for scratches. A protective layer of ophthalmic gel (e.g., Methocel® gel) can be used to lubricate the polished side of the metal eyeshields or the Jaeger plate, respectively, David-Baker retractor. The gel can be rinsed with saline at the end of the operation to check for visual acuity. Despite Stasior's opinion (18) reporting on *wound healing problems* of the transconjunctival incision and even *subconjunctival ointment-containing cysts or granuloma* after using corticosteroids ophthalmic ointment postoperatively, the author and others have not seen delayed wound healing but actually quite good scar quality and faster decreasing of chemosis by using ophthalmic ointments. The use of corticosteroid-containing ophthalmic ointment should be combined with artificial tear fluid to prevent dry eye and complaints related to this aspect. By doing so, even corneal abrasion will heal without sequela in about few days. To avoid delayed wound healing of both skin incisions on the upper eyelid and transconjunctival incisions on the lower eyelid, the surgeon should maintain a focused beam at all times and move it continuously approximately 1 cm/sec. Using the 0.2-mm beam of the $UPCO_2$ laser, the zone of thermal damage measures approximately 115 µm. Therefore, scar quality after laser blepharoplasty is indistinguishable from that produced by cold steel (36).

Burns of the skin outside the surgical field (e.g. nose, eyebrow, and pretarsal skin) are unusual if appropriate backstop material is used (e.g., Jaeger stainless plate to protect the nose, Rabkin spatula or wet cotton-tipped applicator to protect the levator when cutting the septum or during fat resection, DesMarres retractor as backstop for fat resection on the lower lid). However, if this happens, these usually superficial burns will heal under corticosteroid ointment without leaving a scar. Superficial burns with *loss of the eyelashes* will heal without sequela but regrowth of the cilia will take several months to go back to normal. If the follicle is burned as well, the cilia will be permanently lost. A possible cause for burned eyelashes are remainders of inflammable mascara. Therefore, pay attention to removal of all mascara prior to laser surgery.

Resection of the levator aponeurosis is a major intraoperative complication. This white, glistening anatomic structure may undergo an involutional process known as fatty degeneration and inexperienced surgeons may confuse it with the preaponeurotic fat pad and thus resect it. This may lead to a full-thickness eyelid defect with the consequence of a postoperative *ptosis*. It is a very serious complication, which should be recognized and repaired immediately using 6/0 silk to suture the ends of the remaining levator. Secondary repair is not recommended because it is very difficult to recognize the levator aponeurosis in the scar tissue, which develops quite rapidly in this region.

Another anatomical structure, which may be confused with the preaponeurotic fat pad during upper eyelid blepharoplasty is the lacrimal gland. Although this gland lies behind the orbital rim and has a gray color, in certain conditions like inflammation or involutional changes, it may prolapse into the lateral or central portion of the orbit. Its accidental resection will lead to *permanent tear film abnormality* and *keratoconjunctivitis sicca* and, consequently, *the inability to wear contact lenses* (17). However, this complication is less frequent in laser-assisted blepharoplasty because the surgeon may better recognize the anatomic landmarks because of minimal intraoperative bleeding and, thus, superior visualization.

Severe *subconjunctival or even retrobulbar hemorrhage* may occur intraoperatively or postoperatively if the patient has an increased intracranical pressure, e.g., high blood pressure, vomiting, obstipation, and coughing. Antiemetic agents are of great help postoperatively to avoid nausea as well as the need for Valsalva maneuver, especially in patients with a history of similar reactions after general anesthesia. Retrobulbar hematoma is a true emergency and has to be recognized and treated immediately. Common sources of intraoperative bleeding are the vessels located in the medial fat pad and the orbicularis oculi muscle in the upper eyelid blepharoplasty, respectively the vessels in any fat pad or the cut edge of the lower lid retractors in the surgery of the lower eyelid. The source must be located immediately and effective hemostasis using a bipolar cautery should be employed. A unipolar unit should never be used to avoid channeling of the current to the posterior orbit as it may cause spasms of the central retinal, or the posterior ciliary arteries, or injury to the optic nerve itself (37). In laser-assisted blepharoplasty the defocused CO_2 laser beam will simultaneously divide and effectively seal small vessels usually under 0.5 mm, but a bipolar unit should always be available in case a bigger vessel gets away. Larger vessels may be pushed away with the fine tip of the laser hand-piece unit.

A very difficult situation to manage is orbital hemorrhage when a vessel deep within the orbit gets away because of the difficult access to these vessels. This may happen when the fat pad is pulled out with force, twisted, or grasped with a clamp. As the fat pads are connected to the posterior orbit via the orbital connective tissue network (17), an aggressive pulling motion will lead to the twisting and rupturing of the deep vessels. This situation is more common in cold steel surgery. When using the CO_2 beam as a "light scalpel," clamping of the prolapsed fat is no longer necessary, and only the fat pads, which prolapse outside the orbital rim, will be resectioned or vaporized. If retrobulbar hematoma happens postoperatively and the hemorrhage originates in the posterior orbit, the patient will primarily suffer from moderate to severe orbital pain, nausea, vomiting, and visual disturbances like diplopia up to temporary visual loss. Eyelid swelling, periorbital ecchymosis, sometimes even bleeding from the wounds and asymmetric pupils, and even proptosis in extreme cases can be clearly seen. The elevated intraorbital pressure will interrupt the blood flow to the optic nerve and eye, and blindness (less than 0.01% in the literature) can come rapidly (18). In this case, the intraorbital pressure must be decreased immediately, first by opening the surgical wound and evacuating the hematoma. The origin of bleeding should be identified and appropriate hemostasis should be performed. Mannitol and systemic steroids may be administered intravenously to promote orbital decongestion and help reduce edema. The patient should be instructed to sleep with an elevated head and to apply ice compresses. If the increased orbital pressure still cannot be controlled, canthotomy, cantholysis, and vertical splitting of the eyelid may be considered (17). If a diffuse oozing is the source of the bleeding, different hemostatic agents, which should not be left within the orbit, may be used: Gelfoam (absorbable gelatin; Upjohn, Kalamazoo, Michigan, U.S.) or Surgicel (oxidized cellulose; Johnson and Johnson Medical, Arlington, Texas, U.S.) (17).

Other complications that can occur mainly during the transconjunctival approach are injury to the canthal tendons, the inferior oblique muscle, the inferior rectus muscle, and the lacrimal system. Contrary to some surgeons who recommend searching for the inferior oblique muscle if this is not visible, we recommend not doing this. Injury to this muscle or to its connective tissue sheath will produce permanent *diplopia*.

Injury to the levator aponeurosis and even full-thickness eyelid burns may result if a laser-safe instrument (DesMarres retractor, Jaeger plate, etc.) is not appropriately placed as a *backstop* behind the fat pads to be resectioned. If this complication happens, it is necessary to suture the levator aponeurosis but not the orbital septum (actually the orbital septum should never be closed). A skin burn should always be excised and sutured.

Postoperative Complications

Besides orbital hemorrhaging, several other postoperative complications not specifically related to laser-assisted blepharoplasty such as lymphedema and prolonged swelling, entropion, subconjunctival seroma-like fluid collection, and allergic contact reaction may occur.

If the CO_2 laser beam is appropriately used in focus and defocused as described in the operating technique, excessive swelling, postoperatively, is uncommon. By injecting only a small amount of local anesthetic, 1 mL to 2 mL local anesthesia with hyaluronidase, prolonged swelling and lymphedema are avoided. All postblepharoplasty patients will have a slight *blepharoptosis* because of postoperative inflammation and edema. Also, the amount of ptosis is directly related to the height of the lid crease when using the supratarsal fixation (a 10-mm surgical lid crease will create less acquired ptosis than a 13-mm surgical lid crease).

Ectropion or just scleral show or rounding of the lateral portion of the lower eyelid are very commonly seen after transcutaneous lower eyelid blepharoplasty and are not related to the use of the CO_2 laser beam as an incisional tool. These mainly occur because too much skin had been excised, the orbital septum had been seriously violated, or a pre-existing lower eyelid laxity had not been recognized and had not been corrected by a canthoplasty or canthopexy simultaneously. There are many procedures to repair a postoperative ectropion but the description of these procedures is beyond the purpose of this chapter (22,24–26,38–41).

Entropion is a complication related to transconjunctival blepharoplasty and may be avoided by massaging the lower lid upward at the end of the operation. This prevents adhesion of the incision to the orbital rim and thus an overlap of the wound edges producing an entropion. If the patient feels irritation or a *foreign body sensation* postoperatively, one cause may be a subconjunctival collection of a pale yellow, seroma-like fluid visible under the bulbar conjunctiva. This condition disappears by using ice packs, or even spontaneously. Another cause for foreign body sensation—dry eyes and inability to wear contact lenses—may be the persistance of lagophthalmos for over several weeks or a dry eye condition that had not been diagnosed preoperatively. *Lagophthalmos*, the condition of impairment of eyelid closure, is normal for the first three to five days postoperatively. The patient should be well-informed about this condition and instructed to use artificial tears such as lubricating drops during the day and ointment for the night for at least two to three weeks postoperatively.

The use of topical antibiotics-containing ophtalmic ointment may produce *allergic contact reaction* with severe inflammation especially when using on the periorbital skin after laser skin resurfacing. Corticosteroid containing ophthalmic ointments without preservatives are recommended.

Certainly, the patient will not be satisfied with a *dehiscent, hypopigmented* or even *hypertrophic scar* on the upper eyelid but, despite some case reports in the research literature, these complications are very rare. Using the 0.2-mm laser beam of the $UPCO_2$ laser and the UltraPulse® mode, the author has not seen one unacceptable scarring in ten years of experience with innumerable cases. Moreover, using the laser beam to perform the incision on one upper lid and the scalpel on the other in ten cases, not even a slightest difference in scar quality was noted (Figs. 28A and B and 29 A and B). Unacceptable scarring is avoided by using the laser in UltraPulse® mode to cut the skin and by keeping the beam in focus and thus diminishing the zone of thermal damage of the incision's margins. Prophylactically, a weak topical corticosteroid ophthalmic ointment is used two times daily for a maximum of two weeks. A superpotent steroid such as Temovate is not used, to avoid atrophy of the periorbital skin, or even cataract, because glaucoma may develop.

If the incision was performed with the $UPCO_2$ laser beam, a submerged intradermal running suture left in place for at least ten days is recommended. If a continuous wave CO_2 laser beam was used, to compensate for the delayed wound healing, the suture may be removed later (e.g., after two to three weeks). To reduce the period before suture removal, the incision may be alternatively done with the scalpel and the skin-muscle flap excised with the laser beam. In this case, a

(A)   (B)

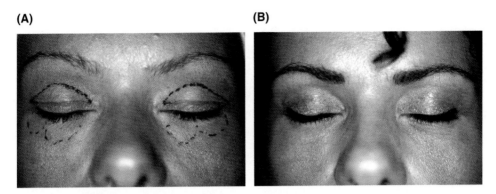

Figure 28
(**A** and **B**) Preoperative view and postoperative result 14 weeks after laser-assisted upper eyelid blepharoplasty: the skin incision on the right upper eyelid was performed using the 0.2 mm laser beam of the UPCO$_2$ laser and the UltraPulse® mode. On the left upper eyelid, the incision was performed with the scalpel.

subcuticular running suture with nonresorbable Prolene 7–0 can be removed after four to five days. Resorbable sutures are not recommended because they produce an inflammatory reaction at the wound edges. In any case, hypertrophic scars are very rare on the upper eyelid even in patients with severe keloid formation and, in the author's experience, are mainly because of the use of bipolar cauterization to close the wound edges. If this situation does not resolve itself, excision in four to six months instead of any kind of laser therapy is recommended.

(A)   (B)

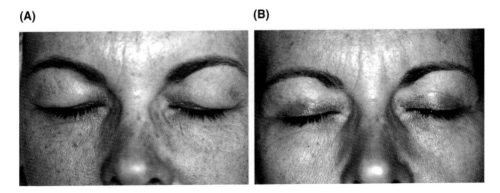

Figure 29
(**A** and **B**) Preoperative view and postoperative result 6 months after laser-assisted upper eyelid blepharoplasty using similar technique as in patient on Fig. 28.

CONCLUSION

Using the $UPCO_2$ laser as a cutting tool in blepharoplasty enhances the surgeon's ability to perform the operation more accurately and judge the necessary amount of fat and skin to be removed. Complication after CO_2 laser blepharoplasty transconjunctivally, like distorting scars, rounded eye, scleral show, and ectropion are only transitory, if any. Therefore, we recommend the transconjunctival blepharoplasty as an important technique, i.e., the golden standard, in eyelid rejuvenation and believe that the majority of young patients will benefit from it. The most frequent complication of the infraciliary approach for lower lid blepharoplasty, the lower eyelid retraction, can thus be avoided. Also, this procedure may be simultaneously combined with $UPCO_2$ laser skin resurfacing or chemical peeling to treat the sun-damaged skin.

ACKNOWLEDGMENTS

The author would like to express her gratitude to her colleagues Dr. Michael Rabkin, and Dr. Thomas Roberts, and Dr. Sterling Baker for their exchange of ideas and technique in the cosmetic rejuvenation of the periorbital region and Dr. Mitch Goldman and Dr. Robert Weiss for editing this manuscript.

REFERENCES

1. Baker SS, Muenzler WS, Small RG, Leonard JE. Carbon dioxide laser blepharoplasty. Ophthalmology 1984; 91:238–244.
2. Baker SS. Editorial. Operative Techniques in Oculoplastic, Orbital, and Reconstructive Surgery 1998; 1:3.
3. Bourguet. Les Hernies Graisseuses De L'Orbite; notre traitement chirurgical. Bulletin De L'Academie Nationale De Medecine (Paris) 1924; 92:1270.
4. Baylis HI, Sutcliffe RT. Conjunctival approach in lower eyelid blepharoplasty. Adv Ophthal Plast Reconstr Surg 1983; 2:43–54.
5. David LM, Sanders G. CO_2 laser blepharoplasty. J Dermatol Surg Oncol 1987; 13: 110–114.
6. David LM. The laser approach to blepharoplasty. J Dermatol Surg Oncol 1988; 14: 741–746.
7. Mittelman H, Apfelberg DB. Carbon dioxide laser blepharoplasty—advantages and disadvantages. Ann Plast Surg 1990; 24:1–6, 1990.
8. Bosniak SL, Cantisano-Zilkha M. Cosmetic Blepharoplasty and Facial Rejuvenation. 2nd ed. Philadelphia: Lippincott-Raven, 1999.
9. Baker TJ, Gordon HL, Stuzin JM. Surgical Rejuvenation of the Face. 2nd ed. St. Louis: Mosby, 1996.
10. Kontis TC, Papel ID, Larrabee WF. Surgical anatomy of the eyelids. Facial Plast Surg 1994; 10:1–5.
11. Putterman AM. Cosmetic Oculoplastic Surgery, 3rd ed. Philadelphia: WB Saunders, 1999.
12. Tardy ME Jr, Thomas JR, Brown RJ. Facial Aesthetic Surgery. St. Louis: Mosby, 1995:237–240.
13. Jelks GW, Jelks EB. Preoperative evaluation of the blepharoplasty patient: bypassing the pitfalls. Clin Plast Surg 1993; 20:213–223.
14. Silkiss RZ. Cosmetic blepharoplasty. Lower eyelid techniques. Cosmet Facial Surg 2000; 12:689–700.
15. Biesman BS. Laser-assisted upper eyelid blepharoplasty. Operative Techniques in Oculoplastic, Orbital, and Reconstructive Surgery 1998:11–18.
16. David LM, Baker SS. David–Baker eyelid retraction. Am J Cosm Surg 1992; 9:147–148.
17. Cole HP, Biesman BS. Laser blepharoplasty: complications and treatment. Operative Techniques in Oculoplastic, Orbital, and Reconstructive Surgery 1998:4–10.
18. Stasior GO. Carbon dioxide laser-assisted transconjunctival lower eyelid blepharoplasty. Operative Techniques in Oculoplastic, Orbital, and Reconstructive Surgery 1998:19–23.
19. Carruthers A, Carruthers J. Clinical indications and injection technique for the cosmetic use of Botulinum A exotoxin. Dermatol Surg 1998; 24:1189–1194.
20. Goldman MP, Skover G, Roberts TL, Fitzpatrick RE, Lettieri JT. Optimizing wound healing in the post-laser abrasion face. J Am Acad Dermatol 2002; 46:399–407.
21. Spinelli HM. Atlas of Aesthetic Eyelid and Periocular Surgery. Philadelphia: WB Saunders, 2004.
22. Flowers RS. Blepharoplasty and brow lifting. In: Roenigk RK, Roenigk HH Jr, eds. Dermatologic Surgery: Principles and Practice. New York: Marcel Dekker, 1989:1215–1238.
23. Cook BE Jr, Lemke BN. Lower eyelid rejuvenation with skin/skin-muscle/fat repositioning techniques. Am J Cosm Surg 2001; 18:237–245.
24. Adamson JE, McCraw JB, Carraway JH. Use of a muscle flap in lower blepharoplasty. Plast Reconstr Surg 1979; 63:359.
25. Adamson PA, Strecker HD. Transcutaneous lower blepharoplasty. Facial Plast Surg 1996; 12:171–183.

26. Adamson PA, Tropper GJ, McGraw BL. Extended blepharoplasty. Arch Otolaryngol Head Neck Surg 1991; 117:606–609.

27. Botti G. Blepharoplasty: a classification of selected techniques in the treatment and prevention of lower lid margin distortions. Aesth Plast Surg 1998; 22:341–348.

28. Labrandter HP. Use of the orbicularis muscle flap for complex lower lid problems: a 6 year analysis. Plast Reconstr Surg 1995; 96:346.

29. Hamra ST. Arcus marginalis relase and orbital fat preservation in midface rejuvenation. Plast Reconstr Surg 1995; 96:354–362.

30. Plaza R, Crus L. The sliding fat pad technique with use of the transconjunctival approach. Aesth Surg J 2001; 21:487–492.

31. Goldberg RA. Transconjunctival orbital fat repositioning: transposition of orbital fat pedicles into a subperiosteal pocket. Plast Reconstr Surg 2000; 105:743–748.

32. Loeb R. Naso-jugal groove leveling with fat tissue. Clin Plast Surg 1993; 20:393–400.

33. Fratila AM. Autologous fat transplantation: my technique of lipofilling. In: Baran R, Maibach HI, eds. Textbook of Cosmetic Dermatology, 3rd ed. London: Taylor & Francis, 2005.

34. Lemke BN, Lucatelli MJ. Anatomy of the ocular adnexa, orbit, and related facial structures. In: Nessi FA, Lisman RD, Levine MR, eds. Smith's Ophthalmic Plastic and Reconstructive Surgery. 2nd ed. St. Louis: Mosby, 1997:55.

35. Barker DE. Dye injection studies of infraorbital fat compartments. Plast Reconstr Surg 1977; 59:82.

36. Biesman BS, Baker SS, Khan J, et al. Effects of defocused carbon dioxide laser beam on human eyelid tissue. Presented at 1997 ASOPRS Annual Meeting, San Francisco, CA, Oct 26, 1997.

37. Callahan MA. Prevention of blindness after blepharoplasty. Ophthalmology 1983; 90:1047–1051.

38. Pham RT, Baker SS. Ectropion repair: carbon dioxide laser-assisted modified tarsal strip procedure. Operative Techniques in Oculoplastic, Orbital, and Reconstructive Surgery. 1998:38–40.

39. Murakami CS, Orcutt JC. Treatment of lower eyelid laxity. Facial Plast Surg 1994; 10:42–52.

40. Shorr N. Madame butterfly procedure with hard palate graft: management of postblepharoplasty round eye and scleral show. Facial Plast Surg 1994; 10:90–118.

41. Rosenberg GJ. Temporary tarsorrhaphy suture to prevent or treat scleral show and ectropion secondary to laser resurfacing or laser blepharoplasty. Plast Reconstr Surg 2000; 106:721–725.

7

Laser Hair Removal

Suzanne L. Kilmer
*Laser and Skin Surgery Center of Northern California,
Sacramento, California, U.S.A.*

Video 9: Hair Removal: Alexandrite Laser

INTRODUCTION

Although the very first laser destruction of hair was noted in the early 1960s by Leon Goldman with a ruby laser (1), its importance went unnoticed; it was not until the mid-1990s that the laser hair removal craze began. Ironically, it was carried out was through the use of a Q-switched 1064 nm Nd:YAG laser purportedly aided by a topical carbon suspension to facilitate absorption of laser light in the hair follicles (2,3). Although this method was later disproved (4,5), the widespread popularity of potentially permanent hair removal with lasers had become appreciated.

The field of laser hair removal has expanded rapidly owing to patient demand. Removal of unwanted hair has long been desired as evidenced by the great number of patients that shave, wax, pluck, use depilatories, seek the service of an electrologist, or, more recently, opt for laser hair removal (6); the use of laser for hair removal appears to be more effective (7,8). Unwanted hair can be in a normal distribution (axilla, bikini, upper lip, and legs) or abnormally distributed and/or excessive, as seen with a hormonal abnormality (e.g., polycystic ovarian disease), medication side effect (e.g., cyclosporin), or hair-bearing skin grafted (9) or flapped (10) onto an area where hair is undesirable. Patients with follicular disorders, such as psuedofolliculitis barbae (11–13), acne nuchae keloidalis, and pilonidal cysts (14), or those desiring hair transplant correction, or male to female transsexuals (15) may also request treatment.

The principle of selective photothermolysis (16), which was initially defined for treatment of vascular lesions, applies to laser hair removal as well. In this case, the target is pigmented hair. The theory predicts that if chosen wavelength is well-absorbed by the target, in this case melanin, the pulse width is shorter than or equal to the thermal relaxation time (TRT) of the target (millisecond range and dependent on hair size), and sufficient energy is delivered, a target can be destroyed without destruction of surrounding tissue.

Development of lasers that directly targeted follicular melanin was underway simultaneously with that of adjunctive carbon suspension modality. The ruby laser was chosen for its high absorption by melanin-laden targets (17–20). Q-switched ruby pulses were used successfully in the treatment of pigment lesions, including nevus of Ota, a dermal melanocytic lesion, and tattoos (21). Because regrowth of hair was noted in initial studies, it was felt that the 25–50 nanosecond pulse width generated by a Q-switched laser was too short to thermally damage larger hair follicles. To better match the target size, the ruby laser, as well as subsequent lasers used for hair removal, utilized pulse widths in the millisecond (msec) domain.

Ruby laser hair removal was initially difficult in darker skin types, occasionally resulting in blistering, hyperpigmentation, and scarring. Unfortunately, the epidermal melanin in darker skin competes with underlying hair melanin; newer strategies were developed to expand the utility of laser hair removal for darker skin types. In an effort to avoid epidermal melanin, lasers emitting longer wavelengths were developed, including the alexandrite at 755-nm, diode at 810-nm, and finally the Nd:YAG laser at 1064-nm. As the wavelength increases, melanin absorption decreases, allowing light to pass through the epidermis with less injury. These longer wavelengths also penetrate deeper, enabling more light to reach the target (Table 1).

In addition to wavelength, as noted above, the pulse width is also important. As stated previously, Q-switched lasers in the nanosecond domain were utilized at first with a topical carbon suspension. One of the reasons for the failure of this modality was that the pulse width was too short to cause sufficient thermal injury to destroy the hair follicle (22). Pulse widths in the millisecond domain were preferred, and the original ruby laser was built with a pulse width of 0.3 msec (17,18), but then extended to 3 msec, which resulted in better efficacy. Alexandrite lasers initially delivered energy with several msec pulse widths. It was discovered that by elongating the pulse width, there was greater thermokinetic selectivity, allowing the finer particles of melanin in the epidermis to dissipate heat more efficiently than the larger collections of melanin found in the hair follicle. For darker skinned patients, it also became apparent that by having very long pulse widths, epidermal melanin was preferentially spared.

The follicular bulge has been discovered to be as important, if not more so, for hair growth, as the hair shaft bulb (23). In its midfollicular location, the bulge area contains presumptive follicular stem cells essential for regenerative follicular activity. Therefore, the true target, the follicular bulge, contains minimal chromophore melanin; consequently, selective photothermolysis, in a classical sense, may not be *the goal with hair removal*. Collateral thermal damage to the regenerative bulge region may be not only desired, but also required for more effective hair removal, hence the need for longer pulse widths.

The phase of hair growth may be important; anagen hairs seem to respond better to laser treatment than telogen hairs (18,24,25). Correlalis

Table 1
Hair Removal Lasers/Light Sources

Device type	Laser name	Laser company	Fluence (J/cm^2)	Pulse width (msec)
Ruby (694-nm)	Epilaser/E2000	Palomar	10–40	3
Alexandrite	GentleLASE	Candela	10–100	3
(755-nm)	Arion	WaveLight	Up to 40	5–40
	Apogee	Cynosure	50	5–40
Diode (810-nm)	Diode laser	Opus	10–40	10–100
	Palomar SLP1000	Palomar	Up to 180	50–1000
	Apex 800	Iriderm	5–60	5–100
	LightSheer ET	Lumenis	10–100	5–400
	Apogee 100	Cynosure	50	50–500
Nd:YAG (1064-nm)	GentleYAG	Candela	10–70	3
	SmartEpil II	Cynosure	16–200	Up to 100
	Profile	Sciton	4–400	0.1–200
	Lyra	Laserscope	15–50	20–200
	CoolGlide excel	Cutera	Up to 300	1–3000
Q-Switched Nd:YAG (1064-nm)	Medlite C6	Hoya/ ConBio	3–3.5	<20
IPL (525– 1200-nm)	EsteLux	Palomar	Up to 27	10–100
	Prolite	Alderm	10–50	N/A
	Lumenis One	Lumenis	30–65	2.5–7
IPL + RF	Aurora DS	Syneron	10–30 Optical 5–20 RF	N/A

Abbreviation: IPL, intense pulsed light.

correlates to the fact that melanin-containing portion is in contact with the regenerative portion of the hair. Alteration in the hair growth cycle may result from repeated treatments (26).

Finally, cooling is a very important adjunctive measure. By sufficiently cooling of the epidermis, the heat that is deposited is delivered mainly to the dermis, where hair follicles are present. It was the significant cooling of the early 0.3-msec ruby laser that allowed it to be utilized in patients that did have some pigment in their skin.

PATIENT-RELATED FACTORS

Skin Type

The darker the skin type, the more epidermal melanin in the epidermis; this is a factor in hair removal. The lighter the skin, and therefore the less

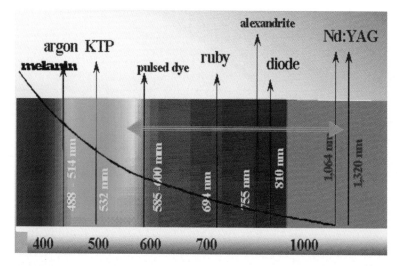

Figure 1
Electromagnetic spectrum melanin absorption curve with lasers labeled that target melanin.

melanin present in the epidermis, the easier it is to perform laser hair removal. The lack of competing chromophore in the epidermis allows the use of higher fluences to better target the follicular melanin. This competing chromophore needs to be avoided to allow less injury to the epidermis and more light delivery down to the target. Also, persons with skin types III to VI should be advised that they are more likely to develop postinflammatory hyperpigmentation, although it is transient and easily treated.

Hair Color

The darker the hair, the better it responds to laser hair removal (27–29). The melanin in hair is the targeted chromophore of which there are two types, eumelanin and pheomelanin. Hair color depends on the amount and type of melanin present (6). Brown or black hairs predominantly contain eumelanin, whereas red hair predominantly has pheomelanin. Blonde hair results from incomplete melanization of melanosomes or production of fewer melanosomes and may contain eumelanin and/or pheomelanin. These lighter hairs are more difficult to target and require the use of shorter wavelength lasers to maximize melanin absorption. Absorption of melanin decreases with increasing wavelength in a linear fashion (Fig. 1), with pheomelanin having significantly less absorption than eumelanin (30). White hair does not respond (29).

Hair Size

Finer hairs have shorter TRTs and thus are better targeted by shorter pulse widths, whereas for larger hairs, most pulse widths will be effective.

(A) **(B)**

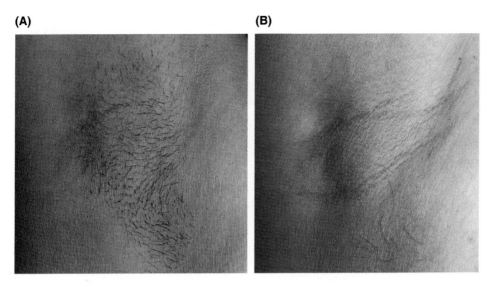

Figure 2
Before (**A**) and three years after (**B**) three treatments with 755-nm alexandrite laser. Note that remaining hairs are finer and lighter.

As hairs become smaller and finer (Fig. 2), which can occur with progressive treatments, shorter pulse widths may be needed. One study documented a decrease in hair diameter three months after ruby laser treatment, however by seven months, the hair shafts had returned to pretreatment size (31). Additional treatments may lead to permanent thinning of the hair.

Hormonal Status

When an increased amount or unusual distribution of hair is seen in women, a hormonal work-up may be warranted. Hirsutism affects approximately 4% to 9% of Caucasian women (32). The most common cause is polycyctic ovarian disease which affects 1% to 4% of reproductive aged women. Other conditions leading to hyperandrogenemia include tumors, congenital adrenal hyperplasia, Cushings disease, and exogenous anabolic steroids or testosterone. Familial tendencies and perimenopausal hormone fluctuations can also lead to increased hair growth, especially in the chin and upper lip regions. Referral to an endocrine specialist is recommended for evaluation prior to laser hair removal, although it is not clear how hormonal imbalances affect treatment efficacy. It is also important to educate these patients about the fact that laser can only target hair that is currently present and will not stop the progression of vellus hair to terminal hair, which is a frequent occurrence in these patients.

PARAMETER SELECTION

Parameters that are important for laser hair removal include wavelength, pulse width, spot size, fluence, and cooling. Each of these has its own set of constraints in any one system; however, in most cases, several parameters can be varied to optimize treatment. Full understanding of these parameters is essential to provide the best possible laser hair removal treatment for any given patient's skin type and hair color and size (Table 2).

Wavelength

In the visible and near-infrared light range, shorter wavelengths have greater melanin absorption (Fig. 1). The relationship is nearly linear with longer wavelengths, with lower absorption requiring more energy to effectively target melanin. Longer wavelengths also penetrate deeper, partially because of less melanin absorption and because they scatter less in the tissue. The greater depth is important as the hair can be as deep as 5 mm below the surface. This declining melanin absorption helps longer wavelengths spare the epidermis where melanin is contained mainly in keratinocytes as well as in melanocytes.

Pulse Width

For selective photothermolysis, pulse widths shorter than or equal to the TRT of the target are desirable. Optimal pulse width is directly related to target size, with larger targets necessitating longer pulse widths. This theory has been expanded to include nonuniformly pigmented targets such as hair (33,34). In this case, the target is actually the larger clumps of melanin in the follicular apparatus with subsequent extension of thermal

---

Table 2
Optimal Treatment Parameters

Wavelength	Avoid skin, but target hair
	Light skin, light hair—use shorter wavelengths
	Light skin, dark hair—any wavelength 694–1064 nm
	Dark skin, dark hair use longer wavelengths to decrease epidermal damage
	Longer wavelengths penetrate deeper
Pulse width	Shorter for finer hairs
	Longer for larger hairs
	Long for darker skin
Fluence	Highest tolerated without blistering
Spot size	Largest possible with effective fluence
	Better depth of penetration and faster treatment time
Use cooling	Especially with darker skin types
	Allows use of higher fluences for better efficacy
	Decreases pain

damage to include the bulge area. Finer hairs may respond best with shorter pulse widths whereas larger, coarser hairs can be treated with even longer pulse widths. There is some evidence that pulse width may not impact efficacy if it is within a reasonable range (35–37), supporting the extended theory of selective photothermolysis.

The theory of thermokinetic selectivity is based on the fact that a smaller target (lower volume) can dissipate heat more easily than larger targets. This principle is what enables the epidermis to suffer less damage with longer pulse widths while hair follicles are still sufficiently thermally destroyed. In other words, while heat accumulates in the pigmented follicular apparatus, the finer granules of epidermal melanin dissipate heat. Super long pulses in the 100- to 1000-msec range were used with the diode laser and found to be helpful for darker skin types. Of note, however, is the fact that the longest pulse at 1000 msec and highest fluences (greater than 100 J/cm^2) were more painful and had higher complication rates (38).

Spot Size

Fluences delivered in larger spot sizes lose relatively fewer photons laterally from scattering and have more forward scattering. Hence, larger spot sizes effectively deliver more photons down into the dermis (39). In other words, the larger the spot size, the deeper the penetration of effective fluence. Larger spot sizes are more efficacious for deeper targets. For a given fluence, use of a larger spot size will more effectively target hair and increase the percent of permanent hair reduction (40). Of note, is the fact that use of a larger spot size may require lowering the fluence to maintain safety, and may also be more painful for a given fluence (41).

Fluence

Sufficient fluence must be delivered to cause enough thermal injury to the hair follicle, to produce permanent destruction. Fluence directly correlates with the percentage of permanent hair reduction (19,25,42),(43). Given the other sets of parameters, the fluence should be high enough to achieve this, yet not so high as to injure the overlying epidermis. Precooling or simultaneous cooling with the laser pulse will help spare the epidermis from thermal injury and allow the use of higher fluences (44).

Cooling

Cooling is an important adjunctive measure to prevent epidermal injury in laser hair removal (45,46) as well as to increase efficacy by allowing the use of higher fluences (44). There are several strategies to cool the epidermis. Cryogen spurts chill the epidermis just prior to the laser pulse, with spurt duration most effective in the 20- to 60-msec range for epidermal preservation (47). Longer spurts are more helpful for reducing pain (47). Concomitant contact cooling occurs by delivering a laser pulse through a chilled sapphire tip or through a glass window containing circulating chilled water. Efficient pre- and postcooling can also be achieved by applying a cold copper plate before and after each laser pulse. With high thermoconductivity, copper quickly chills the epidermal surface and removes heat. Forced cold air also effectively protects the epidermis and can be utilized before, during, and after the laser pulse (44). In addition, use of a gel on the surface will help with cooling, especially if the gel is sufficiently chilled, as well as gliding of the hair removal device along the skin. The anatomic depth of cooling appears to be related to the length of time the cooling is applied (46).

Darker Skin Types, Tanned Skin, and Pseudofolliculitis Barbe

For a given level of skin pigmentation, it is the consensus of skilled practitioners that treating tanned skin is riskier than treating an equally dark, but natural skin color; this is likely because of the difference in melanin distribution. For darker skin types, the longer wavelengths (especially 1064-nm), longer pulse widths, and cooling are very important for successful and safe treatments. Although the alexandrite and diode lasers can be used with dark skin (43,48,49), pulse width needs to be lengthened, cooling maximized, and fluence decreased, which may compromise results. Use of a 1064-nm laser allows maximal fluences with minimal side effects (29,50,51) and the wavelength of this laser best tolerated by tanned and type VI skin, although the super long pulse 810 nm diode can also be used (52,53).

Pseudofolliculitis barbae is very common in darker skin types especially when beard hairs are coarse and curly (Fig. 3). The irritation from a recently shaved hair, unable to exit a follicular opening clearly, can lead to follicular inflammation and even pustules. This often progresses to follicular papules and hyperpigmentation. Laser hair removal can thin hair shaft diameters, facilitating easier exit of the growing hair. Of course, permanent elimination of problematic hair is the ultimate, and frequently achieved, end point (11–13). Parameter constraints are based on a patient's skin type and possibly the follicular hyperpigmentation. In most cases, hyperpigmentation improves with consecutive treatments as the reduction in number and size of the hairs causes less inflammation. Acne nuchae keloidalis is now being effectively treated with this modality.

LASERS

Ruby Laser

The first laser developed to directly target pigmented hairs was the ruby laser, which is shown to produce deep follicular damage in animals (76). Early studies by Dierickx et al. (18) demonstrated effective targeting of pigmented hair using a 694-nm ruby laser (0.3 pulse width, 6 mm spot size). This work confirmed that the 3-msec pulse width was better tolerated and possibly more efficacious than the 0.3-msec pulse width that had been used initially. This work on the 3-msec ruby laser was followed by a multicentered trial (20) confirming the efficacy and safety in 183 patients.

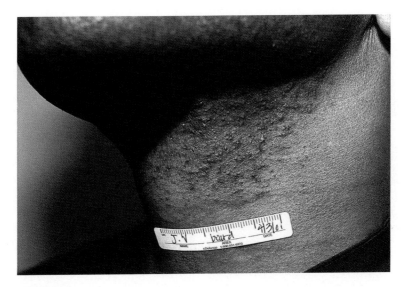

Figure 3
Test site done two days prior to Nd:YAG laser (1064-nm, 10 m, 55 J/cm^2, 30 msec) on darker skin.

The majority of patients had less than 75% hair loss six months after three to six treatments (Fig. 4), and only 2% had less than 25% hair loss. With progressive treatments, hair became finer and lighter. Side effects included 3% hypopigmentation and 6% hyperpigmentation, but not scarring. Histologically, an increase in the number of telogen hairs as well as miniaturization of terminal hairs was noted, (54). Several subsequent studies have demonstrated similar efficacy (7,28,55).

The initial ruby laser, the Epilaser (later replaced by the E2000, Palomar, Burlington, Massachusetts, U.S.A.), utilized a contact cooling sapphire tip. Laser pulses pass through a chilled sapphire window allowing the skin to tolerate the 694-nm ruby pulses as long as there was little pigment in the epidermis. Treatment of darker skin types was limited with this laser (56), and its primary utility remains with its ability to target lighter hairs. Its expense, limited utility, size, and power requirements have led to its progression toward obsolescence.

Alexandrite Laser

Q-switched alexandrite (755-nm) lasers had been utilized for treatment of pigmented lesions and tattoos. This longer wavelength was then explored for hair removal for its deeper penetration and decreased absorption by melanin. Advancements in technology allowed elongation of pulse widths to the millisecond range. Initially an alexandrite laser was developed (Cynosure, Chelmsford, Massachusetts, U.S.A.) with several pulse widths, ranging from 5 to 20 msec, which was later extended to 40 msec.

(A)   **(B)**

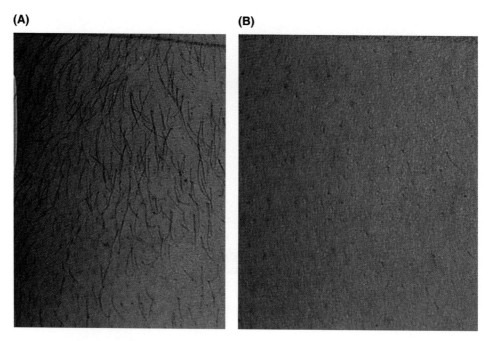

Figure 4
Before (**A**) and six months after (**B**) three treatments with 694-nm at 6 J/cm² (twin pulse).

A second company (Candela, Wayland, Massachusetts, U.S.A.) developed an alexandrite laser with a fixed pulse width of 3-msec. Cooling varied, depending on the model, with the Cynosure model having no cooling initially, and then often being used in association with forced cool air. The Candela version with the 3-msec pulse width had cryogen cooling, to help protect the epidermis. A 2-msec pulse width alexandrite laser was also developed and found to effectively and safely target hair.

These lasers continue to be popular to this day. The 755-nm wavelength has good melanin absorption in the hair follicles, yet epidermal melanin can be spared by increasing pulse widths and cooling. However, alexandrite laser treatment of darker skin types and tanned skin remains limited. A recent study showed (57) hair reduction rates of 32%, 44%, and 55% nine months after one, two, or three treatments respectively with an alexandrite laser [755-nm, 40 msec, 16–24 J/cm²] in 140 Asian patients with skin types III to V (58). Minimal long-term side effects were noted although transient hyperpigmentation was more frequent and the skin type range may have limited the fluence tolerated with some decrease in efficacy noted as compared to other studies (8,35,36,42,59,60) where up to 75% permanent hair reduction has been noted after three treatments. Alexandrite lasers are fairly easy to operate, well-tolerated by patients, and effective for most pigmented hairs (Figs. 2 and 5).

(A)   **(B)**

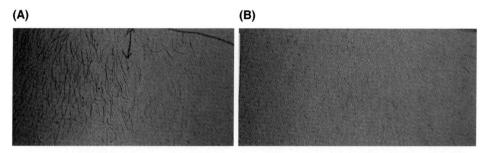

Figure 5
Before (**A**) and six months after (**B**) three treatments with 755-nm alexandrite laser at 25 to 30 J/cm^2.

Diode Lasers

The variable pulse width 810-nm diode laser was developed in an effort to treat a greater breadth of skin types. Its longer wavelength further improves penetration depth and avoids epidermal melanin. A convex sapphire lens with active cooling protects the epidermis. Other similar diode systems have been developed with varying methods of cooling. Dierickx showed excellent (#4 course handout) results; 100% of patients had hair growth delay and averaged 46% permanent hair reduction 6 and 12 months after the second treatment [20 msec, 40 J/cm^2]. The epidermis was more tolerant of this wavelength with few side effects noted. Several studies confirmed this efficacy (61,62) with approximately 70% reduction noted six months after three treatments (Figs. 6 and 7) with one study

(A)   **(B)**

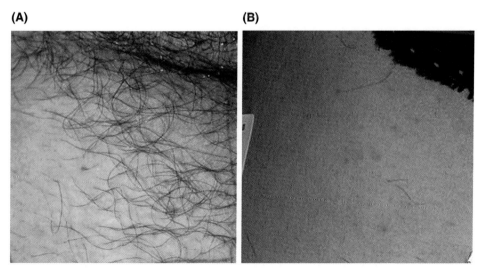

Figure 6
Before (**A**) and six months (**B**) after three treatments with 810-nm diode laser.

(A)   **(B)**

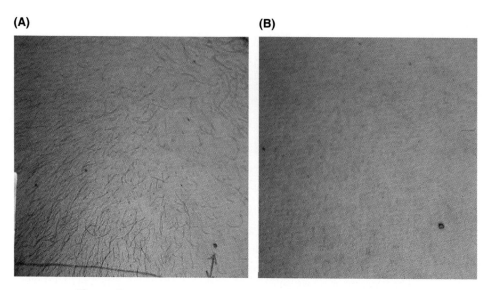

Figure 7
Before (**A**) and six months after (**B**) three treatments with 810-nm diode laser.

histologically noting changes from early catagen induction to follicular destruction (63), however, type V and VI skin and tanned skin still suffered damage from treatment. Super long pulses (100–1000 msec) (53) were developed to further bypass epidermal melanin for treatment in tanned and type VI skin. The optimal pulse width was 400 msec, and the 1000-msec pulse width was associated with more pain and complications (38).

1064 nm Nd:YAG Laser

To further explore an even longer wavelength, 1064-nm laser, which avoids epidermal melanin yet targets follicular melanin was developed. Q-switched 1064-nm pulses effectively treat melanocytes in nevus of Ota and therefore it seemed reasonable that the appropriate pulse width would be able to target the melanin in hair. A concern was that higher fluences would be needed to offset lower absorption by melanin at this wavelength. Initial studies by Kilmer (51) using a 1064-nm laser [50–60 J/cm^2, 15–30 msec pulse width and a chilled copper plate] demonstrated excellent hair reduction nine months after one (38%) and two (50%) treatments (Fig. 8). In that first study, up to skin type V was treated with only minimal hyperpigmentation in three skin type IV and V patients that cleared without treatment in two months. Since then, studies have shown that even tanned and type VI skin can be effectively and safely treated (64). Other 1064-nm devices use cryogen spray, treat through a chilled sapphire window, or use forced cooled air. Several studies corroborate the efficacy and safety of this wavelength (Figs. 9 and 10) (19,50,65–68,65–68).

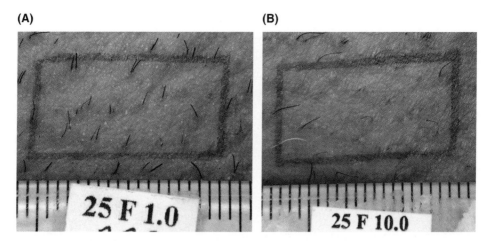

Figure 8
Before (**A**) and 12 months after (**B**) two treatments with 1064-nm CoolGlide.
Note single white hair.

Intense Pulsed Light

Intense pulsed light (IPL) sources typically with cut off filters from 550 to 1200 nm have been used to target hair (69,70). This device is a broadband flash lamp device of high intensity. Cut off filters are placed to block the shorter wavelengths. This device is versatile in that different number of pulses and pulse intervals can be utilized. The shorter wavelengths included

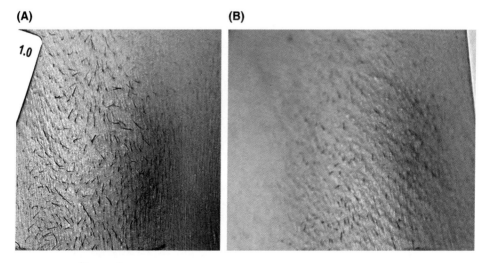

Figure 9
Before (**A**) and six months after (**B**) three treatments with 1064-nm Nd:YAG at 65 J/cm^2, 15 to 20 msec.

(A)   **(B)**

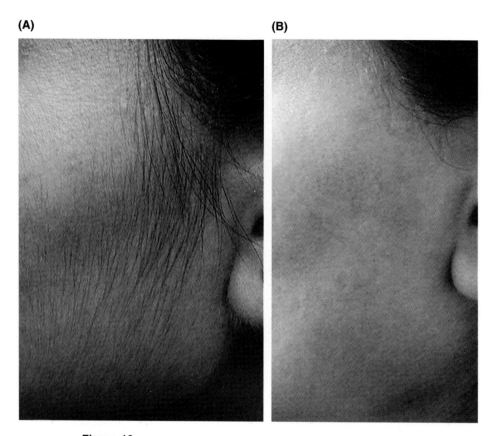

Figure 10
Before (**A**) and after (**B**) three treatments with 1064-nm GentleYAG, at 42 J/cm^2.

in the treatment range, however, increase the likelihood of absorption by epidermal melanin causing occasional burn injuries and pigmentary changes. On the positive side however, the broad spectrum of wavelengths appears to be more beneficial for some of the lighter hairs. Hair reduction rates have been reported to be as high as 76% after 3 treatments (69) as shown in Figure 1.

Radio Frequency + IPL

Most recently, a device utilizing IPL in combination with radio frequency (RF) has been developed to treat hair. This device delivers IPL first to heat hair follicles, and subsequent RF supplies additional thermal energy to the treated area. Preliminary results show efficacy rates similar to the previously mentioned lasers (Kilmer, unpublished results). Other studies are underway to document the efficacy in blond, gray, and white hairs but it appears, at this early stage, that light hairs are affected only if they are coarse in nature.

pulse width lasers, and return of normal pigmentation usually occurs. If there is significant blistering because of inappropriate parameter selection or presence of a significant tan (Figs. 12–14), permanent hypopigmentation can occur. This maybe more likely with the shorter pulse widths that approach the TRT for epidermal melanin (76). Unmasking of vitiligo is also possible with sufficient injury leading to Koebnerization in the treated area. While this hypopigmentation often improves with time (42), sun exposure, phototherapy, and the use of excimer laser (and similar light sources) may be useful for treatment of depigmented areas.

Hyperpigmentation is a transient phenomenon that occurs most commonly in darker skin (19) types, but can occur in any individual who tans easily or has a strong predilection for hyperpigmentation, with minor injury. This is readily treated with broad-spectrum sunscreen (77), preferably zinc oxide and a hydroquinone preparation. Glycolic acid and tretinoin have been added to enhance penetration of the hydroquinone and topical steroids, to decrease any irritation that may be contributing to the hyperpigmentation.

More rarely, scarring, ocular injury, and vessel thrombosis can occur. Scarring usually results from severe blistering and is often accompanied by hypopigmentation. Ocular injury such as retinal damage and uveitis can result from treating within the orbital rim. Colobomas (defect in the iris) have resulted from treating hairs in the eyebrows and possibly the malar region. Although reportedly safe to treat eyelashes, metal eyeshields (78) treatment at the edge of the globe may allow light to scatter in from the side and be absorbed by eye pigment. Also of rare concern is the concomitant thrombosis of an underlying vessel (Kilmer SL, personal

(A)   **(B)**

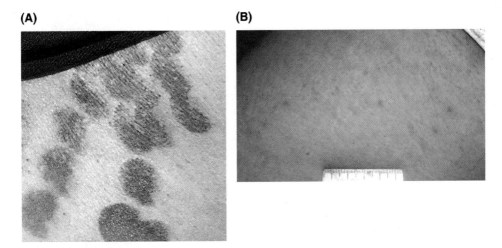

Figure 12
Only erythema was noted immediately post-treatment. However 24 hours later (**A**), crusting appeared, which resulted in (**B**) hyperpigmentation that took six months to clear.

(A)   **(B)**

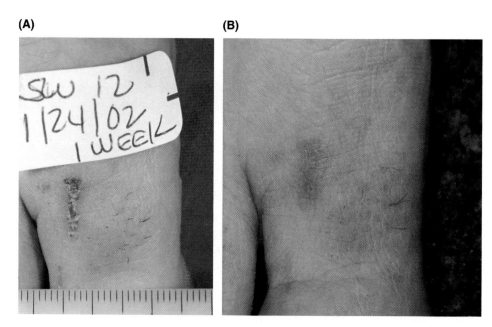

Figure 13
(**A**) Healing ulceration—one week postsingle treatment with Aurora
(22 J/cm^2—20 RF) and (**B**) hyperpigmentation present one month later.

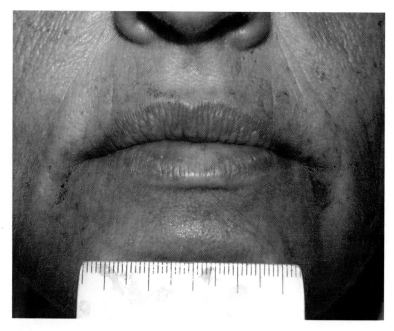

Figure 14
Crusting three days-GentleLASE treatment at 25 J/cm^2.

communication). This presents as a tender chord in the treated area and usually resolves with time; a warm compress and nonsteroidal anti inflammatory agents are helpful.

One final concern is the inadvertent targeting of pigmented lesions present in the treatment field. Accurate diagnosis of these lesions should occur prior to laser hair removal. Laser-treated nevi have characteristic changes and may become easily confused with cytologic atypia (79). This is especially of concern for patients with dysplastic nevi or a history of melanoma.

Who Should Perform the Procedure?

Ideally all laser procedures would be performed by well-trained physicians. Current regulations in many states allow licensed health care workers (exactly which level of training is state determined) to perform these services. Patient safety, not financial considerations, should be of utmost concern. The physician should have appropriate training to evaluate endogenous hypertrichosis, cutaneous lesions in the treatment field, and should choose optimal parameter settings to maximize efficacy and minimize side effects. Under the direct, hands-on training of a physician with laser hair removal expertise, a well-trained registered nurse can perform laser hair removal. Ideally, the supervising physician should be onsite and immediately available to aid with parameter changes and to directly observe any potential adverse events. A recent study (80) confirms this need for appropriate supervision, and both the American Society for Dermatologic Surgery and American Society for Laser Medicine and Surgery recommend following the above guidelines.

REFERENCES

1. Goldman L, Blaney DJ, Kindel DJ, Frinke EK. Effect of the laser beam on the skin. J Invest Dermatol. 1963; 40:121–123.
2. Goldberg DJ, Samady JA. Evaluation of a long-pulse Q-switched Nd:YAG laser for hair removal. Dermatol Surg. 2000; 26(2):109–113.
3. Goldberg DJ, Littler CM, Wheeland RG. Topical suspension-assisted Q-switched Nd:YAG laser hair removal. Dermatol Surg 1997; 23(9):741–745.
4. Kilmer SL, Chotzen VA. Q-switched Nd:YAG laser (1064 nm) hair removal without adjuvant topical preparation. Lasers Surg Med 1997; 9(suppl):145.
5. Nanni CA, Alster TS. Laser-assisted hair removal: optimizing treatment parameters to improve clinical results. Laser Med Surg Suppl 1997; 9:35.
6. Olsen EA. Methods of hair removal. J Am Acad Dermatol 1999; 40:143–155.
7. Polderman MC, Pavel S, le Cessie S, Grevelink JM, van Leeuwen RL. Efficacy, tolerability, and safety of a long-pulsed ruby laser system in the removal of unwanted hair. Dermatol Surg 2000; 26(3):240–243.
8. Gorgu M, Aslan G, Akoz T, Erdogan B. Comparison of alexandrite laser and electrolysis for hair removal. Dermatol Surg 2000; 26(1):37–41.
9. Thomson KF, Sommer S, Sheehan-Dare RA. Terminal hair growth after full thickness skin graft: treatment with normal mode ruby laser. Lasers Surg Med 2001; 28(2):156–158.
10. Moreno-Arias GA, Vilalta-Solsona A, Serra-Renom JM, Benito-Ruiz J, Ferrando J. Intense pulsed light for hairy grafts and flaps. Dermatol Surg 2002; 28(5):402–404.
11. Greppi I. Diode laser hair removal of the black patient. Lasers Surg Med 2001; 28(2):150–155.
12. Kauvar AN. Treatment of pseudofolliculitis with a pulsed infrared laser. Arch Dermatol 2000; 136(11):1343–1346.
13. Rogers CJ, Glaser DA. Treatment of pseudofolliculitis barbae using the Q-switched Nd:YAG laser with topical carbon suspension. Dermatol Surg 2000; 26(8):737–742.
14. Downs AM, Palmer J. Laser hair removal for recurrent pilonidal sinus disease. J Cosmet Laser Ther 2002; 4(3–4):91.
15. Raulin C, Werner S, Harschuh W, Schonermark MP. Effective treatments of hypertrichosis with pulsed light: a report of two cases. Ann Plast Surg 1997; 39(2):169–173.
16. Anderson RR, Parrish JA. Selective photothermolysis: precise microsurgery by selective absorptions of pulsed radiation. Science 1983; 220:524–527.
17. Grossman MC, Dierickx C, Farinelli W, Flotte T, Anderson RR. Damage to hair follicles by normal-mode ruby laser pulses. J Am Acad Dermatol 1996; 35(6):889–894.
18. Dierickx CC, Grossman MC, Farinelli WA, Anderson RR. Permanent hair removal by normal-mode ruby laser. Arch Dermatol 1998; 134(7):837–842.
19. Campos VB, Dierickx CC, Farinelli WA, Lin TY, Manuskiatti W, Anderson RR. Ruby laser hair removal: evaluation of long-term efficacy and side effects. Lasers Surg Med 2000; 26(2):177–185.
20. Anderson R, Burns AJ, Garden J, Goldberg D, Grossman MC, Hruza G, Kilmer SL, Laughlin S, Lui H, Olsen E. Multicenter study of long-pulse ruby laser hair removal. American Society for Laser Medicine and Surgery Inc 1999; 11(suppl):56.
21. Kilmer SL. Laser eradication of pigmented lesions and tattoos. Dermatol Clin 2002; 20(1):37–53.
22. Kilmer SL, Chotzen VA, Calkin JM. Hair removal study comparing the Q-switched Nd:YAG and long pulse ruby & alexandrite lasers. Lasers Surg Med 1998; 10(suppl):41.
23. Sun TT, Cotsarelis G, Lavker RM. Hair follicular stem cells: the bulge activation hypothesis. J Invest Dermatol 1992; 96:77S.
24. Kolinko VG, Littler CM, Cole A. Influence of the anagen:telogen ratio on Q-switched Nd:YAG laser hair removal efficacy. Lasers Surg Med 2000; 26(1):33–40.

25. Dierickx C, Campos VB, Lin WF, Anderson RR. Influence of hair growth cycle on efficacy of laser hair removal. Lasers Surg Med 1999; 24(11):21.

26. McCoy S, Evans A, James C. Histological study of hair follicles treated with a 3-msec pulsed ruby laser. Lasers Surg Med 1999; 24(2):142–150.

27. Liew SH, Ladhani K, Grobbelaar AO, Gault DT, Sanders R, Green CJ, Linge C. Ruby laser-assisted hair removal success in relation to anatomic factors and melanin content of hair follicles. Plast Reconstr Surg 1999; 103(6):1736–1743.

28. Wimmershoff MB, Scherer K, Lorenz S, Landthaler M, Hohenleutner U. Hair removal using a 5-msec long-pulsed ruby laser. Dermatol Surg 2000; 26(3):205–210.

29. Bencini PL, Luci A, Galimberti M, Ferranti G. Long-term epilation with long-pulsed neodimium:YAG laser. Dermatol Surg 1999; 25(3):175–178.

30. Ye, Simon JD. The action spectrum for generation of the primary intermediate revealed by ultrafast absorption spectroscopy studies of pheomelanin. Photochem Photobiol 2002; 77(1):41.

31. Liew SH, Ladhani K, Grobbelaar AO, Gault DT, Sanders R, Green CJ, Linge C. Ruby laser-assisted hair removal reduces the coarseness of regrowing hairs: fallacy or fact? Br J Plast Surg 1999; 52(5):380–384.

32. Liew SH. Unwanted body hair and its removal: a review. Dermatol Surg 1999; 25: 431–439.

33. Ross EV. Extended theory of selective photothermolysis: a new recipe for hair cooking? Lasers Surg Med 2001; 29(5):413–415.

34. Altshuler GB, Anderson RR, Manstein D, Zenzie HH, Smirnov MZ. Extended theory of selective photothermolysis. Lasers Surg Med 2001; 29(5):416–432.

35. Boss WK Jr, Usal H, Thompson RC, Fiorillo MA. A comparison of the long-pulse and short-pulse Alexandrite laser hair removal systems. Ann Plast Surg. 1999; 42(4):381–384.

36. Goldberg DJ, Ahkami R. Evaluation comparing multiple treatments with a 2-msec and 10-msec alexandrite laser for hair removal. Lasers Surg Med 1999; 25(3):223–228.

37. Nanni CA, Alster TS. Long-pulsed alexandrite laser-assisted hair removal at 5, 10, and 20 millisecond pulse durations. Lasers Surg Med 1999; 24(5):332–337.

38. Rogachefsky AS, Silapunt S, Goldberg DJ. Evaluation of a new super-long-pulsed 810 nm diode laser for the removal of unwanted hair: the concept of thermal damage time. Dermatol Surg 2002; 28(5):410–414.

39. Kilmer SL, Farinelli WA, Tearney G, Anderson RR. Use of a larger spot size for the treatment of tattoos increases clinical efficacy and decreases potential side effect. Lasers Surg Med 1994; 6(suppl):51.

40. Baumler W, Scherer K, Abels C, Neff S, Landthaler M, Szeimies RM. The effect of different spot sizes on the efficacy of hair removal using a long-pulsed diode laser. Dermatol Surg 2002; 28(2):118–121.

41. Eremia S, Newman N. Topical anesthesia for laser hair removal: comparison of spot sizes and 755 nm versus 800 nm wavelengths. Dermatol Surg 2000; 26(7):667–669.

42. Eremia S, Li CY, Umar SH, Newman N. Laser hair removal: long-term results with a 755 nm alexandrite laser. Dermatol Surg 2001; 27(11):920–924.

43. Campos VB, Dierickx CC, Farinelli WA, Lin TY, Manuskiatti W, Anderson RR. Hair removal with an 800-nm pulsed diode laser. J Am Acad Dermatol 2000; 43(3):442–447.

44. Raulin C, Greve B, Hammes S. Cold air in laser therapy: first experiences with a new cooling system. Lasers Surg Med 2000; 27(5):404–410.

45. Klavuhn KG, Green D. Importance of cutaneous cooling during photothermal epilation: theoretical and practical considerations. Lasers Surg Med 2002; 31(2):97–105.

46. Zenzie HH, Altshuler GB, Smirnov MZ, Anderson RR. Evaluation of cooling methods for laser dermatology. Lasers Surg Med 2000; 26(2):130–144.

47. Nahm WK, Tsoukas MM, Falanga V, Carson PA, Sami N, Touma DJ. Preliminary study of fine changes in the duration of dynamic cooling during 755-nm laser hair

removal on pain and epidermal damage in patients with skin types III–V. Lasers Surg Med 2002; 31(4):247–251.

48. Nanni CA, Alster TS. Laser-assisted hair removal: side effects of Q-switched Nd:YAG, long-pulsed ruby, and alexandrite lasers. J Am Acad Dermatol 1999; 41(2 Pt 1):165–171.

49. Galadari I. Comparative evaluation of different hair removal lasers in skin types IV, V, and VI. Int J Dermatol 2003; 42(1):68–70.

50. Goldberg DJ, Silapunt S. Hair removal using a long-pulsed Nd:YAG Laser: comparison at fluences of 50, 80, and 100 J/cm. Dermatol Surg 2001; 27(5):434–436.

51. Kilmer SL. Laser hair removal with the long-pulse 1064nm Coolglide laser system. Lasers Surg Med 2000; 12(suppl):84.

52. Rogachefsky AS, Silapunt S, Goldberg DJ. Evaluation of a super long pulsed 810-nm diode hair removal laser in suntanned individuals. J Cutan Laser Ther 2001; 3(2):57–62.

53. Adrian RM, Shay KP. 800 nanometer diode laser hair removal in African American patients: a clinical and histologic study. J Cutan Laser Ther 2000; 2(4):183–190.

54. McCoy S, Evans A, James C. Long-pulsed ruby laser for permanent hair reduction: histological analysis after 3, 4 1/2, and 6 months. Lasers Surg Med 2002; 30(5):401–405.

55. Bjerring P, Zachariae H, Lybecker H, Clement M. Evaluation of the free-running ruby laser for hair removal. A retrospective study. Acta Derm Venereol 1998; 78(1):48–51.

56. Chana JS, Grobbelaar AO. The long-term results of ruby laser depilation in a consecutive series of 346 patients. Plast Reconstr Surg 2002; 110(1):254–260.

57. Eremia S, Li C, Newman N. Laser hair removal with alexandrite versus diode laser using four treatment sessions: 1-year results. Dermatol Surg 2001; 27(11):925–929; discussion 929–930.

58. Hussain M, Polnikorn N, Goldberg DJ. Laser-assisted hair removal in Asian skin: efficacy, complications, and the effect of single versus multiple treatments. Dermatol Surg 2003; 29(3):249–254.

59. Laughlin SA, Dudley DK. Long-term hair removal using a 3-millisecond alexandrite laser. J Cutan Med Surg 2000; 4(2):83–88.

60. McDaniel DH, Lord J, Ash K, Newman J, Zukowski M. Laser hair removal: a review and report on the use of the long-pulsed alexandrite laser for hair reduction of the upper lip, leg, back, and bikini region. Dermatol Surg 1999; 25(6):425–430.

61. Baugh WP, Trafeli JP, Barnette DJ Jr, Ross EV. Hair reduction using a scanning 800 nm diode laser. Dermatol Surg 2001; 27(4):358–364.

62. Lou WW, Quintana AT, Geronemus RG, Grossman MC. Prospective study of hair reduction by diode laser (800 nm) with long-term follow-up. Dermatol Surg 2000; 26(5):428–432.

63. Sadick NS, Prieto VG. The use of a new diode laser for hair removal. Dermatol Surg 2003; 29(1):30–33; discussion 33–34.

64. Lach E. Comparison of alexandrite laser and YAG laser of hair removal in recently tanned individuals and those with darker skin types.

65. Lorenz S, Brunnberg S, Landthaler M, Hohenleutner U. Hair removal with the long pulsed Nd:YAG laser: a prospective study with one year follow-up. Lasers Surg Med 2002; 30(2):127–134.

66. Kilmer SL, Chotzen VA, McClaren ML, Calkin JM, Silva SK. Laser hair removal comparison study with 5 laser/light source systems. Lasers Surg Med 2001; 13(suppl):91.

67. Alster TS, Bryan H, Williams CM. Long-pulsed Nd:YAG laser-assisted hair removal in pigmented skin: a clinical and histological evaluation. Arch Dermatol 2001; 137(7):885–889.

68. Goldberg DJ, Silapunt S. Histologic evaluation of a millisecond Nd:YAG laser for hair removal. Lasers Surg Med 2001; 28(2):159–161.

69. Sadick NS, Weiss RA, Shea CR, Nagel H, Nicholson J, Prieto VG. Long-term photoepilation using a broad-spectrum intense pulsed light source. Arch Dermatol 2000; 136(11):1336–1340.

70. Weiss G, Cohen B. The efficacy of long-term epilation of unwanted hair by noncoherent filtered flashlamp. Lasers Surg Med 2000; 26(4):345.

71. Handrick C, Alster TS. Comparison of long-pulsed diode and long-pulsed alexandrite lasers for hair removal: a long-term clinical and histologic study. Dermatol Surg 2001; 27(7):622–626.

72. Ye JN, Prasad A, Trivedi P, Knapp DP, Chu P, Edelstein LM. Pili bigeminy induced by low fluence therapy with hair removal alexandrite and ruby lasers. Dermatol Surg 1999; 25(12):969.

73. Dover JS, Margolis RJ, Polla LL, Watanabe S, Hruza GJ, Parrish JA, Anderson RR. Pigmented guinea pig skin irradiated with Q-switched ruby laser pulses. Morphologic and histologic findings. Arch Dermatol 1989; 125(1):43—49.

74. Radmanesh M, Mostaghimi M, Yousefi I, Mousavi ZB, Rasai S, Esmaili HR, Khadivi HA. Leukotrichia developed following application of intense pulsed light for hair removal. Dermatol Surg 2002; 28(7):572–574; discussion 574.

75. Moreno-Arias GA, Tiffon T, Marti T, Camps-Fresneda A. Long-term hypopigmentation induced by diode laser photo-epilation. J Cutan Laser Ther 2001; 3(1):9–10 (No abstract available).

76. Moreno-Arias GA, Camps-Fresneda A. Long-lasting hypopigmentation induced by long-pulsed alexandrite laser photo-epilation. Dermatol Surg 2003; 29(4):420–422.

77. Hasan AT, Eaglstein W, Pardo RJ. Solar-induced postinflammatory hyperpigmentation after laser hair removal. Dermatol Surg 1999; 25(2):113–115.

78. Pham RT, Tzekov RT, Biesman BS, Marmor MF. Retinal evaluation after 810 nm Dioderm laser removal of eyelashes. Dermatol Surg 2002; 28(9):836–840.

79. Soden CE, Smith K, Skelton H. Histologic features seen in changing nevi after therapy with an 810 nm pulsed diode laser for hair removal in patients with dysplastic nevi. Int J Dermatol 2001; 40(8):500–504.

80. Brody HJ, Geronemus RG, Farris PK. Beauty versus medicine: the nonphysician practice of dermatologic surgery. Dermatol Surg 2003; 29(4):319–324.

8

Laser Treatment of Vascular Lesions

Arielle N. B. Kauvar
New York University School of Medicine, New York, New York, U.S.A.

INTRODUCTION

Lasers are presently used to treat a wide spectrum of congenital and acquired cutaneous vascular lesions. Before the advent of laser technology, many of these conditions had no acceptable or effective means of treatment. The argon and other continuous wave and quasicontinuous wave lasers were used in the 1970s and in the early 1980s to treat port wine stains. Impressive lightening of mature port wine stains was achieved, but treatment of immature, pale, macular lesions often resulted in scarring (1,2).

In the 1980s, the pulsed dye laser was developed based on the principles of selective photothermolysis (3). Selective injury of the ecstatic port wine stain vessels was produced using a wavelength of light well absorbed by hemoglobin and sufficiently short laser exposure time to spatially confine the thermal injury (4). The pulsed dye laser revolutionized the treatment of port wine stains and was soon thereafter applied to the treatment of a wide variety of congenital and acquired cutaneous vascular lesions.

For two decades since its introduction, the 585-nm, 0.45-millisecond pulsed dye laser remained the standard of care for the treatment of port wine stains, hemangiomas, and facial telangiectasia. Clinical efficacy is high, and side effects are low, with an incidence of scarring less than 1% after multiple, repetitive treatment sessions (5–7).

Despite these successes, lesions with deeper or larger diameter blood vessels, such as hypertrophic port wine stains and leg telangiectasia, could not be successfully treated. Treatment of facial telangiectasia for cosmetic purposes was also hampered by the development of blue–black purpura lasting up to 14 days. More recently, newer vascular lasers have been developed that limit purpura production and effectively target larger caliber vessels. This has been accomplished using a combination of longer wavelengths, millisecond-duration pulses, and epidermal cooling methods.

Longer wavelengths provide deeper penetration into the skin and enable treatment of larger diameter and deeper blood vessels. Longer pulse durations in the millisecond range are required for optimal photocoagulation of vessels greater than 100 μm in diameter. Recent studies have confirmed that, as originally postulated by the theory of selective photothermolysis, pulse durations in the 1- to 50-millisecond range are most effective for thermal destruction of blood vessels with diameters 0.1 to 0.6 mm (8).

The use of very short pulse durations relative to the thermal relaxation time of the targeted blood vessel results in poor lesional clearance. Studies of nanosecond-range pulsed dye lasers for the treatment of port wine stains produced no apparent clinical improvement because of incomplete vessel damage and subsequent revascularization (9). Submillisecond pulses are effective for vessels of diameter 50 to 1000 μm, but produce explosive heating and vessel rupture, leading to red blood extravasation and purpura production. Blood vessels with diameters greater than 1 mm and those deeper than 1 mm from the skin surface require millisecond-duration laser pulses for effective photocoagulation and clearance.

The addition of epidermal cooling during laser treatment helps to conduct heat away from the epidermis (10). Skin-cooling techniques provide analgesia during treatment, protect the epidermis from thermal damage, and minimize the risk of side effects. With the development of longer wavelength lasers that necessitate the use of higher energy fluences, cooling has become an essential component of laser therapy.

Lasers are presently the modality of choice for the treatment of port wine stains, superficial cutaneous hemangiomas, telangiectasia, and poikiloderma. Other lesions that can be improved with vascular lasers include leg telangiectasia and venulectasia (see chap. 9), hypertrophic and erythematous scars, and striae and warts.

LASERS FOR VASCULAR LESIONS (TABLE 1)

Potassium-Titanyl-Phosphate Lasers (Table 2)

Pulsed potassium-titanyl-phosphate (KTP) lasers emit at 532 nm in the green light spectrum. KTP crystals are convenient to work with and are highly reliable. The 532-nm KTP light is absorbed by hemoglobin as well as the 585 nm light is, and roughly has the equivalent depth of penetration through fair skin. With pulse durations in the 1- to 200-nm range, purpura is precluded by the more uniform heating of blood vessels. Most of the available laser systems use grouped nanosecond-domain Q-switched pulses, with millisecond exposure times (Iridex DioLite™, Laserscope Aura™), whereas the Versapulse® (Coherent/Lumenis), produces true millisecond-domain pulses.

These lasers are technically simple to use, and recovery from treatment is fast. Mild edema and erythema accompany treatment and may last 24 hours. The short penetration depth of this wavelength limits its usefulness for deeper lesions. The high absorption by melanin at 532 nm increases the risk of epidermal damage in darker and suntanned skin. As a result, crusting may develop in systems that lack a cooling device. The Aura and Versapulse lasers are equipped with sapphire-cooled laser

Table 1
Lasers and Light Sources for Vascular Lesions

Laser/light source	Wavelength (nm)	Pulse duration (msec)
Pulsed KTP	532	1–200
Pulsed dye	585	0.45
Long-pulsed dye	585, 590, 595, 600	1.5–40
Long-pulsed alexandrite	755	3–20
Diodes	800, 810, 930	1–250
Long-pulsed Nd:YAG	1064	1–100
IPL source	515–1200	0.5–20

Abbreviations: KTP, potassium-titanyl-phosphate; IPL, intense pulsed light.

tips to obviate this problem. Other systems may be used with ice cubes, gels, cold air, or external contact-cooling systems.

Flashlamp Pumped Pulsed Dye Lasers (Table 3)

The flashlamp pumped pulsed dye laser was the first laser developed based on the principles of selective photothermolysis (SPTL) (3,4). The first pulsed dye laser emitted at a wavelength of 577 nm. This wavelength was chosen to correspond with one of the three major absorption peaks for oxyhemoglobin (418, 542, and 577 nm), but was later increased to 585 nm to increase the depth of tissue penetration (11–13). Currently available systems for vascular applications have pulse durations of 0.45 milliseconds. Histologic studies demonstrate agglutinated red blood cells, fibrin, and platelet thrombi within the papillary and superficial reticular dermis immediately following treatment. The epidermis surrounding dermis and adnexal structures remains unaffected. The 585-nm, 0.45-milli second pulsed dye laser effectively photocoagulates blood vessels less than 1.0 mm in diameter and up to 1.0 mm below the skin surface. Treatment results in the immediate appearance of blue–black purpura, lasting

Table 2
Pulsed KTP Lasers

Name	Aura^{TM}	Versapulse$^{®}$	Diolite^{TM}
Manufacturer	Laserscope (San Jose, CA, U.S.A.)	Coherent/Lumenis (Palo Alto, CA, U.S.A.)	Iridex (Mountainview, CA, U.S.A.)
Wavelength (nm)	532	532	532
Pulse duration (msec)	1–50	2–50	1–100
Maximum fluence (J/cm^2)	1–999	0.2–38	0.1–950
Cooling	Contact	Contact	

Abbreviation: KTP, potassium-titanyl-phosphate.

Table 3
Pulsed Dye Lasers

Laser	SPTL-16	C beam	Photogenica V
Manufacturer	Candela (Weyland, MA, U.S.A.)	Candela (Weyland, MA, U.S.A.)	Cynosure (Chelmsford, MA, U.S.A.)
Wavelength (nm)	585	585	585
Pulse duration (msec)	0.45	0.45	0.45
Maximum fluence (J/cm^2)	10	16	10
Cooling		Cryogen	Air

Abbreviation: SPTL, selective photothermolysis.

up to 7 to 14 days, due to the extravasation of red blood cells. Multiple studies have demonstrated the safety and efficacy of the pulsed dye laser for the treatment of port wine stains in infants, children, and adults (14–19).

The pulsed dye laser was subsequently established as the treatment of choice for superficial hemangiomas, telangiectasias (22–24), cherry angiomas (25), and poikiloderma of Civatte (26). Other lesions treatable with the pulsed dye laser include venus lakes (27), pyogenic granulomas (28), angiofibromas (29), erythematous, hypertrophic scars (30,31), striae distensae (32), and warts (33).

Long-Pulsed Dye Lasers (Table 4)

In an effort to optimize the photocoagulation of facial and leg telangiectasia with diameters 0.2 mm and greater, second-generation pulsed dye lasers were introduced with a 1.5 millisecond pulse duration (Cynosure, Chelmsford, Massachusetts and Candela, Nadick, Massachusetts, U.S.A.). These second-generation devices use a rhodamine dye and can be tuned to wavelengths of 585, 590, 595, or 600 nm. The longer pulse duration and wavelengths improve the treatment of larger caliber, deeper vessels. Purpura is still produced at a pulse duration of 1.5 millisecond, but is less intense and of shorter-lived duration (34). These lasers have been successfully applied to the treatment of port wine stains (35,36), hemangiomas (37), and facial and leg telangiectasia (38,39). The 595-nm, 1.5-millisecond pulsed dye lasers can be used in conjunction with cryogen spray cooling or cold air cooling. When used with higher fluences in conjunction with cryogen spray cooling, this laser produces improved clearance of port wine stains and hemangiomas in infants with macular lesions (35) as well as in adults with hypertrophic lesions (36). Larger facial blood vessels that are less responsive to the 585-nm, 0.45-millisecond traditional pulsed dye laser, such as those in the paranasal folds and lateral cheeks, also respond better to these modified pulsed dye lasers. Third-generation pulsed dye lasers are now available with a fixed wavelength

Table 4
Long-Pulsed Dye Lasers

Laser	Sclerolaser®/ Scleroplus®	V beam	Photogenica VLS®	V-Star Photogenica®
Manufacturer	Candela (Wayland, MA, U.S.A.)	Candela (Wayland, MA, U.S.A.)	Cynosure (Chelmsford, MA, U.S.A.)	Cynosure (Chelmsford, MA, U.S.A.)
Wavelength (nm)	585–600	595	585–600	585/595
Pulse duration (msec)	1.5	0.45–40	0.45–1.5	0.5–40
Maximum fluence (J/cm^2)	20	25	10	40
Cooling	Cryogen	Cryogen	Air	Air

of 595 nm, and variable pulse durations of 0.45 to 40 milliseconds. The longer pulse durations permit purpura-free treatment of facial telangiectasia, facial erythema, and poikiloderma.

Long-Pulsed Alexandrite Lasers (Table 5)

Long-pulsed millisecond-domain alexandrite lasers emitting at 755 nm provide deeper penetration into tissue, and preferential hemoglobin absorption based on a small peak in the 800- to 900-nm range. These lasers provide excellent clearance of larger telangiectasia, venulectasia, and feeding reticular veins of the lower extremities (40,41). Treatment of hypertrophic port wine stains, mixed-type hemangiomas, and the superficial component of venous malformations is now being explored with long-pulsed alexandrite lasers.

Table 5
Long-Pulsed Alexandrite

Laser	GentleLase®	Apogee®	Arion Wavelight®
Manufacturer	Candela (Wayland, MA, U.S.A.)	Cynosure (Chelmsford, MA, U.S.A.)	Cynosure (Chelmsford, MA, U.S.A.)
Wavelength (nm)	755	755	755
Pulse duration (msec)	3	5–40	1–50
Maximum fluence (J/cm^2)	100	50	5–70
Cooling	Cryogen	Air	Air

Diode Lasers (Table 6)

Millisecond-domain diode lasers are available at wavelengths of 800, 810, and 930 nm. Like the alexandrite lasers, these systems are effective in treating larger telangiectasia, venulectasia, and feeding reticular veins of the lower extremities (42,43).

Long-Pulsed Nd:YAG Lasers (Table 7)

Compared to the other near-infrared lasers being applied to the treatment of cutaneous vascular lesions, Nd:YAG lasers provide enhanced depth of penetration (up to 5.0 mm in depth) and minimal interference from melanin absorption. Long-pulsed Nd:YAG lasers are effective for the treatment of telangiectasia, venulectasia, and reticular veins of the legs because of their ability to photocoagulate larger diameter, more deeply situated vessels (44,45). Telangiectasia and venulectasia of the face can be successfully treated by using small (1.0–3.0 mm) spot sizes, and by using high fluences to compensate for the decreased absorption coefficient for hemoglobin at this wavelength (46). The pulsed Nd:YAG lasers are equipped with a variety of cooling systems including water-cooled chambers applied directly to the skin (Laserscope Lyra®, Altus Coolglide®, ESC Vasculight®) and cryogen spray cooling (Laser Aesthetics Varia® and Candela Gentle YAG®).

Intense Pulse Light Source (Table 8)

The intense pulsed light (IPL) source was developed by ESC Medical (now Lumenis) in an effort to maximize the efficacy in treating leg veins. This high intensity pulsed flashlamp light source delivers broadband

Table 6
Diode Lasers

Laser	MedioStar®	Apogee®	SkinPulse®	Apex®	Light Sheer®	EpiStar®	SLP 1000®
Manufacturer	Asclepion-Meditec (Jena, Germany)	Cynosure (Chelmsford, MA, U.S.A.)	Dornier (Munich, Germany)	Iridex (Mountainview, CA, U.S.A.)	Lumenis (Santa Clara, CA, U.S.A.)	Nidek (Fremont, CA, U.S.A.)	Palomar (Burlington, MA, U.S.A.)
Wavelength (nm)	810	800	940	800	800	810	810
Pulse duration (msec)	5–30	50–500	10 to continuous	5–100	5–100	200	50–100
Maximum fluence (J/cm^2)	64	50	600	5–60	10–60		179
Cooling	Contact	Air		Contact	Contact		Contact

Table 7
Long-Pulsed Nd:YAG Lasers

Laser	CoolGlide®/ Vantage®	Gentle YAG®	Varia®	Lyra®	Image®	Mydon®
Manufacturer	Cutera (Burlingame, CA, U.S.A.)	Candela, (Wayland, MA, U.S.A.)	ICN (Costa Mesa, CA, U.S.A.)	Laserscope (San Jose, CA, U.S.A.)	Sciton (Palo Alto, CA, U.S.A.)	Wavelight (Erlangen, Germany)
Wavelength (nm)	1064	1064	1064	1064	1064	1064
Pulse duration (msec)	0.1–300	3	0.3–200	10–100	5–200	20–140
Maximum fluence (J/cm^2)	300	10–70	500	200	10–400	15–400
Cooling	Contact	Cryogen	Cryogen/ contact	Contact	Contact/air	Contact/air

light from 515 to 1100 nm (47). Single, double, or triple pulses in the 2- to 20-millisecond domain can be delivered in a synchronized fashion. The broad emission spectrum, in the visible and near infrared region, targets both oxygenated and deoxygenated hemoglobin. The longer wavelengths penetrate deeper into the skin, enabling photocoagulation of deeper vessels, and the longer pulse durations produce uniform heating of larger vessels without inducing vessel rupture. Several IPL sources are now available. This technology has also been applied to the treatment of port wine stains, superficial hemangiomas (48), and facial telangiectasia

Table 8
IPL Sources

Light source	Prolite®	Quantum®	Vasculight®	Estelux®
Manufacturer	Alderm (Irvine, CA, U.S.A.)	Lumenis (Santa Clara, CA, U.S.A.)	Lumenis (Santa Clara, CA, U.S.A.)	Palomar (Burlington, MA, U.S.A.)
Wavelength (nm)	500–900	515–1200	515–1200	500–1200
Pulse duration (msec)		2–7	0.5–2.5	10–100
Maximum fluence (J/cm^2)	10–50	45	90	4–12
Cooling		Contact	Contact	Contact

Abbreviation: IPL, intense pulsed light.

(49) yielding good results. IPL technology presently finds its application mainly in nonablative photorejuvenation to improve the pigmentary, vascular, and textural irregularities of photodamaged skin.

CLINICAL APPLICATIONS

Port Wine Stains

The pulsed dye laser remains the treatment of choice for most port wine stains. Treatment of macular and mildly hypertrophic port wine stains with the 585-nm, 0.45-millisecond pulsed dye laser produces remarkable clinical lightening with minimal side effects. Multiple treatments are required for significant lightening. Early studies demonstrated 75% or more lightening in approximately 36% to 44% of adult patients with port wine stains, and at least 50% lesional lightening in 75% of patients after a total of four treatments (12,14–19,50). The laser has been proven safe and effective, even after 10 to 25 repetitive treatments (7). Treatment may be initiated soon after birth, without adverse effect. Clearing of port wine stain lesions depends on their anatomic location and size. Port wine stains located on the forehead, lateral cheeks, and neck respond better than those located on the central facial regions, specifically areas supplied by the second branch of the trigeminal nerve (51). Smaller lesions with areas less than $20\,cm^2$ respond far more quickly than larger lesions with areas greater than $20\,cm^2$. Head and neck port wine stains respond most favorably. Truncal lesions respond better than port wine stains located on the extremities, with distal extremity lesions being the most resistant.

Newer generation pulsed dye lasers with a wavelength of 595 nm and pulse duration of 1.5 milliseconds enable faster clearance of port wine stains in infants and adults. In studies using this laser in conjunction with cryogen spray cooling to treat 16 infants under 12 months of age with facial port wine stains, there was greater than 75% lightening in 63% of patients after four treatments using energy fluences of 11 to $12\,J/cm^2$ (35). Prospective side-by-side comparison studies of hypertrophic adult port wine stains treated with energy fluences of 12 to $14\,J/cm^2$ using the 595-nm, 1.5-millisecond laser demonstrated increased clearance compared to a fluence of $10\,J/cm^2$, both in conjunction with cryogen spray cooling (36).

Treatment of port wine stains with the 585-nm, 0.45-millisecond laser is usually performed with the largest spot size available to prevent reticulation. Typical treatment fluences using the 7 mm spot are 5.0 to $7.0\,J/cm^2$ and 5.0 to $6.0\,J/cm^2$ with a 10-mm spot size, depending on the age of the patient and the thickness of the lesion. Using the 595-nm, 1.5-millisecond pulsed dye lasers in conjunction with cryogen spray cooling, fluences of 8.0 to $11.0\,J/cm^2$ are used with a 7-mm spot size, and fluences of 5.0 to $6.5\,J/cm^2$ are used with the 10-mm spot size in infants and children. For adults with hypertrophic lesions, fluences up to $13\,J/cm^2$ can be used with a 7-mm spot size and fluences up to $7.5\,J/cm^2$ with a 10-mm spot size.

Determination of the appropriate fluence should be assessed with test performed on the target sites during the initial evaluation.

Immediately after treatment with the 585-nm, 0.45-millisecond pulsed dye laser, intense blue–black purpura develops for approximately 10 to 14 days. The intensity and duration of purpura is significantly lower while using pulse duration of 1.5 milliseconds. If crusting occurs, patients are instructed to apply a topical antibiotic such as bacitracin or polysporin ointment daily until it resolves. Following the resolution of purpura, lesional lightening takes place over a period of four to six weeks. Repeat treatments are performed every 6 to 10 weeks until maximal lesional clearing is achieved. Even after 20 treatment sessions, further lesional lightening may be achieved (7). The development of various skin-cooling methods has obviated the necessity for local or general anesthesia in most cases. With the exception of young children, most infants, teenagers, and adults tolerate the treatment well with the use of a topical anesthetic cream such as Emla or Elamax.

While pulsed dye laser technology remains the standard of care for port wine stain treatment, other technology has been successfully used for this indication. The IPL has been used to lighten port wine stains. Twenty-eight of forty patients treated in one study achieved greater than 75% lesional clearance after an average of four treatments for pink lesions, 1.5 for red ones, and 4.3 for purple-colored port wine stains (52). The lightening of the red or purple port wine stains by the three-millisecond long pulse alexandrite laser has also been found by the author and others (Dierickx C, personal communication) (52).

Hemangiomas

Superficial (capillary) hemangiomas and the superficial component of thin mixed-type hemangiomas respond best to pulsed dye laser therapy. Treatment of thin superficial hemangiomas can often clear these lesions in three to four treatment sessions (20,21,53–56). Thicker lesions may require additional treatments. The pulsed dye laser is also effective in reducing the superficial component of mixed-type hemangiomas; however, the deeper (cavernous) component may continue to proliferate despite laser therapy. Institution of pulsed dye laser therapy during the proliferative phase is helpful in slowing the growth of these lesions. Treatment of superficial hemangiomas helps in minimizing the enlargement of the tumor, prevents the development of complications such as bleeding and ulceration, and achieves improved cosmetic results.

Treatment of proliferating hemangiomas is usually performed at two- to four-week intervals, in an effort to halt further tumor growth. The treatment interval for involuting hemangiomas is usually six to eight weeks. As with port wine stains, the newer 595-nm, 1.5-millisecond pulsed dye lasers, which can be used at higher fluences in conjunction with cryogen spray cooling, appear to achieve faster clearing of hemangiomas compared to historical controls, because of their ability to treat larger diameter and deeper blood vessels. The IPL has also been used for the treatment of superficial hemangiomas and the superficial component of mixed type hemangiomas with some success. Preliminary studies using millisecond-domain pulsed dye, diode, and Nd:YAG lasers show promising results with these wavelengths for thicker lesions.

Telangiectasia

Telangiectasia are capillaries, venules, or arteries that are 0.1 to 1.0 mm in diameter and are visible as superficial cutaneous vessels. Facial telangiectasia are common, and in fair-skinned individuals, they are often associated with rosacea or actinic damage. Other etiologies include collagen vascular disease, genetic disorders, hormonal, primary cutaneous disease, and radiodermatitis. Spider angiomata are telangiectasia with a central feeding arteriole, typically appearing in preschool and school-age children with a peak incidence between the ages of 7 and 10.

Most patients seek treatment for facial telangiectasia because of cosmetic concerns. Techniques used to treat facial telangiectasia have included electrosurgery, sclerotherapy, and treatment with continuous wave and quasi-continuous wave lasers, but these methods may produce textural and pigmentary irregularities. The development of pulsed lasers enabled efficient, effective, and low-risk treatment of these common skin lesions.

A wide variety of vascular laser systems produce excellent clearance of facial telangiectasia. The 585- and 595-nm pulsed dye lasers with 0.45- and 1.5-millisecond pulse durations produce excellent results in one to two treatment sessions, but induce purpura lasting 7 to 14 days (37). Treatment is performed by applying contiguous laser pulses with approximately 10% overlap. The newer, millisecond-duration pulsed dye lasers, used at 6 to 10 milliseconds, clear facial telangiectasia, without purpura production. Effective treatment usually requires stacking of three to four laser pulses with an endpoint of vessel blanching or transient thrombosis. The 532-nm KTP laser produces excellent results for the treatment of facial telangiectasia in one to three treatment sessions (57,58). Contiguous laser pulses are applied directly over the vessels, with additional pulses, if necessary, to achieve visible vessel blanching. Some of the KTP systems are equipped with cooled sapphire hand pieces that enable easy gliding of the laser tip over the skin, when used with cold gel, and relatively painless treatment.

Long-pulsed Nd:YAG lasers, used with spot sizes of 1 to 3 mm and fluences of 120 to 250 J/cm^2, also produce excellent results for facial telangiectasia without purpura production. With the use of higher fluences, proper skin cooling and avoidance of pulse stacking are necessary to prevent epidermal damage, particularly around the nasal ala (46,59,60). The long-pulsed Nd:YAG lasers are particularly useful for the treatment of the larger caliber paranasal vessels that often require multiple, repetitive treatments with the shorter wavelength lasers. Venulectasia commonly seen on the lateral cheeks following rhytidectomy often usually clear in one treatment session. Visible facial veins have also been treated with Nd:YAG lasers, but extreme caution must be exercised to avoid laser exposure within the orbital rim with this deeply penetrating wavelength. The IPL devices also clear facial telangiectasia, and multiple treatment sessions may be necessary (49).

Facial Erythema

Facial erythema with or without associated telangiectasia is a common cosmetic concern. The erythema is usually a manifestation of rosacea or a flushing or blushing disorder. Effective treatment is best achieved with the pulsed dye lasers and IPL sources, using large spot sizes to avoid reticulation (61,62). There is no purpura production with the newer pulsed dye lasers used with 6- to 10-millisecond pulse durations and the IPL devices. Multiple treatment sessions (2–6) may be necessary to achieve good clinical results. An improvement in the associated symptoms or warmth and burning sensation usually accompanies the reduction in erythema.

Poikiloderma

Poikiloderma is treatable with lasers and light sources. Poikiloderma of Civatte is relatively common in fair-skinned, actinically damaged individuals. Clinically, poikiloderma appears as a combination of telangiectasia, irregular pigmentation, and atrophic changes. The treatment of this diffuse condition is best accomplished using the pulsed dye lasers or IPL devices with large spot sizes to avoid reticulation (26,63,64). Overly aggressive treatment with any laser or light source can produce atrophy and hypopigmentation. Compared to the treatment of telangiectasia, fluences should be lowered by approximately 25% to 30% in the treatment of poikiloderma to avoid adverse effects. Treatment of poikiloderma using the 6- to 10-millisecond pulsed dye lasers appears to achieve equivalent results to the shorter pulsed systems without the development of purpura. Contiguous laser pulses are applied without overlap. With the IPL devices, it is often helpful to alternate the axis of the rectangular spot with each treatment to reduce the risk of reticulation.

Scars and Striae Distensae

Pulsed dye laser therapy can be used to improve erythematous and hypertrophic scars. Clinical response rates are 57% to 83% (30,65,66). The pulsed dye laser reduces erythema by eliminating the underlying dilated microvasculative. Scar height and skin surface texture changes are improved, presumably by altering collagen production. Multiple treatment sessions are often necessary, particularly for thicker scars, and adjunctive treatment with intralesional corticosteroid injections is useful. The best results are achieved using 10-mm spot sizes and fluences of 4 to 5 J/cm^2 without skin cooling and 5 to 6 J/cm^2 with skin cooling. Treatment intervals are six to eight weeks.

Low-fluence pulsed dye laser therapy also improves the appearance of striae (32). Striae rubra shows the best response, and can sometimes be entirely eliminated with early laser intervention. The skin textural irregularities in striae alba can be improved with pulsed dye laser treatment and other nonablative lasers and light sources. The mechanism of improvement is presumed to be via fibroblast activation and induction of collagen production.

Warts

Pulsed dye lasers effectively treat cutaneous lesions of human papilloma virus, including plantar warts, periungual warts, flat warts, and verrucae vulgaris (33). Electron microscopic studies suggest that the mechanism of improvement is via thermal alteration of the virally infected tissue (67). Laser treatment appears to be more effective than conventional wart therapy, and carries a minimal risk of scarring, even when used to treat deep plantar warts and subungual and periungual lesions. Treatments are performed following paring of hyperkeratotic lesions, using the 585- or 595-nm pulsed dye laser with pulse duration of 0.45 or 1.5 milliseconds. A 5- or 7-mm spot is used at fluences of 7 to 9J/cm^2 without skin cooling. Recalcitrant warts require three to four repetitive treatments, at two to four week intervals. Uncomplicated warts usually respond in one session.

CONCLUSION

The development of pulsed laser and light source technologies has revolutionized the treatment of cutaneous vascular lesions. Laser therapy remains to be the treatment of choice for port wine stains, superficial hemangiomas, and telangiectasia. These devices have also been successfully applied to the treatment of hypertrophic and erythematous scars, striae, and warts. Unlike other conventional destructive modalities, treatment is noninvasive. Due to the selective deposition and targeting of the light energy, there is little risk of skin wounding or the development of pigmentary or textural irregularities. The development of longer wavelength and longer pulse duration laser technology, along with the skin-cooling methods, has improved the safety and efficacy of vascular lesion therapy.

REFERENCES

1. Silver L. Argon laser photocoagulation of port wine stain hemangiomas. Lasers Surg Med 1986; 6:24–28.
2. Dixon JA, Rotering RH, Huethner SE. Patient's evaluation of argon laser therapy of port wine stains, decorative tattoos, and essential telangiectasia. Laser Surg Med 1984; 4:181–190.
3. Anderson RR, Parrish JA. Selective photothermolysis: precise microsurgery by selective absorption of pulsed radiation. Science 1983; 220:524–527.
4. Anderson RR, Parrish JA. Microvasculature can be selectively damaged using dye lasers: a basic theory and experimental evidence in human skin. Lasers Surg Med 1981; 1:263–276.
5. Glassberg E, Lask GP, Tan EM, Uitto J. The flashlamp-pumped 577 nm pulsed tunable dye laser: clinical efficacy and in vitro studies. J Dermatol Surg Oncol 1988; 14:1200–1208.
6. Levine VJ, Geronemus RG. Adverse effects associated with the 577 and 585 nm pulsed dye laser in the treatment of cutaneous vascular lesions: a study of 500 patients. J Am Acad Dermatol 1995; 32:613–617.
7. Kauvar ANB, Geronemus RG. Repetitive pulsed dye laser treatments improve persistent port wine stains. Dermatol Surg 1995; 21:5151–5521.
8. Dierickx CC, Casparian JM, Venugopalan V, Farinelli WA, Anderson RR. Thermal relaxation of port wine stain vessels probed in vivo: the need for 1–10 msec laser pulse treatment. J Invest Dermatol 1995; 105:709–714.
9. Garden JM, Tan OT, Kerschmann R, Boll J, Furumoto H, Anderson RR, Parrish JA. Effect of dye laser pulse duration on selective cutaneous vascular injury. J Invest Dermatol 1986; 87:653–657.
10. Nelson JS, Majaron B, Kelly K. Active skin cooling in conjunction with laser dermatologic surgery. Sem Cut Med Surg 2000; 19(4):253–266.
11. Tan OT, Murray S, Kurban AK. Action spectrum of vascular specific injury using pulsed irradiation. J Invest Dermatol 1989; 92:868–871.
12. Tan OT, Morrison P. Kurban AK. 585 nm for the treatment of port wine stains. Plast Reconstr Surg 1990; 86:1112–1117.
13. Goldman L, Kerr JH, Larkin M, Binder S. 600 nm flash pumped dye laser for fragile telangiectasia of the elderly. Lasers Surg Med 1993; 13:227–233.
14. Alster TS, Wilson F. Treatment of port-wine stains with the flashlamp-pumped pulsed dye laser: extended clinical experience in children and adults. Ann Plast Surg 1994; 32:478–484.
15. Ashinoff R, Geronemus RG. Flashlamp-pumped pulsed dye laser for port wine stains in infancy: earlier versus later treatment. J Am Acad Dermatol 1991; 24:467–472.
16. Garden JM, Polla LL, Tan OT. The treatment of port wine stains by the pulsed dye laser. Arch Dermatol 1988; 124:889–896.
17. Goldman MP, Fitzpatrick RE, Ruiz-Esparza J. Treatment of port wine stains (capillary malformation) with the flashlamp-pumped pulsed dye laser. J Pediatr 1993; 122:71–77.
18. Reyes BA, Geronemus RG. Treatment of port wine stains during childhood with the flashlamp pumped pulsed dye laser. J Am Acad Dermatol 1990; 23:1142–1148.
19. Tappero JW, Grekin RC, Zanelli GA, Berger TG. Pulsed dye laser therapy for cutaneous Kaposi's sarcoma associated with acquired immunodeficiency syndrome. J Am Acad Dermatol 1992; 27:526–530.
20. Ashinoff R, Geronemus RG. Capillary hemangiomas and treatment with the flashlamp-pumped pulsed dye laser. Arch Dermatol 1991; 127:202–205.
21. Garden JM, Bakus AD, Paller AS. Treatment of cutaneous hemangiomas by the flashlamp-pumped pulsed dye laser: prospective analysis. J Pediatr 1992; 120:555–560.

22. Broska P, Martinho E, Goodman MM. Comparison of the argon tunable dye laser with the flashlamp pulsed dye laser in the treatment of facial telangiectasia. J Dermatol Surg Oncol 1994; 20:749–753.

23. Goldman MP, Weiss RA, Brody HJ, Coleman WP III, Fitzpatrick RE. Treatment of facial telangiectasia with sclerotherapy, laser surgery, and/or electrodesiccasion: a review. J Dermatol Surg Oncol 1993; 19:899–906.

24. Ruiz-Esparaza J, Goldman MP, Fitzpatrick RE, Lowe NJ, Behr KL. Flashlamp-pumped dye laser treatment of telangiectasia. J Dermatol Surg Oncol 1993; 19:1000–1003.

25. Garden JM, Bakus AD. Clinical efficacy of the pulsed dye laser in the treatment of vascular lesions. J Dermatol Surg Oncol 1993; 19:321–326.

26. Wheeland RG, Applebaum J. Flashlamp-pumped pulsed dye laser therapy for poikiloderma of Civatte. J Dermatol Surg Oncol 1990; 16:12–16.

27. Gonzalez E, Gange RW, Momtaz KT. Treatment of telangiectasias and other benign vascular lesions with the 577 nm pulsed dye laser. J Am Acad Dermatol 1992; 27: 220–226.

28. Goldberg DJ, Sciales CW. Pyogenic granuloma in children: treatment with the flashlamp-pumped pulsed dye laser. J Dermatol Surg Oncol 1991; 17:960–962.

29. Hoffman SJ, Walsh P, Morelli JG. Treatment of angiofibroma with pulsed tunable dye laser. J Am Acad Dermatol 1993; 29:790–791.

30. Alster TS. Improvement of erythematous and hypertrophic scars by the 585-nm flashlamp-pumped pulsed dye laser. Ann Plast Surg 1994; 32:186–190.

31. Alster TS, Williams CM. Treatment of keloid sternotomy scars with the 585 nm flashlamp-pumped pulsed dye laser. Lancet 1995; 345:1198.

32. McDaniel DH, Ash K, Zukowski M. Treatment of stretch marks with the 585 nm flashlamp-pumped pulsed dye laser. Dermatol Surg 1996; 22:332–337.

33. Kauvar ANB, Geronemus RG, McDaniel DH. Pulsed dye laser treatment of warts. Arch Fam Med 1995; 4:1035–1040.

34. Kauvar ANB. Long-pulse, high energy pulsed dye laser treatment of port wine stains and hemangiomas. Laser Surg Med 1997; (suppl 9):36.

35. Geronemus R, Quintana A, Lou W, Kauvar ANB. High fluence modified pulsed dye laser photocoagulation with dynamic cooling of port wine stains in infancy. Arch Dermatol 2000; 6:942–943.

36. Kauvar ANB, Lou WW, Zelickson B. Effect of cryogen spray cooling on 595 nm, 1.5 msec pulsed dye laser treatment of port wine stains. Laser Surg Med 2000; (suppl 12):24.

37. West TB, Alster TS. Comparison of the long-pulsed dye and KTP lasers in the treatment of facial and leg telangiectasia. Dermatol Surg 1998; 24:221–226.

38. Hsia J, Lowery JA, Zelickson B. Treatment of leg telangiectasia using a long-pulse dye at 595 nm. Lasers Surg Med 1997; 20:15.

39. Bernstein EF, Lee J, Lowery J, Brown DB, Geronemus R, Lask G, Hsia J. Treatment of spider veins with the 595 nm pulsed-dye laser. J Am Acad Dermatol 1998; 39:746–750.

40. Kauvar ANB, Lou WW. Pulsed alexandrite laser for the treatment of leg telangiectasia and reticular veins. Arch Dermatol 2000; 136:1343–1346.

41. Brunnberg L, Lorenz S, Landthaler M, Hohenleutner U. Evaluation of the long pulsed high fluence alexandrite laser therapy with 755 nm for leg veins. Lasers Surg Med 2002; 31(5):359–362.

42. Dierickx CC et al. Lasers Surg Med 1998; (suppl 10):40.

43. Kaudewitz P, Klovekorn W, Rother W. Treatment of leg vein telangiectases: 1-year results with a new 940 nm diode laser. Dermatol Surg 2002; 28(11):1031–1034.

44. Omura NE, Dover JS, Arndt KA, Kauvar AN. Treatment of reticular leg veins with a 1064 nm long-pulsed Nd:YAG laser. J Am Acad Dermatol 2003; 48(1):76–81.

45. Coles Cm, Werner RS, Zelickson BD. Comparative pilot study evaluating the treatment of leg veins with a long pulse ND:YAG laser and sclerotherapy. Lasers Surg Med 2002; 30(2):149–153.
46. Eremia S, Li CY. Treatment of face veins with a cryogen spray variable pulse width 1064 nm Nd:YAG Laser: a prospective study of 17 patients. Dermatol Surg 2002; 28(3):220–223.
47. Goldman MP, Eckhouse S. Photothermal sclerosis of leg veins. Dermatol Surg 1996; 22:323–330.
48. Schroeter CA, Neumann HAM. An intense light source. The photoderm VL-flashlamp as a new treatment possibility for vascular lesions. Dermatol Surg 1998; 24:743–748.
49. Bierring P, Christiansen K, Troilius A. Intense pulsed light source for treatment of facial telangiectasias. J Cosmet Laser Ther 2001; 3(4):169–173.
50. Tan OT, Sherwood K, Gilchrest BA. Treatment of children with PWS using the flashlamp-pulsed tunable dye laser. New Engl J Med 1989; 320:416–421.
51. Renfro L, Geronemus RG. Anatomical differences of port-wine stains in response to treatment with the pulsed dye laser. Arch Dermatol 1993; 129:182–188.
52. Raulin C, Schroeter CA, Weiss RA, Keiner M, Werner S. Treatment of port wine stains with a non-coherent pulsed light source: a retrospective study. Arch Dermatol 1999; 135:679–683.
53. Barlow RJ, Walker NPJ, Markey AC. Treatment of proliferative hemangiomas with the 585 nm pulsed dye laser. Br J Dermatol 1996; 134:700–704.
54. Maier H, Neumann R. Treatment of strawberry marks with flashlamp-pumped pulsed dye laser in infancy. Lancet 1996; 347:131–132.
55. Ricci RM, Finley EM, Grimwood RE. Treatment of cutaneous hemangiomas in preterm neonatal twins with the flashlamp-pumped pulsed dye laser. Lasers Surg Med 1998; 22:10–13.
56. Sherwood KA, Tan OT. Treatment of a capillary hemangioma with the flashlamp-pumped dye laser. J Am Acad Dermatol 1990; 22:136–137.
57. Adrian RM, Taughetti EA. Long pulse 532 nm laser treatment of facial telangiectasia. Dermatol Surg 1998; 24(1):71–74.
58. Goldsberg DJ, Meine JG. Treatment of facial telangiectases with the diode-pumped frequency-doubled a-surbled Nd:YAG laser. Dermatol Surg 1998; 24:828–832.
59. Major A, Brazzini B, Campolmi P, Bonan P, Mavilia L, Ghersetich I, Hercogova J, Lottit T. Nd:YAG 1064 nm laser in the treatment of facial and leg telangiectasias. J Eur Acad Dermatol Venereol 2001; 15(6):559–565.
60. Kauvar A, Mafong E, Friedman P, Bernstein L, Alexiades-Armenakas M, Geronemus R. Treatment of facial telangiectasia with a long pulsed ND:YAG laser. Laser Surg Med 2002; (suppl 14):135.
61. Angermeier MC. Treatment of facial vascular lesions with intense pulsed light. J Cutan Laser Ther 1999; 1(2):95–100.
62. Lowe NJ, Behr KL, Fitzpatrick R, Goldman M, Ruiz-Esparza J. Flashlamp pumped dye laser for rosacea-associated telangiectasia and erythema. J Dermatol Surg Oncol 1991; 17(6):522–525.
63. Raulin C, Greve B, Grema H. IPL technology: a review. Lasers Surg Med 2003; 32(2): 78–87.
64. Weiss RA, Goldman MP, Weiss MA. Treatment of essential telangiectasias with an intense pulsed light source (PhotoDerm VL). Dermatol Surg 1996; 23(10):941–945; discussion 945–946.
65. Alster TS, Kurban, AK, Grove GL, Grove MJ, Tan OT. Alteration of argon laser-induced scars by the pulsed dye laser. Lasers Surg Med 1993; 13:368–373.

66. Alster TS, Williams CM. Improvement of hypertrophic and keloidal median sternotomy scars by the 585 nm flashlamp-pumped pulsed dye laser: a controlled study. Lancet 1995; 345:1198–1200.

67. Ross EV, McDaniel DH, Anderson RR, Kauvar ANB, Geronemus RG. Pulsed dye (585 nm) treatment of warts: a comparison of single versus multiple pulse techniques examining clinical response, fast infrared thermal camera measurements, and light electron microscopy. Lasers Surg Med 1995; (suppl 7):59.

9

Laser Treatment for Leg Veins

Neil S. Sadick

Weill Medical College of Cornell University, New York, New York, U.S.A.

Video 10: Leg Veins
Video 11: Leg Veins: Gemini® Device

INTRODUCTION

The incidence of unsightly venulectasias and/or telangiectasias on the legs occurs in up to 41% of women and 15% of men (1). The utilization of lasers and intense pulsed light (IPL) sources for the treatment of lower extremity veins has gained increased popularity over the past five years. This technology, driven by consumer demand, has been shown to be effective in treating vessels that are refractory to sclerotherapy, vessels that arise from prior surgical treatment or sclerotherapy (telangiectatic matting or angiogenic flushing), and needle-phobic patients.

Initial problems involving laser/IPL technologies have centered on the fact that it is inherently more difficult to get photons safely and in sufficient numbers through several layers of blood vessel wall into the target chromophore, that is oxygenated and deoxygenated hemoglobin. Injections directly into the target are inherently more efficient.

However, a greater recent understanding of photoendothelial interaction has led to improved efficiency of light modalities in this setting (2,3). The choice of wavelength(s), degree of energy fluence, and pulse duration of light exposure are all related to the type and size of the target vessel treated. Deeper vessels require a longer wavelength to allow penetration to their depth (4). However, even at a penetrating wavelength, pulse duration must be matched to the vessel size. As the depth and size of the vessel change, so do the absorption characteristics. Larger diameter vessels require longer pulse duration to allow sufficient time for diffusion of heat evenly throughout the cylindrical vessel lumen (5). In addition, deliverance of this energy should occur with a shock wave producing gentle cavitation, to prevent posttreatment hemorrhage and purpura. It should also produce an epidermal bypass to protect this structure from deleterious thermal effects. Optimal laser/IPL parameters for treatment of lower extremity vessels are present in Table 1 (6).

In this regard, shorter (500–600 nm) wavelengths may be used to treat Class I superficial oxygenated reddish telangiectasias while a longer wavelength (755–1100 nm) may be used to treat Class II to III deeper

Table 1
Optimal Laser/IPL Parameters for Treatment of Lower Extremity Vessels

	Wavelength (nm)	Pulse duration (msec)	Beam diameter (mm)
Diameter of vessels			
100 μm	580	1	–
300 μm	590	10	–
600 μm to 1 mm	600	20–100	–
Vessel depth			
Less than 1 mm	>500	–	Small (2–6 mm)
Greater than 1 mm	>600	–	Large (6–12 mm)

deoxygenated bluish venulectasias and reticular veins up to 4 mm in diameter (7). This "bimodal" wavelength approach to the treatment of lower extremity veins produces results superior to previously described treatment paradigms for photothermolytic eradication of lower extremity vessels (8).

When and How to Choose Laser/IPL vs. Sclerotherapy

The utilization of light sources for the treatment of leg veins is efficacious for treating telangiectasia/venulectasia or reticular veins less than 3 mm in diameter (9,10).

It is commonly used for the patient who is needle-phobic or requests laser as a primary modality of treatment.

It is very effective in the treatment of noncannulizable or sclero-resistant vessels. Areas of neovascularization with telangiectatic matting or angiogenic flushing are primary indications for this approach (3,11).

Practical Tips in Laser Treatment of Leg Veins

- Rule out areas of reflux by means of physical examination and Duplex ultrasound,
- treat larger diameter vessels by foam sclerotherapy or ambulatory phlebectomy,
- sclerotherapy of cannulizable vessels,
- laser treatment of residual veins,
- a varied monomodal approach to treatment of leg veins is the major approach utilized by most phlebologic vein laser surgeon (Table 2).

This incorporates utilizing one of the 1064 neodymium–yttrium–aluminum–garnet (Nd:YAG) technologies using small spot sizes (1.0–2.0 mm), high fluences (150–400 J/cm^2), and short pulse durations (15–30 milliseconds) for treatment of small red vessels of less than 1 mm in diameter which contain a high degree of oxygenated hemoglobin.

Table 2
Varied Mode Monomodal Approach to Leg Veins

	Vessel <1 mm (red)	Vessel 1–3 mm (blue)
Spot size	1–2 mm	3–6 mm
Fluence	150–400 J/cm^2	100–250 J/cm^2
Pulse duration	15–30 msec	30–50 msec

In a similar fashion, the same long wavelength laser can be employed with larger spot sizes (3–6 mm), more moderate fluences of 100 to 250 J/cm^2, and more extended pulse durations of 30 to 50 milliseconds for treatment of blue vessels (1–3 mm) which are deeper in location and have a higher degree of deoxygenated hemoglobin (Figs. 1 and 2).

Compression is usually not necessary following laser/IPL/RF treatment of nonbulging vessels (12).

A summary of recent technologic advances in laser/IPL treatment of lower extremity veins is presented in Table 3. A compilation of laser and IPL sources utilized in this setting is present in the following discussion and listed in Table 4.

It is important to explain to the patient that this technology like sclerotherapy, takes multiple treatments to see progress. In addition, it is important during the initial consultation to explain to the patient that forces of hydrostatic pressure and reflux must be addressed prior to laser therapy to optimize therapeutic efficacy and to minimize side effects.

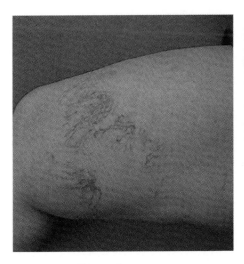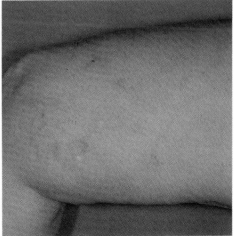

Figure 1
Pre-/post-1064 Nd:YAG (Laserscope Lyra) three treatments: blue vessels 3 mm spot size, F-200 J/cm^2, PD 40 milliseconds; red vessels 1.5 mm spot size, F-350 J/cm^2, PD 20 milliseconds.

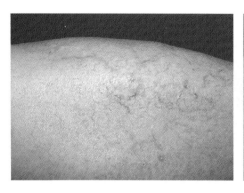 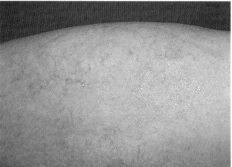

Figure 2
Pre-/post-diode laser/RF Syneron Polaris treatment of blue and red vessels
two treatments: λ 915 nm; spot size 5 × 8; LE 90 J/cm^2; RF 90 J/cm^3.

A comparison of laser/IPL treatments for telangiectasia of less than
0.5 mm versus sclerotherapy is presented in Table 5.

CONTINUOUS WAVE ND:YAG LASERS

The Nd:YAG laser at 1064 nm has also been used to treat leg telangiectasias in a continuous mode (13). Absorption by blood is relatively poor
at this wavelength (up to 3.7 nm) leading to much nonspecific damage.
Therefore, the continuous wave Nd:YAG laser has no role in the treatment of leg vessels (14).

578 nm Copper Bromide (CuBr) Yellow Light Laser

A new yellow light laser utilizing a copper bromide medium has shown
efficacy in the treatment of red lower extremity telangiectasia of less than
2 mm. An average of 1.7 patient treatment sessions produced significant
clearing of 75% to 100% in 71.8% of patients. Positive results are confined
to the treatment of red vessels (1 mm) (15).

Table 3
Recent Technologic Advances in Laser/IPL Treatment of Lower Extremity Veins

---

Cooling technologies
Longer wavelengths
Extended pulse durations
Monomodal varying pulse duration/spot size/___ fluence technology (1064 nm Nd:YAG)
Captured pulsing
Larger beam diameter (spot size)
Higher energy fluences

Abbreviation: Nd:YAG, neodymium–yttrium–aluminum–garnet.

Table 4
Lasers for Leg Veins

Device (company)	Wave length (nm)	Pulse duration (msec)	Spot size (mm)	Maximum fluence (J/cm)	Maximum speed (Hz)	Cooling device	Comments
E2000 (Palomar/ ConBio)	694	3 or 100	10 mm hexagon; 20 mm square	50	1	Sapphire contact	Employs photon recycling
EpiTouch Ruby (Lumenis)	694	1.2	4–6	40	1–1	Gel	Q-switched mode available
RubyStar (Aesculap Meditec)	694	2	3–14	35	1	Contact plate precooling	Q-switched mode available
GentleLASE (Candela)	755	3	7–18	100	1	DCD	2×7 mm spot for leg veins
EpiTouch Plus Alex (Lumenis)	755	2–40	5–10	50	5	Gel	Scanner available
LPIR/ Apogee (Cynosure)	755	5040	7–16	50	1	Cold air flow	Scanner available
LightSheer (Lumenis)	800	5–30	9–9	60	1	Sapphire contact	Diode array in handpiece
CoolGlide (Cutera)	1064	10–100	9–9	100	2	Copper contact precooling	FDA approval pending, scanner
Lyra (Laser- scope)	1064	10–50	3–5	100	4	Contact cooling	Carbon makes no difference
Softlight (Thermo- lase)	1064	10–20	7	2–3	10	Not needed	Sequence of multiple pulses
Flashlamp (Lumenis)	Variable from 550 to 1200	Variable	8–33 or 10–45	30–65	<1	Circulating cooling device	Combine diode laser + radio-frequency
Polaris (Syneron)	900 + RF	250	5–8	RF: 100 J/cm³; diode: 140 J/cm	1	Contact + cooling gel	

Abbreviation: DCD, dynamic cooling device.

Table 5
Sclerotherapy vs. Laser/IPL for Treatment of Telangiectasia

	Microsclerotherapy	Laser flashlamp
Number of treatments	=	=
Bruising	−	+
Discomfort	−	+
Clinical efficiency	−	+
Purpura	+	−
Pigmentation	=	=
Ulceration	−	+
Cost	+	−
Patient satisfaction	−	+
Physical skill	=	=

CONTINUOUS WAVE LASERS

Argon and Continuous Wave Dye Lasers

Argon (488 and 514 nm) and continuous wave dye lasers (515 to 590 nm) are well-absorbed by hemoglobin, and they penetrate to the depth of mid-dermal vessels, more than 1 mm within the skin. Results with this short-wave technology have overall been disappointing with improvement reported in less than 50% of individuals in previous studies (17). Synergistic treatment with sclerotherapy have yielded improved results (18).

PULSED LASERS AND LIGHT SOURCES

Potassium-Titanyl-Phosphate Lasers

Early attempts to treat vessels with the continuous wave potassium-titanyl-phosphate (KTP) crystal laser were mostly unsuccessful. At 532 nm, hemoglobin ablation is excellent. However, the depth of penetration limits the use of this laser to superficial leg telangiectasias of less than 1 mm in diameter.

Although the results of treatment of facial vessels have been excellent, the results of treatments utilizing small spot sizes and pulse durations of less than 10 milliseconds have been more variable (9,19–21).

More updated technologies including Versapulse KTP laser (Lumenis, Santa Clara, California, U.S.) using larger spot sizes (3–5 mm) and longer pulse durations (10–50 milliseconds) at fluences of 14 to 20 J/cm^2 have been more promising. A 4°C chilled tip provides epidermal protection. In published studies, two to three treatments have yielded maximal vessel improvement, although pigment dyschromia including temporary hyperpigmentation has been reported in darker-or tanned-skin individuals. Other technologies including the Aura (Laserscope, San Jose, California, U.S.) have produced comparable results.

Patient acceptance of this laser treatment is high with minimal treatment discomfort of the longer penetrating wavelengths and a relatively uncomplicated postoperative course (22).

Flashlamp-Pumped Pulsed Dye Laser

Newer innovations in flashlamp-pumped pulsed dye laser technology have produced improved treatment of leg telangiectasia (23). The traditional pulsed dye laser (POL)(585-nm, 450-microsecond pulse duration) has been shown to be highly effective in the management of port wine stains and facial telangiectasias. This technology was shown to be less effective in the management of leg veins. Although 585-nm light can penetrate 1.2 mm to reach the typical depth of leg telangiectasias, the pulse duration is inadequate for effective damage of all but superficial fine vessels approximately 0.1 mm or smaller in diameter (24).

Variable results, persistent purpura, and a high incidence of both hyper- and hypopigmentation limited the widespread usage of this technology.

Long-Pulsed Dye Lasers

Based on the theory of selective photothermolysis, the predicted pulse duration ideally suited for thermal destruction of leg veins (0.1 to several millimeters in diameter) is the 1- to 50-millisecond domain (25). Four long-pulsed dye lasers, two with 1.5 millisecond pulse durations (Sclero Plus, Candela, Wayland, Massachusetts, U.S., VLS, Cynosure, Chelmsford, Massachusetts, U.S.) and two with variable pulse durations as long as 40 milliseconds (V-beam, Candela, V-Star, Cynosure), are now available. Each device uses a Rhodamine dye to produce wavelengths of 585, 590, 595, or 600 nm. These longer pulse durations and wavelengths theoretically improve the ability to treat deeper, larger caliber vessels (25).

More recent modifications to the pulsed dye laser have included the addition of the dynamic cooling device (DCD) (Candela), a method of cryogen spray cooling capable of generating higher fluences (up to 25 J/cm^2).

Six studies reported in the literature have assessed the effectiveness of these long-pulsed dye lasers in the treatment of leg veins, with variable results (26–29). Most of these studies achieved 50% to 60% clearing of treatment sites after three treatment sessions with an incidence of both hyper- and hypopigmentation approaching 50%. The delivery of equivalent laser fluences over extended pulse durations have helped to eliminate posttreatment purpura.

Longer Wavelength Pulsed Lasers

Based upon the deeper penetration of longer wavelength visible and near-infrared light and a small peak of hemoglobin absorption in the

700-to 900-nm range, long-pulsed alexandrite and Nd:YAG lasers have been developed to treat moderately deep, larger caliber spider and feeding reticular veins of the lower extremities.

The alexandrite lasers have wavelength of 755 nm with pulse durations of 3 to 20 milliseconds. The Nd:YAG lasers have a wavelength of 1064 nm and pulse durations up to 100 milliseconds. Diode lasers with a wavelength of 800, 810, and 930 nm and pulse durations of 10 to 250 milliseconds may also be used.

Long-Pulsed Alexandrite Lasers

Long-pulsed alexandrite lasers have recently been applied to the treatment of leg telangiectasia and reticular veins, less than 3 mm in diameter, with good results. The longer wavelength provides deeper tissue penetration and an ability to treat larger diameter and more deeply situated vessels. Although hemoglobin absorption of this wavelength is lower than that of the 532 and 595 nm wavelengths, it is sufficient to achieve photocoagulation of a wide range of vessel sizes with the use of higher fluences. To penetrate tissue more deeply and to allow greater thermal diffusion time to treat larger vessels, the alexandrite laser has been modified to provide pulse duration of up to 20 milliseconds. Optimal treatment parameters for long-pulsed alexandrite lasers seem to be 20 J/cm^2, double pulsed at a repetition rate of 1 Hz.

In two reported trials, the laser has been shown to be effective in the treatment of mid-sized leg veins. Sixty-three percent clearance of leg veins after three treatments (0–4 mm 0 1 mm) was reported (30). The best response in this study was seen with sclerotherapy performed as a supplemental technique, confirming the importance of sclerotherapy for leg veins.

In a second study, patients with Fitzpatrick skin types I and III and leg veins measuring 0.3 to 2.0 mm in diameter were treated utilizing an 8-mm spot size and fluences of 60 to 80 J/cm^2 with concomitant cryogen cooling. Seventy-five percent or greater clearance was noted in treated site after a single treatment. Patient discomfort and temporary hypopigmentation were reported in one-third of the treated sites (31).

Diode Lasers

Diode lasers (800 nm at 5- to 250-millisecond pulse duration) have been used to treat superficial telangiectasias and reticular veins. These devices with near-infrared wavelengths allow deeper tissue penetration with decreased absorption by melanin. In addition, their wavelength matches a tertiary hemoglobin absorption peak at 915 nm. Two methods of delivery for diode lasers are available: filler optic transmission of an 810-nm laser (gallium-arsenide) and an overlapping 800-nm diode array with a fixed spot size of 9 mm×9 mm up to 12 mm×12 mm.

The longer wavelength (940 nm) diode laser offers better vessel clearance and fewer complications when compared to its predecessors. In one study with short-term (16 weeks) follow up, the best results were obtained in a subset of patients who had vessels ranging from 0.8 to 1.4 mm. Eighty eight percent of these patients had greater than 75% vessel clearance, with one-third of those patients obtaining complete vessel clearance (32). A long-term (12 months) study showed even more improvement, with 75% of all patients had greater than 75% vessel clearance (33).

Goldman describes the advantages of the 1064 nm Nd:YAG laser for the treatment of leg veins are due to the longer wavelengths ability to penetrate more deeply into the tissue and offer more effective thermosclerosis of small to medium blood vessels. Another advantage is the minimal melanin absorption at this wavelength, allowing for the treatment of all skin types and patients with tanned skin (34).

In a study comparing the 1064 nm Nd:YAG, 810 nm diode and 755 nm Alexandrite lasers for the treatment of 0.3–3.0 mm leg veins the overall best results and fewest complications were obtained with the 1064 nm Nd:YAG laser. Greater than 75% improvement was seen with 88% of patients treated with this laser. The authors reported their results with the 810 nm diode laser as "unpredictable" and the 755 nm Alexandrite laser induced too much purpura, inflammation, and matting at the treatment sites (35).

In one study, using an 810-nm quasi-continuous diode laser with vessel size of 0.2 to 0.5 mm, 60% mean vessel clearance was obtained after a mean of 2.2 treatment sessions (36).

More recently, the introduction of higher fluence capability diode lasers has occurred, providing enhanced efficacy in this treatment setting (10,37).

IPL Sources

High IPL sources emanating from a filtered flashlamp (Photoderm VL, Vasculight IPL, Lumenis, Palo Alto, California, U.S.) were developed to treat leg veins. Other manufacturers of pulsed light devices include Energis Technology (Energis Elite IPL)(Swansea, JK) and Danish Dermatologic Development (Elipse)(Hoersholm, Denmark).

The Energis System is a low-output device with 5 to 19 J/cm^2 output, a spot size of 10 mm×50 m, a pulse train of 15 to 40 milliseconds, and four or five pulses per train with a delay of 1.5 milliseconds. The Lumenis device is a high-output system with up to 90 J/cm^2 output, a spot size of 8 mm×35 mm, variable pulse lengths of 2 to 40 milliseconds, and a variable of 1 to 1000 milliseconds.

Selectivity for IPL is obtained by manipulating pulse widths to match the thermal relaxation times of vessels larger than 0.2 mm and by using a filter to remove lower wavelengths of visible light. High fluences of up to 90 J/cm^2 can be delivered. Segmented pulsing of 1 to 25 millisecond duration separated and synchronized with 1 to 100 millisecond test intervals delivers wavelengths of 515 to 1000 nm. The IPL devices are most commonly used with the 550- and 570-nm filters to deliver primarily the yellow and red wavelengths with a minor component of infrared.

The main advantages of IPL technology in the treatment of leg veins has been the use of large spot sizes, causing minimal purpura. The shorter wavelengths have not been shown to be effective in the treatment of larger, deeper, and bluish-colored vessels.

IPL (515–1000 nm range) with various fluences from 5 to 90 J and varied pulse durations of 2 to 25 milliseconds have been used to treat venulectasias of 0.4 to 2.0 mm in diameter. Clinical trials utilizing the IPL with multiple pulses of variable duration have demonstrated efficacy of up to 90% clearance in vessels of smaller than 0.2 mm in diameter, 80% in vessels (0.2–0.5 mm), and 70% in vessels of 0.5 to 1 mm in diameter. Few studies have shown the 90% clearance rate in initially reported cases (38). In one study, 73.6% of patients with leg telangiectasias up to 1 mm in diameter had 73.6% clearance immediately posttreatment and 84.3% after one month. Hyperpigmentation was noted in 3% to 4% of patients. The most successful treatment parameters were a single 3 millisecond pulse at a fluence of 22 J/cm^2 for vessels of less than 0.2 mm in diameter to a double pulse of 3j at a fluence of 40 J/cm^2, 2.4/4.0 millisecond with a 10-millisecond delay. Vessels with 0.2 to 0.5 mm diameter were treated with the same double pulse parameters or with a 3.0- to 6.0-millisecond pulse at a fluence of 35 to 45 J/cm^2 with a 20-millisecond delay.

In a more recent study, the utilization of a short-pulse long-pulse protocol using 2.4 or 3 millisecond and 6 to 7 millisecond pulses separated by a 10- to 20- millisecond delay employment. The 570-nm filter has yielded the best results using the IPL device in treating leg vessels. Seventy-four percent clearance with 8% incidence of hyper- or hypopigmentation has been reported (39). By combining short and long pulses, theoretically, both superficial and larger diameter vessels should be targeted.

Newer contact epidermal cooling devices have allowed deliverances of higher fluence with less epidermal absorption.

LONG-PULSED ND:YAG LASER (1064 nm)

Millisecond domain, 1064 nm, lasers have been utilized to treat both blue venulectasias and large caliber subcutaneous reticular veins (40). The deeper penetrating wavelength and the absence of absorption by melanin allow treatment of dark skin phenotypes and larger diameter vessels allowing uniform pan-vessel heating.

The newer pulsed 1064 nm lasers have pulse durations between 1 and 200 milliseconds [Vasculight Lumenis, (Palo Alto, California, U.S.A.), Cool Touch Varian (San Jose, California, U.S.A.), Cool Glide Altus (Burlingame, California, U.S.A.), and the Scion Profile, Sciton (Palo Alto, California, U.S.A.)].

Penetrating wavelength (1064 nm) technologies are more painful, requiring adequate cooling and sometimes topical anesthesia. Larger, bluer vessels greater than 0.5 mm in diameter respond best to treatment, requiring lesser treatment sessions.

In consideration of the recently described bimodal approach to treatment of lower extremity veins, smaller spot sizes and higher fluences have been shown to be efficacious in the treatment of smaller red vessels of less than 1 mm in diameter (41–43).

Vessels up to 3 to 4 mm in diameter can be treated with the long-pulsed Nd:YAG laser. Minor effects of hydrostatic pressures may be addressed by treating these larger vessels. Pain increases with treatment of vessels of greater than 2 mm in diameter.

The Lyra uses contact cooling. Seventy-five percent improvement of veins of all colors and sizes has been reported with this technology (44).

The Sciton Image has been utilized predominantly for treatment of lower extremity telangiectasias and reticular veins up to 3 mm in diameter (45). Its high energy fluence and large spot size have increased its efficacy in treating both large diameter vessels (i.e., reticular veins) and small capillary mats less than 1 mm in diameter. A static cooling device is employed.

The Vasculight has also been utilized for treatment of both smaller vessels and larger reticular veins up to 4 mm in diameter. The operator applies a coupling cooling gel in addition to an internal DCD (1–4°C) and applies the laser tip directly to the treatment vessel under consideration. Superficial red telangiectasias less than 1 mm in diameter may be treated with the handpiece coagulated and defocused off the skin and a lower energy fluence of 90 to 100 J/cm^2 with a pulse duration of 10 to 12 milliseconds delivered as a single pulse.

Weiss et al. (35) achieved 75% improvement at three-month follow-up of 0.3 to 3.0 mm vessels documented by Duplex closure. Settings in this study including fluence of 80 to 120 J/cm^2 and single-pulse durations of 10 to 30 milliseconds were utilized.

Sadick et al. (46) treated 20 Fitzpatrick skin type II to IV patients with a similar technology. A mean of 25 treatments produced 100% clearance in 88% of patients.

Mild purpura was noted in 20% of patients, and postlaser hyperpigmentation was noted in 10% of patients.

SKIN COOLING DEVICES

The CoolGlide utilizing a contact cooling tip has been found to produce 70% vessel clearance for vessels of all colors and sizes (150–250 J/cm^2). The only complication at three months was postinflammatory hyperpigmentation.

The Varia has been utilized exclusively for the treatment of leg veins 4. This technology has recently been shown to be particularly effective in the treatment of lower extremity vessels in type V skin (47). Pulsed cooling with the "Cool Tube" cryogen spray lowers epidermal skin temperature to about 25°C and delivers a more precise specific cooling effect compared to the "continuous cooling" of topical gel and contact chill tips. Delivery of active cooling immediately postlaser can quench any heat approaching the surface through back scattering of conduction. Postcooling may improve efficacy because one does not have to reheat targets affected by precooling. A brief precooling pulse can be added for additional protection, if significant surface pigment is present.

The Role of Cooling

The cooling plays an integral role in the management of laser treatment for leg veins in an effort to maintain epidermal protection, prevent damage to adjacent vascular structures, and diminish patient discomfort (44).

Several approaches are presently utilized including water-cooled chambers applied directly to the skin through which the laser beam is directed (Chess Chamber, VersaPulse, Chill Tip, and IPL Chiller), cooling coupling gels, and refrigerated-spray cooling devices (e.g., DCD) or cryogen spray.

Such cooling accomplishes two goals: it minimizes epidermal damage and allows the laser surgeon to employ higher fluence thus creating more potential to produce pan-endothelial vascular destruction (48).

COMBINED LASER/RADIOFREQUENCY TECHNOLOGIES

Combined diode laser bipolar radiofrequency application (Fig. 3) has recently been shown to be effective in the treatment of lower extremity vessels.

This technology can generate light fluences from 50 to $100 \, J/cm^2$ and radiofrequency energies of 10 to $100 \, J/cm^3$. Further studies are in progress substantiating the efficacy. The theory behind this technology is that lower amounts of light energy may be introduced into the target chromophore, i.e., hemoglobin, which may have synergistic effects with the bipolar radiofrequency component. This has been referred to as electro-optical synergy.

Endpoint of Therapy

The endpoint of therapy utilizing all laser technologies for treatment of leg veins is immediate contraction and late erythema. Overtreatment is to be avoided as is prolonged blanching as this may eventuate in epidermal necrosis leading to pigment dyschromia or epidermal irregularities. Because of the high upregulation of cytokines after laser-endothelial interaction, it is recommended that the laser surgeon wait for 8 to 12 weeks between treatment sessions to assess results, and let the laser-induced inflammatory mediator expression subside. Photoprotection both pre- and posttreatment for at least three to four weeks is indicated.

Complications

Prolonged erythema pigmentation and epidermal surface irregularities (scarring) are the main side effects associated with laser/IPL treatment of lower extremity veins.

Overtreatment is the major etiologic factor. Immediate vessel contraction and urticaria remain the endpoints of therapy and, if proper guidelines are followed, will help to minimize these adverse sequelae. Prolonged vessel contraction and whitening are signs of overtreatment. Cooling technology should be an integral part of all laser/IPL vessel treatment protocols. Conservative settings and "spot test" sessions in dark skin phenotypical individuals as well as fastidious photoprotection are other caveats of importance in minimizing side effects.

In the author's experience with all the aforementioned systems, postlaser hyperpigmentation has been noted in 15% to 30% of treated individuals. It represents melanin versus post-sclerotherapy hemosiderin as seen following sclerotherapy. Compassion has been shown to play no role in this postlaser treatment of lower extremity vessels (45,49). In the majority of cases, pigment dyschromia usually resolves in 8 to 12 weeks, but may last up to six months. Three to four percent hydroquinone derivatives or 20% azelaic acid preparations may be employed in this setting. In refractory cases, the Q-switched ruby or alexandrite laser, or IPL source, can improve this pigmentation. Persistent erythema may be managed by twice-a-day application of potent Class I corticosteroids such as clobetasol proprionate and betamethasone diproprionate (50).

Indications for Laser Treatment

Sclerotherapy remains the gold standard for treatment of lower extremity telangiectasia and reticular veins; however, improved parameter lasers and IPL sources have certainly gained a role in the phlebologist's armamentarium. Expense as well as variable response to previous technologies remains an issue. Patients who are needle-phobic or have had poor clinical outcomes or unusual complication profiles are good candidates for the utilization of the above-described technologies for treatment of lower extremity vessels.

When small linear new-arborizing vessels, which are difficult to cannulate, are present or the blushing associated with telangiectatic matting is present, there are also primary indications for choosing a laser/IPL technology for treating such vessels. A comparative assessment of microsclerotherapy and laser/IPL treatment of lower extremity vessels in the author's experience is presented in Table 5.

CONCLUSIONS

Although sclerotherapy remains the gold standard for treatment of lower extremity telangiectasias, improved cooling technology, longer wavelength devices and variable pulsing modes have allowed more consistent results in the management of lower extremity vessels of less than 3 mm in diameter. Addressing hydrostatic forces and understanding venous anatomy, appropriate wavelength pulse diameter considerations, optimal treatment intervals, and emphasis upon strict photoprotection will lead to improved clinical outcomes and greater patient satisfaction in employing this evolving technology.

REFERENCES

1. Kauvar ANB. The role of lasers in the treatment of leg veins. Sem Cutan Med Surg 2000; 19:245–252.
2. Sadick NS. Updated laser approaches to the management of cosmetic leg veins. Phlebol 2003; 18:54–53.
3. Lupton J, Alster T, Romero P. Clinical comparison of sclerotherapy versus long-pulsed Nd:YAG laser treatment for lower extremity telangiectasias. Dermatol Surg 2002; 28:694–697.
4. Dover JS, Sadick NS, Goldman MP. The role of lasers and light sources in the treatment of leg veins. Dermatol Surg 1999; 25:328–336.
5. Goldman MP. Treatment of leg veins with lasers and intense pulsed light. Dermatol Clin 2001; 19:467–473.
6. Sadick NS, Weiss RA, Goldman MP. Advances in laser surgery for leg veins: bimodal wavelength approach to lower extremity vessels, new cooling techniques and longer pulse durations. Dermatol Surg 2002; 28:16–20.
7. Sadick NS. A dual wavelength approach for laser/intense pulsed light source treatment of lower extremity veins. J Am Acad Dermatol 2002; 46:66–72.
8. Goldman MP, Weiss RA. Treatment of leg telangiectasia with laser and high-intense pulsed light. Dermatol Ther 2000; 13:38–49.
9. Fournier N, Brisot P, Murdon S. Treatment of leg telangiectasias with a 532 nm KTP laser in multi-pulse model. Dermatol Surg 2002; 28:564–571.
10. Passeron T, Ollivier V, et al. The new 940 nanometer diode laser. An effective treatment for leg venulectasia. J Am Acad Dermatol 2003; 48:768–774..
11. Coles C, Werner R, Zelickson B. Comparative pilot study evaluating the treatment of leg veins with a long-pulse Nd:YAG laser and sclerotherapy. Lasers Surg Med 2002; 30: 154–159.
12. Sadick NS. Laser treatment with a 1064 nm laser for lower extremity class I-III veins employing variable spots and pulse width parameters. Dermatol Surg 2003; 29:916–919.
13. Apfelberg DB, Maser MR, et al. Study of three laser systems for treatment of superficial varicosities of the lower extremity. Lasers Surg Med 1987; 7:219–223..
14. Weiss RA, Dover JS. Laser surgery of leg veins. Dermatol Clin 2002; 20:19–36.
15. Sadick NS, Weiss RA. The utilization of a new yellow light laser (578 nm) for the treatment of Class I red telangiectasia of the lower extremities. Dermatol Surg 2002; 28:21–25.
16. Apfelberg DB, Maser MR, et al. Use of the argon and carbon dioxide lasers for treatment of superficial venous varicosities of the lower extremity. Lasers Surg Med 1984; 4:221–231.
17. Dixon JA, Rotering RH, Huether SE. Patient's evaluation of argon laser therapy of port-wine stain, decorative tattoos, and essential telangiectasia. Lasers Surg Med 1984; 4: 181–184.
18. Coros L, Longo L. Classification and treatment of telangiectases of the lower limbs. Laser 1988; 1:22–27.
19. Keller GS. KTP laser offers advances in minimally invasive plastic surgery. Clin Laser Mon 1991; 10:141–144.
20. West TB, Alster TS. Comparison of the long-pulse dye (590–595 nm) and KTP (532 nm) lasers in the treatment of facial and leg telangiectasias. Dermatol Surg 1998; 24:221–226.
21. Spendel S, Prandl EC, et al. Treatment of spider leg veins with the KTP (532 nm) laser. A prospective study. Lasers Surg Med 2002; 31:194–201..
22. Adrian RM. Treatment of leg telangiectasias using a long-pulse frequency-doubled neodymium:YAG laser at 532 nm. Dermatol Surg 1998; 24:19–23.
23. Goldman MP, Fitzpatrick RE. Pulsed-dye laser treatment of leg telangiectasia: with and without simultaneous sclerotherapy. J Dermatol Surg Oncol 1990; 16:338–344.

24. Garden JM, Tan OT, et al. Effect of dye laser pulse duration on selective cutaneous vascular injury. J Invest Dermatol 1986; 87:653–657.

25. Dierickx CC, Casparian JM, et al. Thermal relaxation of port-wine stain vessels probed in vivo: the need for 1–10 millisecond laser pulse treatment. J Invest Dermatol 1995; 105: 709–714.

26. Hsia J, Lowery JA, Zelickson B. Treatment of leg telangiectasia using a long-pulse dye laser at 595 nm. Lasers Surg Med 1997; 20:1–5.

27. Alora MB, Herd RH, Szabo E. Comparison of the 595 nm long pulse (1.5 ms) and the 595 nm ultra-long pulse (4 ms) laser in the treatment of leg veins. Lasers Surg Med 1998; 10(suppl):38.

28. Lee PK, Lask G. Treatment of leg veins by long-pulsed dye laser (sclerolaser). Lasers Surg Med 1997; 9(suppl):40.

29. Reichert D. Evaluation of the long-pulse dye laser for the treatment of leg telangiectasias. Dermatol Surg 1998; 24:737–740.

30. McDaniel DH, Ash K, et al. Laser therapy of spider leg veins: clinical evaluation of a new long-pulsed alexandrite laser. Dermatol Surg 1999; 25:52–58.

31. Kauvar AN, Lou WW. Pulsed alexandrite laser for the treatment of leg telangiectasia and reticular veins. Arch Dermatol 2000; 136:1371–1375.

32. Passeron T, Oliver V, Duteil L, Desruelles F, Fontas E, Ortonne J. The new 940-nanometer diode laser: An effective treatment for leg venulectasia. J Am Acad Dermatol 2003; 48(5):768–774.

33. Kaudewitz P, Klovekorn W, Rother W. Treatment of leg vein telangiectases:1-year results with a new 970 nm diode laser. Dermatol Surg 2002; 28:1031–1034.

34. Goldman M. Laser treatment of leg veins with 1064 nm long-pulsed lasers. Cosm Dermatol 2000:27–30.

35. Eremia S, Li C, Umar S. A Side-by-side comparative study of 1064 nm Nd:YAG, 810 nm diode and 755 nm alexandrite lasers for treatment of 0.3–3 nm leg veins. Dermatol Surg 2002; 28:224–230.

36. Garden JM, Bakus AD, Miller ID. Diode laser treatment of leg veins. Lasers Surg Med 1998; 10(suppl):38.

37. Kaudewitz P, Klorekorn W, Rother W. Treatment of leg vein telangiectasias. One years results with a new 940 nm diode laser. Dermatol 2002; 28:1031–1034.

38. Goldman MP, Eckhouse S. Photothermal sclerosis of leg veins. ESC Medical Systems, LTD Photoderm VL Cooperative Study Group. Dermatol Surg 1996; 22:323–330.

39. Weiss RA, Weiss MA, et al. Non-coherent filtered flashlamp intense pulsed light source for leg telangiectasias: long pulse durations for improved results. Lasers Surg Med 1998; 10(suppl):40.

40. Groot D, Rao J, Johnston P, Nakatsuc I. Algorithm for using a long-pulsed Nd:YAG laser in the treatment of deep cutaneous vascular lesions. Dermatol Surg 2003; 29:35–42.

41. Omura N, Dover J, Arndt K, Kauvar A. Treatment of reticular leg veins with a 1064 nm Nd:YAG laser. J Am Acad Dermatol 2003; 48:76–81.

42. Major A, Brazzini B, et al. Nd:YAG 1064 nm laser in the treatment of facial and leg telangiectasias. Eur Acad Dermatol Venereol 2001; 15:595–565..

43. Lic Y, Eremia S. Treatment of leg and face veins with a cryogen spray, variable pulse with 1064 nm Nd:YAG laser—a prospective study of 47 patients. Am J Cosmet Surg 2002; 19:3–8.

44. Bencini PL, Lucci A, Galimberti M, Ferranti G. Long-term epilation with long-pulsed Neodymium:YAG laser. Dermatol Surg 1999; 25:175–178.

45. Eremias LICV. Treatment of leg and face veins with a cryogen spray variable pulse width 1064 nm Nd:YAG laser—a prospective study of 47 patients. J Cosmetic Laser Ther 2001; 3:147–153.

46. Sadick NS. Long-term results with a multiple synchronized pulse 1064 nm Nd:YAG laser for the treatment of leg venulectasias and reticular veins. Dermatol Surg 2001; 27:365–369.

47. Reguchefsky A, Silapunt S, Goldberg DJ. Nd:YAG laser 1064 nm irradiation for lower extremity telangiectasias and small reticular veins: efficacy as measured by vessel colors and size. Dermatol Surg 2002; 28:220–223.

48. Waldorf HA, Alster TS, et al. Effect of dynamic cooling on 585-nm pulsed dye laser treatment of port-wine stain birthmarks. Dermatol Surg 1997; 23:657–662.

49. Eremias LIC, Umars H. A side-by-side comparative study of 1064 nm Nd:YAG, 310 nm diode and 755 nm alexandrite lasers for treatment of 0.3–3.0 mm leg veins. Dermatol Surg 2002; 28:224–230.

50. Goldman MP, Sadick NS, Weiss RA. Cutaneous necrosis, telangiectatic matting and hypersensitivity following sclerotherapy. (CME article) Dermatol Surg 1993; 21:19–29.

10

Laser Resurfacing with the UPCO$_2$ + Er:YAG Lasers

Mitchel P. Goldman

Department of Dermatology/Medicine, University of California, San Diego, California, U.S.A. and La Jolla Spa MD, La Jolla, California, U.S.A.

INTRODUCTION

Cutaneous rejuvenation through the use of laser vaporization of the skin has been demonstrated to be safe and effective since its introduction in 1994, with the ultrapulse CO$_2$ laser (1). It is estimated that over one million patients have been treated with laser resurfacing (LR) with over 100 medical articles on this procedure having been published. Despite its demonstrated effectiveness in treating extensive cutaneous changes due to solar damage, including lentigines, precancerous lesions, and wrinkles, adverse effects can occur (2). Prolonged erythema, dyspigmentation, delayed healing, and potential complications of infection and scaring have been reported (3,4). These adverse effects have been sensationalized in the media leading to an increase in the public's apprehension about this useful procedure. Many patients present with first-hand knowledge of friends, who have undergone the procedure only to be left with three to six months of erythema and permanent hypopigmentation (especially along the mandibular angle). Many of these erythematous and hypopigmented patients have been treated by physicians, who rent a LR machine and do not use optimal postoperative care or techniques to decrease nonspecific thermal damage. Fortunately, newer wound healing techniques, which limit nonspecific thermal damage by sequential use of erbium: YAG (Er:YAG) LR after carbon dioxide LR, as well as optimized postoperative dressings have dramatically reduced these adverse effects (5,6). Unfortunately, a less-than-optimal result provides far more publicity than an optimal result.

Another drawback of LR, even with the most advanced techniques, has been that it alone does not correct vascular ectasia, secondary to photodamage. This inability of LR to treat telangiectasia has been solved by performing vascular-specific laser ablation simultaneously with LR (7). Obviously, this requires the laser surgeon to have multiple lasers in

219

the operating room—a luxury very few laser centers have. However, even though modern techniques, utilizing a variety of lasers and optimal postoperative wound care, have addressed many of the adverse sequelae of LR "down-time" still and will always exist. This has led to the popularization of minimally invasive nonablative rejuvenation techniques.

Minimally invasive "rejuvenative" techniques including the intense pulsed light (IPL) that originally developed to treat telangiectasia, are effective in treating dyspigmentation, dark hair, and perhaps, shallow wrinkles and enlarged pores (8); other lasers that have been specifically developed to produce selective dermal scarring with minimization of wrinkles include the CoolTouch^{TM} (CoolTouch Corporation, Roseville, California, U.S.) (9) and SmoothBeam^{TM} (Candela Laser Corporation, Wayland, Massachusetts, U.S.); pulse dye lasers that were developed to treat vascular lesions and the Q-switched 532 and 1064 nm Nd:YAG lasers developed to treat tattoo and deep pigmented lesions have also been demonstrated to stimulate dermal collagen remodeling (10,11). There is presently a debate as to which system is best or whether a combination of nonablative lasers used during the same treatment session (such as the CoolTouch^{TM} followed by the IPL) is necessary.

Although these minimally invasive lasers rejuvenate the skin to some extent, none do so as predictably and effectively as true LR. So, where is this procedure today? As the "hype" of LR has calmed down with a decreasing public demand and fewer companies renting lasers to physicians, a rational use of this technique is present. LR is now being used mainly by physicians, who are expert in this technique and who perform hundreds of procedures each year. Importantly, these physicians also have staff dedicated to provide optimal pre- and postoperative care, which is nearly as important as performing LR itself. Thus, far fewer complications occur, and patient "downtime" is minimized.

I believe that LR with either the CO_2 and/or Er:YAG lasers is the optimal technique for treating severe photodamage, premalignant lesions, and wrinkles. Tissue tightening and debulking with these lasers cannot be accomplished to a similar degree as with minimally invasive techniques. LR will produce a 60% to 70% improvement in wrinkles in one procedure as compared to at most 30% to 40% improvement requiring multiple (3–6) nonablative procedures. Improvement is immediate and continues for 6 to 12 months. LR will also remove seborrheic keratoses, nevi, benign adnexal growths, and sebaceous hyperplasia that cannot be removed with nonablative procedures. So, for the patient who wants to achieve maximal rejuvenation/improvement and has a week to stay at home and another week before going to a "black-tie" affair, LR is the optimal procedure. Minimally invasive, nonablative techniques are most appropriate for patients, who have minimal photoaging and do not have the luxury of any "down-time." Both techniques are useful. This chapter will describe ablative LR with the CO_2 and Er:YAG lasers. Techniques to minimize adverse sequelae and to maximize therapeutic outcome will be presented.

The most common and also the most easily avoidable adverse sequelae from LR are prolonged erythema and delayed wound healing. Avoidance of these two adverse effects requires intensive patient education as well as close postoperative surveillance and early intervention when signs first appear. We have previously demonstrated that when prolonged erythema and delayed healing is not secondary to bacterial, viral, or candidal infection, or to an irritant reaction for a topical ointment or cream, these adverse effects are secondary to nonspecific thermal damage present after LR (5,12).

Histologic evaluation immediately after LR with various microsecond pulsed CO$_2$ laser systems (10,600 nm wavelength) shows 80–140 µm of nonspecific damage (13–15). Er:YAG laser vaporization at the usual 350-µsec pulse (2940-nm wavelength) leaves far less thermal damage (5–10 µm) as well as thinner ablation (20 µm), because the 2940-nm wavelength has an affinity for water 10 times stronger than the 10,600-nm wavelength of the CO$_2$lasers (16,17). This shorter depth of ablation makes the Er:YAG more time-consuming and less efficacious than the UPCO$_2$ laser in treating significant photodamage (wrinkling). However, we have found that its sequential use after CO$_2$ LR will decrease the extent of nonspecific damage and will result in decreased postoperative erythema and improved wound healing.

We therefore recommend combining these two lasers as well as minimizing the risks inherent in their combination. A step-by-step method will be presented of our technique. Or, novel laser systems combining the CO$_2$ laser modality with the Er:YAG in a near simultaneous exposure Derma-K^{TM} (Lumenis, Santa Clara, California, U.S.) and two systems combining normal Er:YAG laser parameters with a second near simultaneous nonablative long-pulsed Er:YAG pulse Contour^{TM} (Sciton, Palo Alto, California, U.S.) and CO$_3$ (Cynosure, Chelmsford, Massachusetts, U.S.) are also recommended, as they encompass both the thermal effects of the standard CO$_2$ lasers and the ablative aspect of the Er:YAG laser.

Theoretical Considerations

Before re-epithelialization of a wound, inflammatory cells and macrophages that occur over the wound were recovered to eliminate potential contaminants (bacteria/yeast) as well as nonviable tissue. In this process, inflammatory mediators stimulate angiogenesis, attract additional inflammatory cells, and stimulate production and release of various growth factors. The total effect stimulates wound healing through epidermal migration and proliferation as well as dermal remodeling (18–20). Wound healing occurs through a balance of inflammatory mediators and cells. If excessive inflammation occurs then persistent and /or excessive angiogenesis results, leading to prolonged clinical erythema and delayed wound healing. As the extent of inflammation is proportional to the extent of nonviable tissue in the wound (21), it is reasonable to expect a disruption of optimal wound healing when nonviable tissue is present in the wound.

Immediately after CO_2 LR in patients treated in our series with three passes of the UPCO$_2$ laser at 300 mJ with a computer pattern generated (CPG) density setting of 6, followed by 5 and 4, the average extent of nonspecific thermally damaged dermal tissue for UPCO$_2$ laser–treated skin was 80 μm ($\pm$20 μm) (Fig. 1). The average extent of thermal damage of dermal tissue in patients treated with two passes of the UPCO$_2$ laser at 300 mJ with a CPG density of 6, followed by 5, and with two passes of the Er:YAG laser at approximately 15 J/cm^2, was 20 μm($\pm$10 μm) (Fig. 2). Thus, the erbium laser removed about 75% of this nonviable tissue.

At 48 to 72 hours, a mixed inflammatory infiltrate with polymorphonucleoctyes and eosinophils was present with nuclear debris. Less inflammation was present in the UPCO$_2$/Er:YAG laser–treated patients. Angiogenesis, with a similar density of superficial blood vessels, was present in both treatment groups at this time.

The epidermis reformed one to two days faster with combination of UPCO$_2$/Er:YAG treatment than with UPCO$_2$ treatment alone. At one week, all specimens of both groups showed complete re-epithelialization with a mild mixed inflammatory infiltrate, which was greater in the UPCO$_2$ laser–treated areas than the UPCO$_2$/Er:YAG laser–treated areas. The density of blood vessels in the superficial papillary dermis was also increased in the UPCO$_2$ laser group.

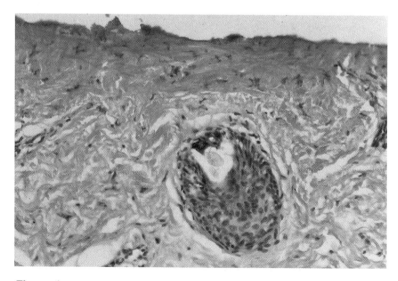

Figure 1
Immediately after laser resurfacing with three passes of the UPCO$_2$ laser as previously described. The epidermis is completely vaporized. A zone of nonspecific thermal damage extends approximately 80 μm beneath the vaporized layer (hematoxylin–eosin 200×). *Source*: From Ref. 5.

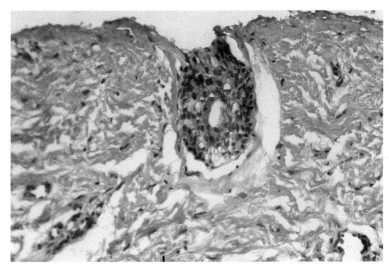

Figure 2
Immediately after laser resurfacing with two passes of the UPCO$_2$ laser and two passes of the Er:YAG laser as previously described. The epidermis is completely vaporized. A zone of nonspecific thermal damage extends approximately 10 μm beneath the vaporized layer (hematoxylin–eosin 200×). *Abbreviation*: Er:YAG, erbium:YAG. *Source*: From Ref. 5.

Method for Resurfacing with UPCO$_2$/Er:YAG Lasers

To maximize patient comfort and efficiency of treatment, we have our patients placed under general anesthesia. Appropriate internal eye shields are placed, and the patient's face draped with wet towels. The skin is first resurfaced with the UPCO$_2$ with two passes with the CPG at 300 mJ at settings of 596 and 595 nm. (Where 5 is the rectangular pattern, 9 the size of the pattern with 5 being the smallest and 9 being the largest, and the last number (6 and 5) representing the density overlap of the individual spots as explained below.) The first pass at a density of 6 (30–35% overlap) results in complete removal of the epidermis with minimal vaporization of the superficial papillary dermis. Some collagen contraction occurs in thin-skinned areas like the periorbital region. The charred epidermal debris is then wiped off with saline-soaked cotton gauze. A moderate amount of pressure is necessary to remove the proteinaceous debris completely (Fig. 3). The second pass at a density of 5 (25–30% overlap) produces collagen contraction (Fig. 4). The treated area is again wiped off any additional debris with saline-soaked gauze, but little debris is present except in areas skipped by the first laser pass.

If more significant photodamage is present in some areas, such as the glabellar, perioral areas, and cheeks, an additional CO$_2$ pass may be performed selectively in these areas at a density of 4 or 5 to achieve deeper ablation as well as further collagen tightening. The 3-mm diameter spot may also be used cautiously to achieve further tightening in small

(A)   **(B)**

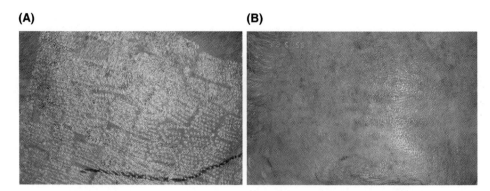

Figure 3
A moderate amount of pressure is necessary to remove the proteinaceous debris completely after one pass with the UPCO$_2$ laser 300 mJ with the CPG at a setting of 596. (**A**) Immediately after the first pass of the laser; (**B**) immediately after wiping off epidermal debris.

areas as well as to better define the vermilion border at a fluence of 300 to 500 mJ.

The Er:YAG laser is then used at maximal power settings with a focused 4-mm diameter spot size (15–20 J/cm^2). We have found that two passes at these settings are necessary to vaporize the nonspecific thermal damage left by the UPCO$_2$ laser (Fig. 5). We do not wipe the treated areas between passes because proteinaceous debris is not apparent.

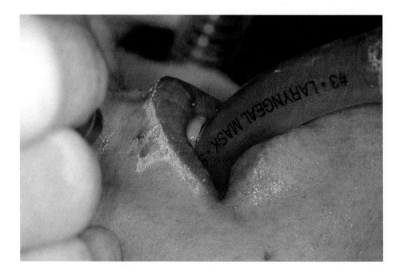

Figure 4
The second pass with the UPCO$_2$ laser 300 mJ at a density of 5 produces collagen contraction. A line of 3-mm impacts is placed along the vermillion border to enhance the lipline and along the shoulders of persistent wrinkle lines of the upper lip. These impacts are generally overlapped 50% in this application.
Source: From Ref. 3.

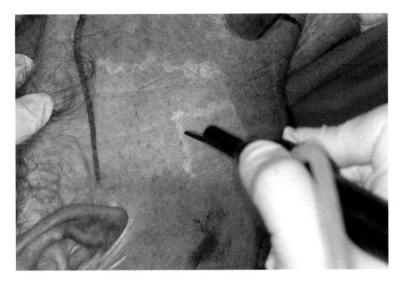

Figure 5
After two passes with the UPCO₂ laser, the Er:YAG laser is then used at maximal power settings with a 4 mm diameter spot size and 1.7 J (approximately
16 J/cm²). *Abbreviation*: Er:YAG, erbium:YAG.

In addition, we have found that it is easier to treat the area in surface
units of 2 to 4 cm × 2 to 4 cm (Fig. 6). This dermabrasion-like method
maintains focus on the treated area so that the entire surface area can
be evenly resurfaced (21).

The focused handpiece when moved away from the skin will give a
larger spot size that will decrease the energy fluence. (The same energy is
distributed onto a larger area of the skin.) When the handpiece is moved
closer to the skin, a smaller spot size is produced that increased the relative energy density on the skin. Therefore, controlling the diameter of the
laser spot size on the skin allows for both feathering at the borders of the
treated area and sculpting of individual lesions.

Next, additional passes with the Er:YAG laser permits the surgeon
to sculpt acne scars (Fig. 7) as well as to sculpt a cupids bow on the upper
lip (Fig. 8) and, more completely, plane wrinkles. These can be done with
a 0.2-mm diameter focusing handpiece that allows the surgeon to vary the
fluence from 5 to 50 J/cm², as necessary.

As we have previously reported (23), patients treated with the combination UPCO₂/Er:YAG laser had erythema resolved within two to three
weeks as compared to eight weeks when treated with the UPCO₂ laser alone.

Clinically, there was no difference in the extent or time of edema
between the two techniques. There was also no difference in the improvement rating between the two treatment groups at the eight-week
follow-up time of the first study. We have evaluated our initial 20 patients
for over a year and have found that over 75% of the combination patients
had improvement as good or better as noncombination UPCO₂ laser
patients (Fig. 9).

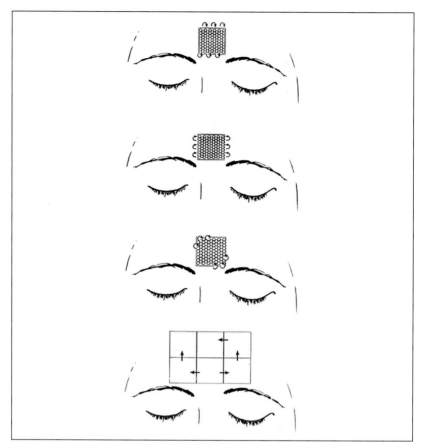

Figure 6
The Er:YAG laser is easily used to uniformly vaporize a given area through
the use of a dermabrasion-like technique treating the area in surface units
of 2 to 4 cm × 2 to 4 cm. *Source*: From Ref. 22.

Another advantage of combination laser treatment is that the usual
demarcation line between cheek and neck at the mandibular angle was
less apparent. This may be because of the ability to extend LR onto
the upper neck with the Er:YAG laser and to blend the resurfaced skin
more gradually onto nonresurfaced areas.

Combined Er:YAG + CO₂

One laser manufacturer has combined the CO_2 laser with the Er:YAG
laser in a near-simultaneous beam. The Er:YAG portion is identical to
all other Er:YAG lasers in its fluence and pulse-duration, which can be
varied based on both the energy output and the beam diameter. The
CO_2 portion comprises a standard, low power continuous CO_2 laser that
does *not* operate within the microsecond-domain pulse mode. Thus, the
CO_2 laser is not utilized to vaporize tissue, but to heat tissue beneath
the Er:YAG vaporized tissue (Fig. 10).

(A)   **(B)**

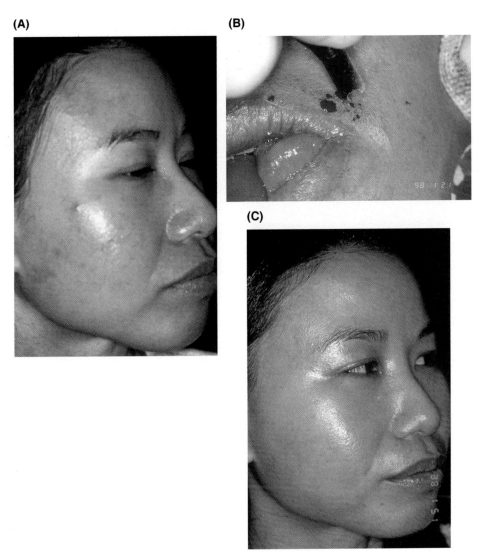

(C)

Figure 7
Additional passes with the Er:YAG laser allow the surgeon to sculpt acne
scars. (**A**) Before treatment, (**B**) sculpting acne scars after first removing
the epidermis as described in the text, and (**C**) clinical appearance 11 months
after treatment with resolution of acne scarring. *Source*: From Ref. 3.

We have found excellent safety and efficacy when using the Derma-
K™ at the following parameters: Er:YAG 1.7 J with a 4-mm diameter
spot (approximately 16 J/cm^2) and the CO$_2$ at 5 W with a 50-msec pulse
at a rate of 10 Hz. At this setting, we have found efficient vaporization of
skin to a similar depth as when the Er:YAG is used alone, but with better
hemostasis. Four passes at this setting do not produce excessive bleeding,
which usually would occur while performing four passes with the
Er:YAG alone at these fluences (Fig. 11).

(A)   **(B)**

(C)   **(D)**

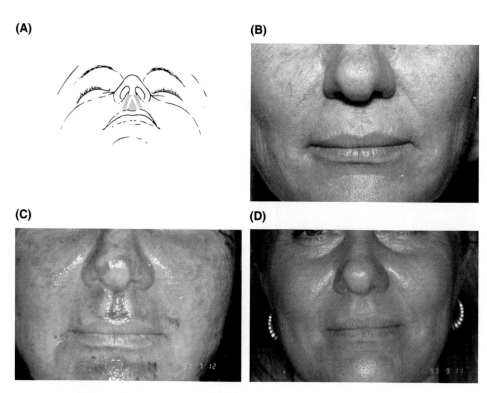

Figure 8
A cupids bow can be sculpted on the upper lip with the Er:YAG laser. (**A**) Diagram of technique, (**B**) appearance before sculpting, (**C**) immediately after sculpting as described in text, and (**D**) appearance two months after cupids bow sculpting. *Abbreviation*: Er:YAG, erbium:YAG. *Source*: From Ref. 3.

We evaluated 10 patients treated with four passes at these parameters (22). We measured photoaging scores as well as thermal damage and new collagen formation immediately before and after treatment as well as at two weeks and three months postoperatively. The average pretreatment periorbital score was 6.2. The average posttreatment periorbital scores were 4.2 ($p = 0.0239$) at two weeks postoperatively (32% improvement) and 3.8 ($p = 0.0028$) at three months postoperatively (38% improvement). The average pretreatment perioral score was 5.9. The average post-treatment perioral scores were 3.0 ($p = 0.0001$) at two weeks postoperatively (49% improvement) and 3.3 ($p = 0.0009$) at three months postoperatively (44% improvement). The average pretreatment cheek score was 4.7. The average posttreatment cheek scores were 2.7 ($p = 0.0066$) at two weeks postoperatively (43% improvement) and 3.8 ($p = 0.0152$) at three months postoperatively (36% improvement). The average pretreatment forehead score was 4.7. The average posttreatment forehead scores were 3.8 ($p = 0.0340$) at two weeks postoperatively (33% improvement) and 3.6 ($p = 0.0147$) at three months postoperatively (37% improvement). The average depth of collagen measured in the dermis pretreatment was 29 μm. The average depth of collagen at three months posttreatment was 54 μm. This is an average increase of 25 μm or an 86% increase in collagen ($p = 0.006$). The average thermal damage immediately posttreatment was 20 μm. This limited study demonstrated that the Derma-K^{TM} at these settings was comparable at four passes to the UPCO$_2$ laser used at three passes (1) or to the UPCO$_2$ at two passes followed by two passes with the Er:YAG (23,25).

(A)   (B)

(C)   (D)

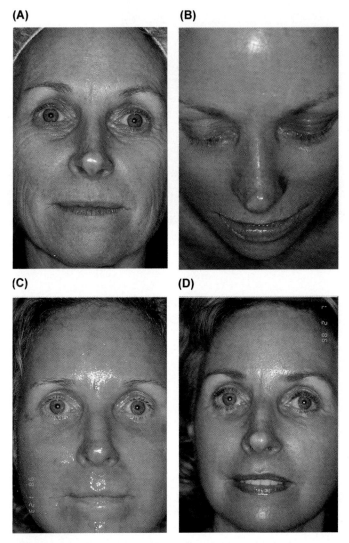

Figure 9
Combination UPCO$_2$/Er:YAG (*right side*) showed equal improvement as the left side treated with the UPCO$_2$ laser alone. (**A**) Before treatment, (**B**) immediately after treatment as described in the text, (**C**) seven days after laser resurfacing, (**D**) three weeks after resurfacing, (**E**) two months after resurfacing. *Source*: From Ref. 3. (*Continued next page*)

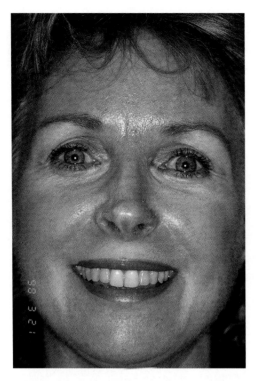

Figure 9 (*Continued*)

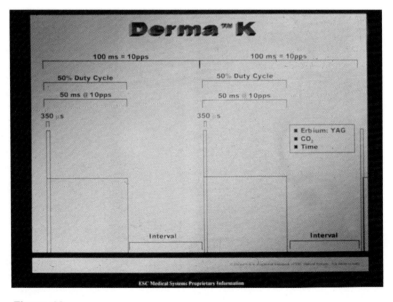

Figure 10
Schematic representation of the energy profile for the Derma-K™ laser.
Source: Courtesy of ESC Energy Systems, Inc.

(A) **(B)**

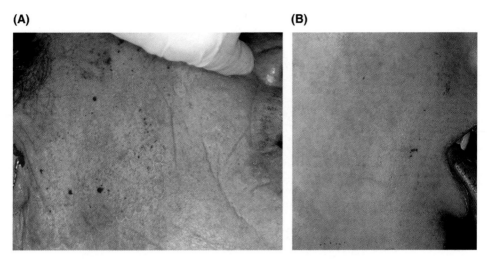

Figure 11
(**A**) Immediately after four passes with the Er:YAG laser alone at 1.7 J with a 4 mm diameter spot and 10% to 20% overlap. Note bleeding from superficial papillary vessels. (**B**) Immediately after four passes with the Derma-K™ at identical Er:YAG settings but with the addition of the CO₂ laser at 5 W and 50 msec pulse duration. There is much less if any bleeding. *Abbreviation*: Er:YAG, erbium:YAG. *Source*: From Ref. 3.

At the above-mentioned settings, there appears to be a decreased depth of nonspecific thermal damage than when the UPCO₂ laser is used alone (14.8 μm with the Derma-K™ vs. 27–59 μm with the UPCO₂ laser or in sequence with the Er:YAG laser 23–37 μm) (Fig. 12). In addition, the duration of erythema is also longer than when the Er:YAG laser is used alone to vaporize to a similar depth, but shorter than when the UPCO₂ laser at similar depths of vaporization. It also appears that the efficacy is also at a level between the Er:YAG and UPCO₂ lasers. Thus, the Derma-K™ appears to be a unique laser with properties of both previous systems (advantages and disadvantages).

CO₃ LR

The CO₃ laser (Cynosure, Chelmsford, Massachusetts, U.S.) contains a single Er:YAG laser head that has been optimized to provide extended pulse durations from 0.5 up to 10 msec. Long-pulse treatment combines both ablation as well as thermal effects. This laser has an average power of 15 W with an energy of each pulse of 2 J. The repetition rate can be adjusted from 2 to 10 Hz. Three handpieces of 3, 5, and 7 mm in diameter are available. It can also be operated with a scanner. The scanner provides a variable overlap with a 5-mm spot size and a 1 in. × 1 in. scanning area. The scanner also has the usual number of scanning shapes.

Thermal effects are reported to be 30 to 40 μm with 10-msec pulses less than 10 μm with the short pulse at 5 J/cm². This allows the CO₃ laser

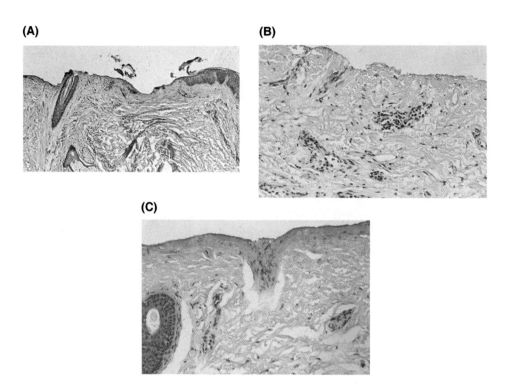

Figure 12
Histologic examination immediately after (**A**) eight passes with the Er:YAG laser alone at 1.7 J with a 4 mm diameter spot and 10 to 20% overlap. (**B**) Immediately after three passes with the Derma-K™ at identical Er:YAG settings but with the addition of the CO_2 laser at 10 W and 50 msec pulse duration. (**C**) Immediately after four passes with the Derma-K™ at identical Er:YAG settings but with the addition of the CO_2 laser at 5 W and 50 msec pulse duration (hematoxylin–eosin 200×). Note minimal amount of non-specific thermal damage at these laser fluences. *Abbreviation*: Er:YAG, erbium:YAG. *Source*: From Ref. 3.

to be used by combining short- and long-pulse passes to ablate and provide thermal effects relatively independently.

Adrian and Colleagues reported a side-by-side comparison with the $UPCO_2$ laser on periorbital and perioral areas. They compared the $UPCO_2$ laser set at a density of 5×3 passes with 10, 10-msec pulses of the Er:YAG at $5 \, J/cm^2$ with a 5-mm diameter spot size on the other side. Postoperative discomfort, erythema, and time for re-epithelialization were similar. Patients treated with the $UPCO_2$ laser had a better response on deeper wrinkles (13).

Sciton Contour™ LR

This Er:YAG laser combines two separate laser heads to combine independent thermal and ablative effects by having one laser head operate in a short pulse (0.5 msec) with the other head operating in a long pulse mode (1–10 msec). In this manner, the Sciton Contour^{TM} laser ablates tissue with a sequential thermal seal.

This laser provides 45 W of power with a 50-Hz repetition rate. At 50% overlap of 3-mm diameter spots, fluences of up to $100 \, J/cm^2$ can be generated. The ablative mode has a short 200 μsec suprathreshold pulse. A coagulative pulse immediately follows the ablative pulse.

The Sciton Contour^{TM} pattern generator gives a 4-mm spot diameter with a scanning field variable to 3.5 cm × 3.5 cm. Spots can be overlapped from 10% to 50%. The pattern has an autorepeat mode of 0.5 to 2.5 seconds delivering 1 to 50 pulses/sec in the single pulse mode. All of the standard patterns are available.

Typical settings that we have found useful are two passes with a 30% overlap at $16 \, J/cm^2$ plus coagulative settings of 100 μm coagulation (machine presets that lengthen the pulse width and adjust fluence to achieve measured coagulation depth). The third pass is given as an ablative pass only at $6 \, J/cm^2$. In a side-by-side comparative study of 18 patients with one side treated with these settings and the other side treated as described above with the CO_2 laser with 2 passes at 10 msec and 2 passes at 0.5 msec we found no apparent clinical difference between the two sides of the face (Fig. 13). Patients had a slightly quicker healing rate, decreased degree

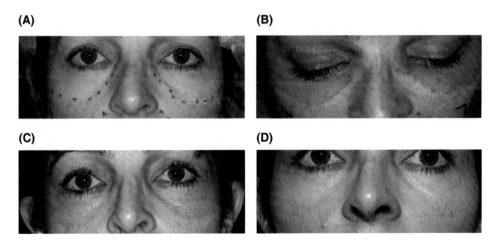

(A) **(B)**

(C) **(D)**

Figure 13
Side-by-side comparison of ling pulsed Er:YAG laser treatment: Sciton versus CO_3. (**A**) Before treatment and (**B**) immediately after treatment. The right side was treated with two passes of the Sciton laser given with a 50 μm coagulation depth, at $15 \, J/cm^2$ followed by two passes with zero coagulation at $15 \, J/cm^2$. The left side was treated with two passes of the CO_3 at 10 msec pulse with $15 \, J/cm^2$ followed by two passes at 0.5 msec at $5 \, J/cm^2$. Both lasers were used with a 4 mm diameter spot size. Note equal clinical appearance between the two sides (**C**) seven weeks after treatment. Note slight erythema with equal clinical appearance in the two sides. (**D**) Six months after treatment. Note equivalent results between the two sides.

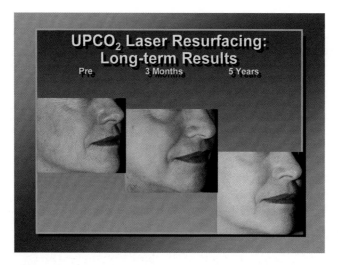

Figure 14
Long-term follow-up of laser resurfacing. (*Left*) Immediately before full face laser resurfacing. (*Middle*) Three months after laser resurfacing with three passes of the UPCO$_2$ laser at 300 mJ, density pattern of 6 followed by 5, followed by 4. (*Right*) Five years after resurfacing. Note continued improvement without recurrence of rhytids.

of erythema, and other postoperative adverse sequelae at one and two weeks postoperatively with the Sciton laser (46). This was associated with slightly less nonspecific thermal effects. However, the same degree of new collagen formation as well as clinical improvement was seen with the Sciton followed by Er:YAG laser (23). Thus, we believe that the Sciton Contour^{TM} laser functions as two separate lasers. These observations are similar to those reported by Chris Zachary and Roy Grekin, who perform resurfacing with the Contour^{TM} at varying parameters ranging from 25 to 100 μm of coagulation and 10 to 16 J/cm^2 with 20% to 50% overlap (LaserNews.net, 1999). Thus, the ideal parameters are not yet apparent. What is apparent is the safety and efficacy of this laser.

Recommendations

The goal of LR is to replace the photodamaged epidermis with nonphotodamaged cells and the elastotic dermis with healthy collagen and elastin fibers. This combined technique has also been demonstrated to result in both a contraction of existing collagen fibers as well as formation of new dermal collagen. Unfortunately, many patients develop prolonged erythema, pigmentary changes, and delayed healing with aggressive CO$_2$ LR. We have shown that the beneficial effects of LR can be maintained with a reduction of adverse sequelae through minimizing the extent of nonspecific thermal damage by using a combination of UPCO$_2$ laser followed by Er:YAG laser. Using the Sciton Contour^{TM} or Cynosure CO$_3$ lasers, first with thermal necrosis settings approximating that of pulsed CO_2 LR and then following passes with pure ablative Er:YAG settings, approximates the clinical results seen with sequential CO_2/Er: YAG resurfacing.

There appears to be a slightly superior efficacy in combining the UPCO₂ laser with the Derma-K^{TM} laser. However, patients must be prepared to live with a few more weeks of erythema. We therefore reserve the combination CO_2/Derma-K^{TM} laser for severely photodamaged and wrinkled patients and/or those with severe acne scars and/or for neck resurfacing. All other patients were treated with the combination UPCO₂/Er:YAG laser, except those with minimal photodamage who can be treated with the Er:YAG laser alone, single pass UPCO₂ laser alone, or single to double pass Derma-K^{TM} laser alone.

Other techniques using the Er:YAG laser alone or an ultrashort CO_2 laser (Tru-Pulse) (24), or the Derma-K^{TM} laser (25–27), which produce a decrease in nonspecific thermal damage, have been found to result in a decreased extent and duration of erythema and pigmentary changes with quicker re-epithelialization. Unfortunately, these lasers are more time-consuming and tedious to perform than standard CO_2 LR with the UPCO₂ or other short-pulsed CO_2 laser systems. Therefore, the combination technique for resurfacing appears superior. This technique takes advantage of the predictable thermal effects of the UPCO₂ laser resulting in heating dermal collagen to 60 to 65°C causing its contraction, and adds to it the highly specific effect of the Er:YAG laser to reduce the resulting nonspecific thermal damage yielding the best and most predictable results in our practice. Combination long-pulsed Er:YAG systems may also work as well as the UPCO₂ laser followed by the Er:YAG laser without the need to purchase or rent two laser systems.

Long-Term Efficacy (Fig. 14)

The duration of improvement that can be expected following LR: We have followed a significant number of our patients since first performing this procedure in 1993. Our impression is that although patients continue to age, the wrinkles that have been softened or eliminated at the three month follow-up look the same at 5 to 10 years. We have performed a detailed study of 104 patients, followed for 12 to 44 months (average 24 month) that confirm our impression (4). We found a 31% improvement in perioral wrinkles at three months that persisted at a rate of 85% and an average of two years. An average 38% improvement in perioral wrinkles at three months showed 96% persistence at an average of two years. More importantly, histologic evaluation of our patients showed an increase in both the epidermal thickness of 20 μm at both 3 and 24 months and the Grenz zone from 25 to 75 μm at 3 months and 170 μm at 5 years associated with a decrease in solar elastosis from 850 μm before treatment to 300 μm at three months, 750 μm at one year and 650 μm at two years. This argues for not only persistent improvement clinically but also continuing improvement histologically. Naturally, after undergoing full face LR, patients are motivated to avoid excessive sun exposure and to continue with a topical rejuvenation program consisting of retinoids, alpha and beta hydroxyacids, and others. The histologic improvement is probably secondary to a combination of continued topical treatments with sun-avoidance and perhaps stimulation from LR.

LR in Patients with Dark Skin

In fair-skinned patients, the most common indication for skin resurfacing is to treat chronic sun-damage, wrinkles, traumatic scars, surgical scars, and acne scars. In nonwhite-skinned patients, acne scarring is the most common indication for this procedure. Unfortunately, the risk of prolonged or permanent dyspigmentation, especially postinflammatory hyperpigmentation parallels the degree of the patient's constitutive skin color or pigment; the darker the skin color, the greater the potential for pigmentary dysfunction (28,29). Postinflammatory hyperpigmentation, the most common complication seen following cutaneous CO_2 LR in nonwhite patients, usually develops around the first month after treatment in 25% of Hispanic patients (skin phototypes II–V) (30). This was compared to a 3% to 7% incidence of hyperpigmentation after CO_2 LR in skin phototypes I to IV where hyperpigmentation occurred only in patients with skin phototypes III and IV (28,29).

Studies on CO_2 (30–35) and Er:YAG (34,36–39)LR in nonwhite skin (skin phototypes III–V) have shown that these procedures can be performed effectively and safely. Pre- and postoperative treatment regimens have been recommended to reduce the incidence of postinflammatory hyperpigmentation (28,30,31,40,41). In addition to topical retinoic acid applied each night, patients with skin phototypes III to VI are given topical preparations of hydroquinone, kojic acid, azelaic acid, or vitamin C to be used for one to two months preoperatively. Although an arbitrary minimum preoperative treatment time of two weeks is often recommended, achieving maximum benefit may require months of use.

Although we believe in its efficacy, the advantage of the preoperative treatment remains debatable. A study by West and Alster noted no significant difference in the incidence of post-CO_2 LR hyperpigmentation between subjects who received pretreatment with either topical glycolic acid cream or combination tretinoin/hydroquinone cream and those who received no pretreatment regimen (42). In our experience, postinflammatory hyperpigmentation may occur in spite of careful preoperative treatment. From a retrospective review of 22 of our Fitzpatrick Type IV patients, who underwent full face LR, a 68% incidence of PIH beginning one month postoperative and lasting 3.8 months was found (43). Preoperative treatments did not prevent or minimize PIH. PIH did respond to appropriate treatments once it has developed.

The application of broad-spectrum sunscreen and sun-avoidance pre- and postoperatively would seem necessary to minimize hyperpigmentation. The advantage of sun-avoidance has been demonstrated in a study showing that pre- and postoperative ultraviolet exposure on laser-treated skin resulted in a poor cosmetic appearance including textural change and hyperpigmentation (44).

Although postoperative hyperpigmentation and prolonged erythema seem to occur at roughly the same rate among patients with darker skin after Er:YAG LR, it is often less severe and resolves more quickly compared with that which results after CO_2 laser treatment (37). The Er:YAG laser or other techniques that limit nonspecific thermal damage appear to be better suited for resurfacing of nonwhite skin. The favorable result of UPCO₂ followed by Er:YAG (as described previously) has also been confirmed by a study on treatment of atrophic scars in Korean patients with skin phototypes IV to V (45).

In conclusion, LR is effective in treating photodamaged skin and acne scars in patients with skin phototypes III to V. Methods to limit nonspecific thermal damage appear to be important in this population of patients. The effect of pre- and postoperative treatment regimens, and sun-avoidance to limit the incidence and severity of PIH, although logical, is not clear at this writing. A test patch may be used when considering skin resurfacing for this group of patients. However, this is not always a reliable predictor of postoperative complications.

REFERENCES

1. Fitzpatrick RE, Goldman MP, Satur NM, Tope WD. Ultrapulse CO_2 laser resurfacing of photoaged skin. Arch Derm 1996; 132:395–402.
2. Goldman MP, Fitzpatrick RE. Cutaneous Laser Resurfacing: The Art and Science of Selective Photothermolysis. 2d. St. Louis: Mosby, 1999.
3. Goldman MP, Manuskiatti W, Fitzpatrick RE. Combined laser resurfacing with the ultraplulse carbondioxide and Er: YAG lasers. In: Fitzpatrick RE, Goldman MP, eds. Cosmetic Laser Surgery. St. Louis: Mosby, 2000.
4. Manuskiatti W, Fitzpatrick RE, Goldman MP. Long-term effectiveness and side effects of carbon dioxide laser resurfacing for photoaged facial skin. J Am Acad Dermatol 1999; 40:401–441.
5. Goldman MP, Manuskiatti W, Fitzpatrick RE. Combined laser resurfacing with the $UPCO_2$ & Er:YAG lasers. Derm Surg 1999; 25:160–163.
6. Goldman MP, Skover G. Optimizing wound healing in the post-laser abrasion face. Cosmet Dermatol 1999; 12:25–29.
7. Manuskiatti W, Fitzpatrick RE, Goldman MP. Treatment of facial skin using combinations of CO_2, Q-Switched alexandrite, flash lamp-pumped pulsed dye, and Er:YAG lasers in the same treatment session. Dermatol Surg 2000; 26:114–120.
8. Bitter Jr P. Noninvasive rejuvenation of photodamaged skin using serial, full-face intense pulsed light treatments. Dermatol Surg 2000; 26:835.
9. Trelles MA, Allones I, Luna R. Facial rejuvenation with 1320 nm Nd:YAG laser. Dermatol Surg 2001; 27:111.
10. Bjerring, et al. Non-ablative laser rejuvenation J Cutan Laser Ther 2000; 2:9.
11. Goldberg DJ, Silapunt S. Q-switched Nd:YAG laser non-ablative dermal remodeling. J Cutan Laser Ther 2000; 2:157.
12. Goldman MP, Marchell N. Laser resurfacing of the neck with the combined CO_2/Erbium:YAG laser. Dermatol Surg 1999; 25:923–925.
13. Fitzpatrick RE, Goldman MP, Satur NM, et al. Pulsed carbon dioxide laser resurfacing of photoaged skin. Arch Dermatol 1996; 132:395–402.
14. Cotton J, Hood AF, Gonin R, et al. Histologic evaluation of preauricular and postauricular human skin after high-energy, short-pulse carbon dioxide laser. Arch Dermatol 1996; 132:425–428.
15. Stuzin JM, Baker TJ, Baker TM, et al. Histologic effects of the high energy pulsed CO_2 laser on photoaged facial skin. Plast Reconstr Surg 1997; 99:2036–2050.
16. Walsh Jr JT, Deutsch TF. Er:YAG laser ablation of tissue: measurement of ablation rates. Lasers Surg Med 1989; 9:327–337.
17. Tse Y, Manuskiatti W, Detwiler SP, et al. Tissue effects of the erbium:YAG laser with varying passes, energy, and pulse overlap. Lasers Med Surg 1998; 10(suppl):70.
18. Woodley DT, O'Keefe EJ, Prunieras M. Cutaneous wound healing: a model for cell–matrix interactions. J Am Acad Dermatol 1985; 12:420–433.
19. Clark RA. Biology of dermal wound repair. Dermatol Clin 1993; 11:647–666.
20. Pollack SV. Wound healing 1985: an update. J Dermatol Surg Oncol 1985; 11:296–300.
21. Brody HJ. Chemical peeling and resurfacing. 2nd edn. St. Louis: Mosby-Year Book, Inc., 1997:29–38.
22. Goldman MP. Techniques for erbium:YAG laser skin resurfacing: initial pearls from the first 100 patients. Dermatol Surg 1997; 23:1219–1225.
23. Rostan ER, Fitzpatrick RE, Goldman MP. Laser resurfacing with a long pulse erbium:YAG laser compared to the 950 msec pulsed CO_2 laser. Laser Surg Med 2001; 29:136–141.

24. Smith KJ, Skelton HG, Graham JS, Hamilton TA, et al. Depth of morphologic skin damage and viability after one, two and three passes of a high-energy short-pulse CO$_2$ laser (Tru-Pulse) in pig skin. J Am Acad Deramtol 1997; 37:204–210.

25. Goldman MP, Marchell N, Fitzpatrick RE, Tse Y. Laser resurfacing of the face with the combined CO$_2$/Er:YAG Laser. Dermatol Surg 2000; 26:102–104.

26. Greene D, Egbert BM, Utley DS, Koch RJ. In vivo model of histologic changes after treatment with the superpulsed CO$_2$ laser, erbium:YAG laser, and blended lasers: a 4 to 6 month prospective histologic and clinical study. Lasers Surg Med 2000; 27:362–372.

27. Trelles MA, Mordon S, Benitez V, Levy JL. Er:YAG laser resurfacing using combined ablation and coagulation modes. Dermatol Surg 2001; 27:727–734.

28. Bernstein LJ, Kauvar ANB, Grossman MC, Geronemus RG. The short- and long-term side effects of carbon dioxide laser resurfacing. Dermatol Surg 1997; 23:519–525.

29. Ruiz-Esparza J, Barba Gomez JM, Gomez de la Torre OL, Huerta Franco B, Parga Vazquez EG. UltraPulse laser skin resurfacing in Hispanic patients. A prospective study of 36 individuals. Dermatol Surg 1998; 24:59–62.

30. Khatri KA, Ross V, Grevelink JM, Magro CM, Anderson RR. Comparison of erbium:YAG and carbon dioxide lasers in resurfacing of facial rhytides. Arch Dermatol 1999; 135:391–397.

31. Ho C, Nguyen Q, Lowe NJ, Griffin ME, Lask G. Laser resurfacing in pigmented skin. Dermatol Surg 1995; 21:1035–1037.

32. Alster TS, West TB. Resurfacing of atrophic facial acne scars with a high-energy, pulsed carbon dioxide laser. Dermatol Surg 1996; 22: 151–154; discussion 154–155.

33. Kim JW, Lee JO. Skin resurfacing with laser in Asians. Aesthetic Plast Surg 1997; 21:115–117.

34. Cho SI, Kim YC. Treatment of atrophic facial scars with combined use of high-energy pulsed CO$_2$ laser and Er:YAG laser: a practical guide of laser techniques for the Er:YAG laser. Dermatol Surg 1999; 25:959–964.

35. Song MG, Park KB, Lee ES. Resurfacing of facial angiofibromas in tuberous sclerosis patients using CO$_2$ laser with flashscanner. Dermatol Surg 1999; 25:970–973.

36. Kye YC. Resurfacing of pitted facial scars with a pulsed Er:YAG laser. Dermatol Surg 1997; 23:880–883.

37. Polnikorn N, Goldberg DJ, Suwanchinda A, Ng SW. Erbium:YAG laser resurfacing in Asians. Dermatol Surg 1998; 24:1303–1307.

38. Yu DS, Kye YC. Cutaneous resurfacing of pitted acne scars with Er:YAG laser. J Kor Soc Laser Med 1999; 3:59–61.

39. Kwon SD, Kim SN, Kye YC. Resurfacing of pitted facial acne scars with a pulsed erbium:YAG laser. Ann Dermatol 1999; 11:5–8.

40. Lowe NJ, Lask G, Griffin ME. Laser skin resurfacing: pre- and posttreatment guidelines. Dermatol Surg 1995; 21:1017–1019.

41. Fitzpatrick RE. Laser resurfacing of rhytides. Dermatol Clin 1997; 15:431–447.

42. West TB, Alster TS. Effect of pretreatment on the incidence of hyperpigmentation following cutaneous CO$_2$ laser resurfacing. Dermatol Surg 1999; 25:15–17.

43. Sriprachya-anunt S, Marchell NL, Fitzpatrick RE, Goldman MP. Facial resurfacing in patients with Fitzpatrick skin type IV. Masers Surg Med 2002; 30:86–92.

44. Haedersdal M, Bech-Thomsen N, Poulsen T, Wulf HC. Ultraviolet exposure influences laser-induced wounds, scars and hyperpigmentation: a murine study. Plast Reconstr Surg 1998; 101:1315–1322.

45. Cho SI, Kim YC. Treatment of facial wrinkles with char-free carbon dioxide laser and erbium:YAG laser. Kor J Dermatol 1999; 37:177–184.

46. Goldman MP, Skover G, Roberts TL, Fitzpatrick RE, Lettieri JT. Optimizing wound healing in the post-laser abrasion face. J Am Acad Dermatol 2002; 46:399–407.

11

The Role of Pulse Dye Laser in Photorejuvenation

Steven Q. Wang
*Department of Dermatology, University of Minnesota School of Medicine,
Minneapolis, Minnesota, U.S.A.*

Brian D. Zelickson
*Department of Dermatology, University of Minnesota School of Medicine and
Skin Specialists Inc., Abbott Northwestern Hospital Laser Center, University of
Minnesota, Minneapolis, Minnesota, U.S.A.*

INTRODUCTION

Cutaneous aging is an inevitable process that is influenced by individual genetic factors and accelerated by exogenous toxins such as cumulative solar UV exposure. Environmental photodamage can lead to (1) epidermal proliferation such as actinic keratosis and squamous cell carcinoma, (2) uneven increase in melanin production resulting in solar lentigenes, (3) dermal vascular dilatation producing flushing and telangiectasias, and (4) dermal collagen and elastin breakdown causing wrinkles and skin textual changes.

Many treatment modalities are available to halt and even reverse signs of cutaneous aging. Photorejuvenation employing light energy sources is an effective treatment option in the physicians' armamentarium. Initially, ablative lasers, such as the CO_2 and Erbium laser, were used for treating irregular pigmentation and facial phytids. These ablation systems remove the epidermis and caused superficial dermal injury. As part of the wound healing process, a subsequent rebuilding of dermal collagen and regeneration of the epidermis ensue. This healing and remodeling process also corrects the skin defects brought on by cumulative photodamage. Because of longer healing time and the potential complications associated with ablative photorejuvenation, there has been a growing demand in the research and development of equally effective nonablative photorejuvenation techniques using lasers, intense pulsed light, and radiofrequency devices (1–4). Although the mechanism of nonablative photorejuvenation is still unclear, selective thermal injury to the dermis resulting in subsequent wound healing with an activation of

(A)   **(B)**   **(C)**

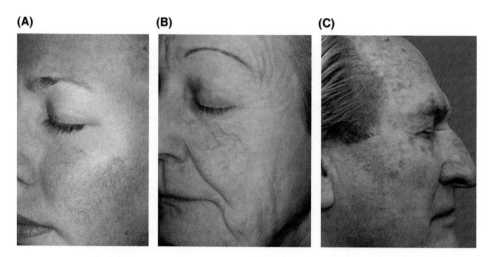

Figure 1
Note the clinical signs of photodamage **(A)** mild telangiectiasia and pigmentation, **(B)** extensive telangiectasia, dischromia and moderate rhytids and facial
laxity, **(C)** multiple actinic keratosis.

fibroblast and collagen synthesis remains as the primary explanation.
Other mechanisms include the inhibition of matrix metalloproteinase
and positive influence of cytokinins on production of extracellular matrix
proteins (5,6).

Currently, nonablative photorejuvenation has been classified into
several categories. Type 1 tackles pigmentary and vascular changes; this
corrects defects such as solar lentigenes, hyperpigmentation, telangiectasias, and erythema (Fig. 1A). Type 2 addresses skin changes in the dermal
collagen and connective tissue; this corrects rhytides and fine surface irregularities (Fig. 1B). Type 3 addresses precancerous changes such as actinic keratosis (Fig. 1C). This chapter describes the role of pulsed dye laser
(PDL) in photorejuvenation, specifically the second type.

PULSE DYE LASER

PDL emits wavelengths in the yellow color spectrum between 585 and
600 nm. These wavelengths have good absorption for melanin and oxyhe-
moglobins. Compared to 595 nm, 585 nm is preferentially absorbed by
both chromophores. By preferentially targeting the hemoglobin, the
PDL is an effective laser therapy for treating vascular lesions, erythema,
and telangiectasias. The literature is replete with studies documenting the
effectiveness of PDL in treating vascular lesions and skin changes
associated with photodamage. Hence, it is not a surprise that PDL is also
effective in relieving telangiectasias and diffuse erythema exacerbated by
photodamage (Fig. 2). Although, the PDL wavelengths are also absorbed

(A) **(B)**

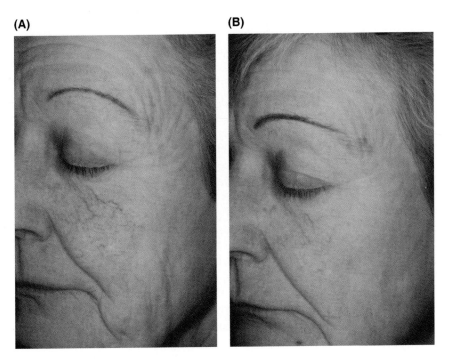

Figure 2
Long pulsed dye laser (**A**) Pretreatment and (**B**) Three months after two non-purpuric V-Beam treatments. Note improvement of erythema and tela-niectasia with mild improvement in facial rhytids.

by melanin and have some benefit in lightening irregular pigmentation; lasers and light sources with shorter wavelengths are generally better at treating epidermal melanin.

TYPE II PHOTOREJUVENATION

In the recent years, PDL has been shown to modulate collagen and elastin in the dermis. Its effectiveness in this arena was first demonstrated by Alster et al. (7) for treating scars induced by Argon lasers. In a follow-up study where 14 patients were treated with a flashlamp-pumped PDL (Candela Laser Corporation, Wayland, Massachusetts, U.S. and a wave-length of 585 nm, pulsed duration of 400 microsecond, fluence of between 6.5 and 6.75 J/cm^2), Alster (8) demonstrated a 57% to 83% lightening of the scar coloration after one to two treatments, respectively. In addition, some of the patients showed smoothing of the skin texture comparable to that of the normal surrounding skin. Subsequent studies (9–11) using simi-lar lasers with comparable treatment setting have confirmed the efficacy of PDL for treating hypertrophic scars and keloids in improving texture, color, and pliability. It is now generally recognized that PDL serves as an excellent treatment option (12). Although the exact mechanism of the PDLs ability in reducing hypertrophic scars is still unclear, it is thought that PDL selectively damages the microvasculature of the scars. This selective photothermolyses of the capillaries may induce hypoxia and reduce cellular nutrient supply within the scar, which leads to subsequent involution of the scar. In addition, PDL promotes mast cell granulation, leading to the subsequent degradation of connective tissue matrix.

The investigation of PDL in reducing rhytides has been prompted by the success of PDL in treating scars (13–15). Initial investigations (16) were performed with the original 0.45 millisecond, short-pulsed, and high-energy PDLs. To avoid the common side effect of purpura and at the same time to deliver the comparable thermal injury to the dermis, later studies were performed with PDLs that have (1) low energy and short–pulse duration (3,17,18) and (2) longer pulse duration.

The early study using the original, short-pulsed, 585 nm laser (Photogenica V, Cynosure, Massachusetts, U.S. and SPTL-1b, Candela, Massachusetts, U.S.) was published by Zelickson et al. (16) who treated 20 patients with mild to severe sun-induced perioral-and periocular wrinkles. The laser with a fluence of 3 to 6.5 J/cm^2, a pulse duration of 450 microseconds, and a 7 or 10 mm spot size with a 10% to 15% overlap was used. After receiving one treatment, 90% (16) of the mild to moderate and 40% (16) of the moderate to severe wrinkled patients showed clinical improvement. As expected, nearly all patients developed swelling and purpura that resolved after one to two weeks. Comparison of routine histology taken prior and after the treatment showed replacement of degenerated elastic fibers with well-organized elastin and collagen fibers in the treated area. This histologic finding supports the thought that PDL stimulates collagen synthesis via nonspecific, thermal injury to the dermis upon heating the surrounding vessels.

A follow-up study using low-energy 585 nm PDL (N-Lite, ICN Pharmaceuticals, Inc, Costa Mesa, California, U.S.) for the treatment of sun-induced wrinkles was first published by Bjerring et al. (3). Unlike original PDL, N-Lite uses low energy of 2.5 to 3 J/cm^2, with pulse duration of 350 microseconds and a spot size of 5 mm. It is the first PDL device approved by the Food and Drug Administration for nonablative photorejuvenation of periocular rhytides (3). After a single treatment, Bjerring et al. (3) showed an average cosmetic improvement of 1.88 reduction in wrinkle appearance as measured on the Fitzpatrick Wrinkle Severity scale. More importantly, the investigators demonstrated an increase of aminoterminal propeptide of type III procollagen-72 hours after a single treatment. In addition, there were no changes in epidermal barrier function as measured by the pre-, post-treatment measurement of skin transepidermal water loss. Collectively, the data are consistent with the stimulation of collagen remodeling via nonspecific thermal damage, which is thought to be the main mechanism of PDL photorejuvenation. However, the clinical improvement was not as dramatic in a subsequent study by Goldberg et al. (18) who treated 10 patients with the same setting. A study by Moody et al. (17) using the similar N-Lite setting showed an increase in dermal collagen accumulation via ultrasound measurement.

Unfortunately, the study did not assess the clinical improvement. A multi-center study presented by Van Laborte et al. (19), treated 58 subjects with one or two N-Light treatments. This study showed increased mRNA collagen expression by Northern Blot analysis as well as a statistically significant difference in skin texture between the treated and nontreated sides as measured by Primos analysis; however, there were no discernable differences in treated and nontreated sides upon photographic analysis (Figs. 3–5). Hence, caution is needed to extrapolate the data from ultrasound measurement to clinical outcomes.

Adopting a different strategy to avoid purpura, the long-pulsed, 595-nm PDL (Vbeam, Candela, Wayland, Massachusetts, U.S. and Vstar, Cynosure, Helmsford, Massachusetts, U.S.) was used to stimulate the thermal remodeling effect on the dermis at low energy with longer pulse duration of 2 to 40 milliseconds. Recently, the Candela V-Beam PDL has also been approved by the Food and Drug Administration for nonablative photorejuvenation. The long–pulse duration is not achieved by a single continuous pulse, but rather by stacking a number of small pulselets together. In addition to avoiding the purpuric side effects, this long pulse setting have the theoretic advantage of slowly heating the vessel and thereby allowing more thermal energy to dissipate from the vessels to the surrounding extracellular matrix. Using the longer

(A)   **(B)**

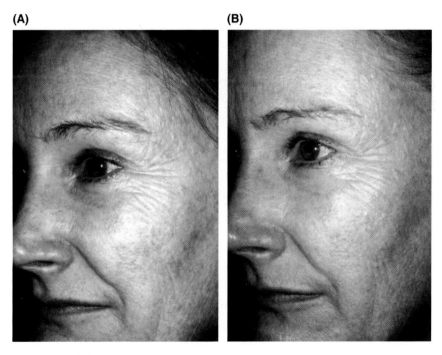

Figure 3
Images showing pretreatment (**A**) and four weeks after two N-Light treatments (**B**). Note mild improvement in periorbital rhytids.

(A)   **(B)**

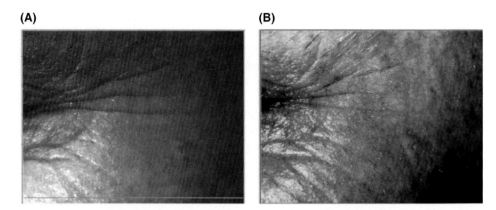

Figure 4
Images showing pretreatment (**A**) and four weeks after two N-Light treatments (**B**). Note mild improvement in periorbital rhytids.

PDL, Rostan et al. (20) demonstrated clinical efficacy in treating facial wrinkles in 15 patients with moderate to severe rhytides. After four treatments at one-month interval, 11 of the 15 patients demonstrated improvement on the treated side, comparing to 3 of the 15 patients on

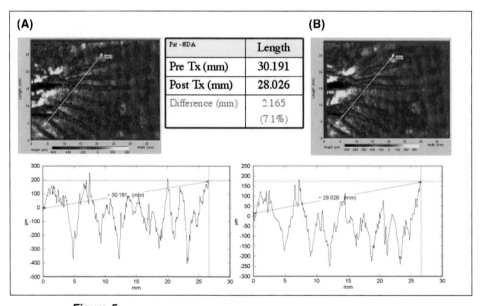

Pat -SDA	Length
Pre Tx (mm)	30.191
Post Tx (mm)	28.026
Difference (mm)	2.165 (7.1%)

Figure 5
Primos colorometric and topographical graph showing a 7.1% reduction in surface roughness. Images showing pretreatment (**A**) and four weeks after two N-Light treatments (**B**).

the placebo-treated side. A histologic evaluation showed a significant increase in the activated fibroblasts, collagen build up, and dermal thickening in the treated side. The results of the study was confirmed by Dahiya et al. (21) who demonstrated increase in dermal thickening, collagen band width, and increase in cellular hypertrophy in a porcine model after a single PDL treatment.

PATIENT TREATMENT PROTOCOL

In the following, an outline of our approach to the patient being treated with the PDL for photorejuvenation is discussed. As there are many different approaches to the patient with photodamage as well as many different protocols for these treatments, this outline is to be used only as a starting point and not as a cookbook approach for treatment.

The following segment will cover several key issues for treatment including patient selection, setting patient expectations, and pre-, during,

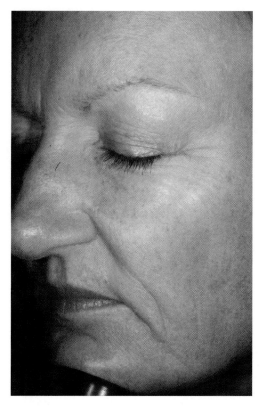

Figure 6
Good candidate for PDL photorejuvination.

and post-treatment protocols. Due to the focus of this chapter, it is assumed that the reader has some experience with the use of the PDL.

Patient Selection

For selecting of the most appropriate patient for PDL photorejuvenation, one must have a realistic expectation of what the device can do. The strengths of the PDL are treating vascular lesions and to a lesser extent superficial pigmentation and improving fine lines and skin texture. With that in mind, it is clear that those best suited to get a good to excellent response to PDL photorejuvenation are those individuals with significant erythema and vascularity, some superficial pigmentation, and mild textural change and fine lines (Fig. 6). As the PDL does have good melanin absorption it is best not to treat patients with dark skin types, greater than IV or with a tan to avoid significant epidermal damage and scarring (Fig. 7). Aside from this there are several contraindications for treatment:

1. pregnant,
2. exposure to Accutane® within the past six months,
3. active infection, other than acne, in or adjacent to the treatment area,
4. photosensitivity to visible light, and
5. unrealistic expectations.

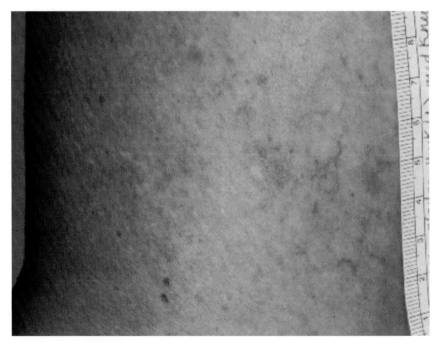

Figure 7
Tanned patient with PDL induced scarring.

Treatment Protocol

Pretreatment

1. Obtain informed consent: The treatment should be explained in detail to the patient and an informed-consent form should be signed which also includes consent for photographs.
    a. Realistic expectations should be set which include a 30% improvement in erythema and pigmentation per treatment and a 10% to 20% improvement in fine lines and texture after several treatments. These results can vary between individuals.
    b. There will be a mild discomfort felt during the treatment, which may feel like multiple snaps of a rubber band.
    c. After the treatment, there may be redness and swelling which can last for several hours to several days. There may be occasional bruising and scabbing which may last for one to two weeks.
2. Scarring which includes transient or permanent pigmentary changes or raised or depressed texture changes may occur less than 1% of the time.
3. Photographs should be taken (Fig. 8).
4. All the patient's make-up should be removed.
5. The patient and all personnel in the laser suite should have protective goggles on.

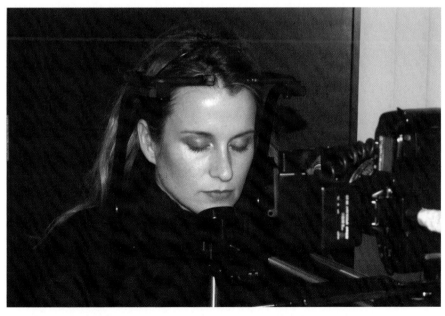

Figure 8
Patient having images taken with Canfield photographic system.

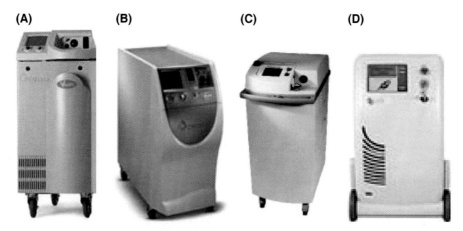

(A)   **(B)**   **(C)**   **(D)**

Figure 9
(**A**) V-Beam, (**B**) C-Beam, (**C**) V-Star, and (**D**) N-Light.

Treatment

Choosing treatment settings and treatment protocol: There are many different PDLs, and there are many ways to use each of them (Fig. 9**A**–**D**). There is currently no consensus as to the best PDL system, set of parameters, or treatment protocol for photorejuvenation.

a. Treatment parameters: Although, we have given a set of starting parameters for each PDL device in Table 1 these are just rough estimates, and the main issue is to look for the immediate tissue response. The tissue response that seems to give the best clinical response while avoiding prolonged purpura and risk of side effects is the one that gives rise to a transient cyanosis of the tissue which resolves within seconds.

b. Treatment protocols: Again, while there are no good scientific studies confirming the best treatment protocol, we perform multiple treatments from six to eight weeks apart until the desired amount of improvement is obtained.

Post-Treatment Care

1. Do not use Retin-A, alpha-hydroxy, or vitamin C products for 24 hours.
2. Avoid direct sun exposure to the treated area for one to two days. Use a total sun block that includes the ingredient zinc oxide.
3. Do not exfoliate the treated area for three to four days following treatment.
4. Cleanse, tone, and moisturize for the next 24 hours.

Table 1
Summary of Clinical Studies Using the Pulsed Dye Laser in the Treatment of Rhytides

Investigators	Lasers	Settings (wavelength, fluence, pulse duration, spot size)	No. of patients	Evaluation	Reference
Zelickson et al.	Photogenica V (Cynosure, Massachusetts, U.S.)	585 nm 3–5 J/cm^2 450 microsec 10 mm	10	Clinical Histologic	8
	SPTL-1b (Candela, Massachusetts, U.S.)	585 nm 5–6 J/cm^2 450 microsec 7–10 mm	10		
Bjerring et al.	N-Lite, (ICN Pharmaceuticals Inc., California, U.S.)	585 nm 2.5–3 J/cm^2 350 microsec 5 mm		Clinical Histologic	9
Moody et al.	N-Lite (ICN Pharmaceuticals Inc., California, U.S.)	585 nm 2.4–3 J/cm^2 350 microsec 5 mm	10	Clinical Ultrasound measure-ment	10
Goldberg et al.	N-Lite (ICN Pharmaceuticals Inc., California, U.S.)	585 nm 2.5 J/cm^2 350 microsec 5 mm	10	Clinical Histologic	11
Zelickson et al.	N-Lite (ICN Pharmaceuticals Inc., California, U.S.)	585 nm 2.4–2.9 J/cm^2 350 microsec 7 mm	57	Clinical Histologic	12
Rostan et al.	V beam (Candela Corp., Massachusetts, U.S.)	595 nm 6 J/cm^2 6 msec 10 mm	15	Clinical Histologic	13

5. If blistering occurs, apply antibiotic ointment to affected area and keep it moist.
6. Do not tweeze or wax the area after treatment for two to three days.

What may happen following a treatment:

1. Redness normally occurs following a treatment. This usually subsides within the first few hours, but it may last for one to two days.

2. Blistering rarely occurs, but if it does occur, keep the area clean and apply a topical antibiotic ointment.
3. You may notice the brown spots becoming darker in appearance after treatment. It is imperative to avoid sun exposure and wear sun block. Do not become alarmed, they will gradually flake off or lighten up.
4. Over a period of time, you may notice improvement in the texture of the skin, diffused redness, and/or hyperpigmentation.

SUMMARY

The clinical efficacy of PDL in treating vascular lesions, telangiectasias, and erythema has been well documented. With the development of longer PDL, 2 to 40 millisecond devices, it can certainly play a vital role in type 1 photorejuvenation, specifically reducing erythema and facial telangiectasias, without the side effect of purpura and swelling associated with the original 0.45 millisecond devices. As for its role in type 2 nonablative photorejuvenation, specifically, dermal collagen and elastin remodeling, basic and clinical research have provided the evidence to support its potential efficacy, although the clinical outcome in reducing facial rhytides is often subtle.

The mechanism of PDL in nonablative photorejuvenation is still unclear. The leading explanation is the diffusion of heat from the capillaries to the surrounding tissue resulting in nonselective thermal injury. As a part of remodeling and wound healing process, there is an increase in collagen and elastin deposition to the dermis. Evidence from histologic analysis supports this explanation. However, troubling questions still remain. For one, how can the original 585 nm PDLs with the same fluence and pulse duration be effective in reducing hypertrophic scars/keloids, stimulating collagen proliferation, and improving facial rhytides? This seemingly contradictory effect of PDL points out the complexity of tissue interaction with PDL nonablative treatment.

In addition to the need for further exploration on the mechanism, clinical research aimed to elucidate the optimal treatment parameters, and protocol for treating rhytides will be welcomed. Lastly, efforts are needed that move beyond routine morphologic analysis to the molecular and genetic level to promote the knowledge base and the understanding in the field of nonablative photorejuvenation.

REFERENCES

1. Kelly KM, Majaron B, Nelson JS. Nonablative laser and light rejuvenation: the newest approach to photodamaged skin. Arch Facial Plast Surg 2001; 3:230–235.
2. Goldberg DJ, Samady JA. Intense pulsed light and Nd:YAG laser non-ablative treatment of facial rhytides. Lasers Surg Med 2001; 28:141–144.
3. Bjerring P, Clement M, Heickendorff L, Egevist H, Kiernan M. Selective non-ablative wrinkle reduction by laser. J Cutan Laser Ther 2000; 2:9–15.
4. MacReady N. Radiofrequency devices offers nonsurgical face lift. Skin Allergy News 2002; 33:30.
5. Wong WR, Kossodo S, Kochevar IE. Influence of cytokines on matrix metalloproteinases produced by fibroblasts cultured in monolayer and collagen gels. J Formos Med Assoc 2001; 100:377–382.
6. Weiss RA, McDaniel DH, Geronemus RG. Review of nonablative photorejuvenation: reversal of the aging effects of the sun and environmental damage using laser and light sources. Semin Cutan Med Surg 2003; 22:93–106.
7. Alster TS, Kurban AK, Grove GL, Grove MJ, Tan OT. Alteration of argon laser-induced scars by the pulsed dye laser. Lasers Surg Med 1993; 13:368–373.
8. Alster TS. Improvement of erythematous and hypertrophic scars by the 585-nm flashlamp-pumped pulsed dye laser. Ann Plast Surg 1994; 32:186–190.
9. Alster TS, Nanni CA. Pulsed dye laser treatment of hypertrophic burn scars. Plast Reconstr Surg 1998; 102:2190–2195.
10. Manuskiatti W, Fitzpatrick RE, Goldman MP. Energy density and numbers of treatment affect response of keloidal and hypertrophic sternotomy scars to the 585-nm flashlamp-pumped pulsed-dye laser. J Am Acad Dermatol 2001; 45:557–565.
11. Kono T, Ercocen AR, Nakazawa H, Honda T, Hayashi N, Nozaki M. The flashlamp-pumped pulsed dye laser (585 nm) treatment of hypertrophic scars in Asians. Ann Plast Surg 2003; 51:366–371.
12. Alster TS, Handrick C. Laser treatment of hypertrophic scars, keloids, and striae. Semin Cutan Med Surg 2000; 19:287–292.
13. Alster TS, McMeekin TO. Improvement of facial acne scars by the 585 nm flashlamp-pumped pulsed dye laser. J Am Acad Dermatol 1996; 35:79–81.
14. Patel N, Clement M. Selective nonablative treatment of acne scarring with 585 nm flashlamp pulsed dye laser. Dermatol Surg 2002; 28:942–945; discussion 945.
15. McDaniel DH, Ash K, Zukowski M. Treatment of stretch marks with the 585-nm flashlamp-pumped pulsed dye laser. Dermatol Surg 1996; 22:332–337.
16. Zelickson BD, Kilmer SL, Bernstein E, Chotzen VA, Dock J, Mehregan D, Coles C. Pulsed dye laser therapy for sun damaged skin. Lasers Surg Med 1999; 25:229–236.
17. Moody BR, McCarthy JE, Hruza GJ. Collagen remodeling after 585-nm pulsed dye laser irradiation: an ultrasonographic analysis. Dermatol Surg 2003; 29:997–999; discussion 999–1000.
18. Goldberg D, Tan M, Dale Sarradet M, Gordon M. Nonablative dermal remodeling with a 585-nm, 350-microsec, flashlamp pulsed dye laser: clinical and ultrastructural analysis. Dermatol Surg 2003; 29:161–163; discussion 163–164.
19. Van Laborte S, Dover J, Pon K, Arndt K, Zelickson B, Burns J, Kilmer S, Hruza G, Waner M. Use of the N-Light laser for non-ablative wrinkle reduction. Presented at the ASMLS meeting in Atlanta, Georgia, April 11–14, 2002.
20. Rostan E, Bowes LE, Iyer S, Fitzpatrick RE. A double-blind, side-by-side comparison study of low fluence long pulse dye laser to coolant treatment for wrinkling of the cheeks. J Cosmet Laser Ther 2001; 3:129–136.
21. Dahiya R, Lam SM, Williams EF III. A systematic histologic analysis of nonablative laser therapy in a porcine model using the pulsed dye laser. Arch Facial Plast Surg 2003; 5:218–223.

12

Nd:YAG (1064 nm) Laser

David J. Goldberg
*Skin Laser & Surgery Specialists of New York & New Jersey, and Mount Sinai
School of Medicine, New York, New York, U.S.A.*

Video 12: Nd:YAG Laser: YAG5®
Video 13: Nd:YAG Laser: CoolGlide®
Video 14: Nd:YAG Laser: Lyra®
Video 15: Nd:YAG Laser: Varia®

INTRODUCTION

All nonablative lasers and light sources attempt to induce new collagen formation by either a direct effect on upper dermal vasculature (with a secondary effect on the surrounding dermis) or a direct thermal effect on the dermis.

The Q-switched Nd:YAG laser with its 1064 nm wavelength was introduced in the late 1980s for tattoo and pigmented lesion removal. Their absorption in the skin can lead to a specific nonspecific photomechanical effect in the dermis. This may lead to new collagen formation with resultant dermal remodeling and skin toning.

The Q-switched Nd:YAG laser was the first laser evaluated for nonablative remodeling. Goldberg et al. (1) treated 11 subjects with perioral and periocular rhytides using a Q-switched Nd:YAG laser at 5.5 J/cm^2 and a 3-mm spot size with overlapping passes and a clinical endpoint of pinpoint bleeding. No surface cooling was used. Results following treatment with the Q-switched Nd:YAG laser were compared to the results obtained when the contralateral side was treated with a pulsed CO_2 laser. Both perioral and periorbital regions were treated. Clinical results were evaluated at three months after treatment. In three patients (two perioral and one periorbital), the Q-switched Nd:YAG laser produced results clinically indistinguishable from that of a pulsed CO_2 laser. In six subjects (three perioral and three periorbital), clinical improvement was noted with the Q-switched Nd:YAG laser, but the improvement was not as marked as that seen with a CO_2 laser. In two subjects (one perioral and one periorbital), no improvement with the Q-switched Nd:YAG laser was noted. Complete re-epithelialization of the skin surface was noted in all subjects for on average of three to five days after treatment with the Q-switched Nd:YAG laser as compared with 6 to 11 days after treatment with the CO_2 laser. At one and three months posttreatment, no pigmentary changes were noted in any subject. At one month post-operation, 3 of the 11 subjects treated with the Q-switched Nd:YAG laser exhibited erythema. Of note, these were the three subjects who showed clinical results similar to that seen with the CO_2 laser.

Although the above study was limited by the small sample size, this pilot-study showed that the Q-switched Nd:YAG laser might be efficacious in the treatment of some perioral and periorbital rhytides (Figs. 1 and 2). This was thought to occur due to dermal remodeling with increased Type I collagen formation.

In an expanded follow-up study, Goldberg and Metzler (2) utilized a Q-switched Nd:YAG laser with a topical carbon-assisted solution as an added chromophore. Two hundred forty-two solar-damaged anatomical sites on 61 human subjects with Fitzpatrick skin phenotypes I–II were treated with three laser treatments at two study centers. The treatment involved applying a carbon suspension to the skin surface and irradiating the exogenous chromophore with a Q-switched Nd:YAG laser. In this study, a cosmetically desirable, nonpetechia-producing low fluence of $2.5 \, J/cm^2$ was utilized. The treatment sites were evaluated at baseline, 4, 8, 14, 20, and 32 weeks for skin texture, skin elasticity, and rhytid reduction. All sites were treated at baseline, four, and eight weeks. Skin replicas taken prior to treatment and at the conclusion of the study were analyzed for wrinkle and cosmetic improvement. Adverse events were recorded throughout the study.

At eight months, the investigators reported improvement in skin texture and skin elasticity, as well as rhytid reduction compared to that at baseline. In self-assessments, subjects also reported noticeable skin texture and cosmetic improvement, but assessed wrinkle reduction less favorably

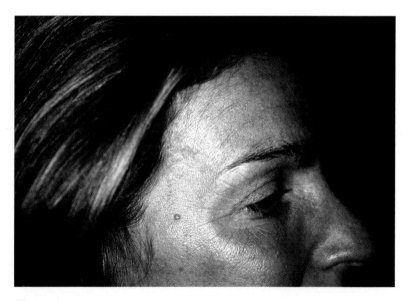

Figure 1
Before treatment with high fluence, Q-switched Nd:YAG laser.

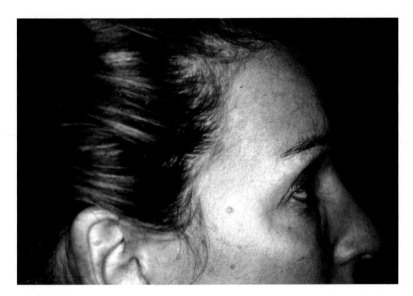

Figure 2
After treatment with high fluence, Q-switched Nd:YAG laser.

than the investigators' assessments of wrinkle and cosmetic improvement. The majority of adverse events were limited to mild, brief erythema.

Pretreatment skin replicas were obtained from 47 random subjects for comparison with posttreatment replicas utilizing profilometric analyses. As described above, the investigators and subjects completed evaluation forms at baseline, 4, 8, 14, 20, and 32 weeks by recording their assessments of skin texture, elasticity, and cosmetic improvement of rhytides. Skin elasticity was evaluated with a routine dermatologic pull test. Skin texture and elasticity were rated on a relative scale. Texture was expressed as a percentage, with larger numbers representing rougher textures. Elasticity was recorded as a number between 1 and 100, with 1 representing minimal elasticity and 100 representing optimal elasticity. Cosmetic improvement was expressed as a percent improvement over baseline.

The investigators recorded adverse effects throughout the study. At the conclusion of the study, posttreatment skin replicas were produced for the 47 subjects who had pretreatment replicas. The results of the pre- and posttreatment skin replicas were analyzed for wrinkle and cosmetic improvement.

Because the Study Center 1 entered predominantly Class I rhytid individuals and Study Center 2 entered predominantly those with Class II rhytid, the reported results in skin texture, elasticity, and wrinkle reduction varied slightly at each center. At eight months, 210 of the 242 anatomic sites were evaluated for improvement in skin texture and elasticity. The following sections summarize the results for each of the parameters evaluated.

The investigators at both the study centers and the subjects at Study Center 2 observed marked improvements in skin texture at eight months.

Table 1
Average Skin Texture Scores (0 = Smooth, 100 = Rough; *N* = 210 Sites)

Study center	Investigator		Subject	
	Baseline	8 months	Baseline	8 months
2	42	27	48	30
1	20	9	32	32
Combined average	31	18	40	31
Average % change		42%		22%

However, the subjects at the Study Center 1 did not report improvement in this category. Table 1 summarizes the results of skin assessments for 210 treatment sites.

At eight months, Study Center 1 investigators observed significantly greater improvement in skin elasticity than did their Study Center 2 counterparts. The subjects did not evaluate skin elasticity in their self-assessments. Table 2 summarizes the results of skin elasticity assessments.

Investigators categorized facial rhytides as Fitzpatrick classification I or II prior to the first treatment. Of the 210 evaluated eight-month sites, 150 sites were on the face. These sites were evaluated for rhytid reduction.

A total of 78 Class I rhytid sites were evaluated. Table 3 summarizes the eight-month data in this group.

A substantial improvement in fine wrinkles was observed. Investigators reported that 97% of fine wrinkles had at least slight improvement. Subjects reported a lesser, but nevertheless significant, or slightly greater improvement in Class I rhytides (71%).

A total of 72 Class II rhytid sites were evaluated. Table 4 summarizes the eight-month data in this group.

Both the subjects and investigators noted an improvement in Class II rhytides. The subjects and investigators found at least slight improvement in 49 of 72 (68%) versus 62 of 72 (86%) of the treatments,

Table 2
Average Skin Elasticity Scores (0 = Poor, 100 = Excellent; *N* = 84 Sites)

Study center	Investigator	
	Baseline	8 months
2	54	59
1	35	62
Combined average	45	60
Average % change		25%

Table 3
Class I Rhytides

	Investigator	Subject
Worse	0	4
No Change	2	19
Slightly improved	17	26
Improved	46	17
Much improved	13	12
Total	78	78

respectively. This finding is consistent with the historical observation that treated subjects tend to be more critical of cosmetic results than the investigators.

An analysis of 47 random sets of pre- and posttreatment skin replicas supported the investigator and subject assessments of wrinkle improvement. The optical profilometric analyses provided measurement of the degree of wrinkling, roughness, and other surface irregularities. The Rz profilometric value system was utilized. The Rz value reflects the difference between the minimum and maximum heights of five equally spaced sections of a profile. Table 5 presents the baseline and eight-month values.

The mean difference of the Rz component, which represents the average difference between minimum and maximum heights in the skin replica data, was significant ($p = 0.01$).

The posttreatment data presented in Table 6 indicate that mild transient erythema was the most common adverse event seen after each of the treatment sessions. Purpura occurred in five sites following the initial treatment; three cases of pinpoint bleeding were recorded (one following the initial treatment and two at eight weeks), and one instance of postinflammatory hyperpigmentation was reported at eight weeks.

This study was the first to show that the low fluence, topical carbon suspension–assisted Q-switched Nd:YAG laser offered a safe and effective treatment of solar-damaged skin (Figs. 3 and 4). However, because

Table 4
Class II Rhytides

	Investigator	Subject
Worse	0	1
No change	10	23
Slightly improved	30	23
Improved	28	21
Much improved	4	5
Total	72	72

Table 5
Skin Replica Analysis Results ($N = 47$)

	Rz-Value
Pretreatment	34.50
At 8 Months	30.331

of the messy topical carbon suspension and increasing anecdotal evidence that similar clinical results could be obtained without the use of a topical adjuvant, topical carbon-assisted Q-switched Nd:YAG nonablative dermal remodeling is rarely used.

Cisneros et al. (3) in a study of 22 subjects with facial rhytides noted improvement after two Q-switched Nd:YAG laser treatments. The investigators used the following parameters: 3-mm spot size and a fluence of 6 to $7 \, J/cm^2$. They also noted improvement in postacne scarring.

In a more recent study, the efficacy and safety of multiple Q-switched Nd:YAG laser treatments in the nonablative treatment of facial rhytides were evaluated (4).

Eight female subjects ranging in age from 40 to 63 years (average 51.6 years) were enrolled in this study; five subjects had Fitzpatrick skin type II, two subjects had skin type IV, and one subject had skin type III. The periorbital area was treated in five of eight subjects; the perioral area was treated in the remaining three subjects. Two subjects were noted to have Class I rhytides; three subjects had Class II rhytides; three subjects had Class III rhytides. Treatments were undertaken with a Q-switched Nd:YAG laser at fluences of $7 \, J/cm^2$ and a 3 mm spot size. Two laser passes were used in all subjects in an attempt to promote petechiae as the typical visible endpoint. All subjects used bacitracin ointment for posttreatment care. All subjects received three treatments, once a month, over a consecutive three-month period. Photographs were taken before treatment and three months after the third treatment. A nontreating, independent physician evaluated the photographs. Every effort was made

Table 6
Adverse Effects

Description	Initial treatment ($N = 242$)	% of Total	Week 4 ($N = 234$)	% of Total	Week 8 ($N = 210$)	% of Total
Erythema	146	60	131	56	114	54
Pigmentation change	0	0	0	0	1	0
Pinpoint bleeding	1	0	0	0	2	1
Purpura	5	2	0	0	0	0
Other	0	0	0	0	0	0

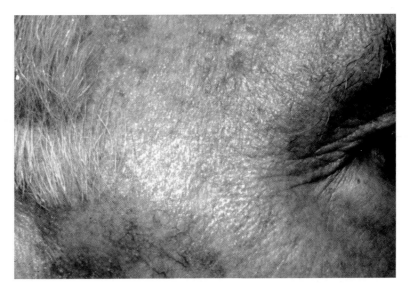

Figure 3
Before treatment with low fluence, carbon-assisted, Q-switched Nd:YAG laser.

to have the quality, exposure, lighting, and angle of the camera consistent for each photograph. Subjects filled out a questionnaire at 24 hours and 7 days after each treatment. Subjects quantified and recorded the level of discomfort as a result of the laser treatment as follows: (i) no pain at all, (ii) mild pain, not requiring any pain medication (iii) moderate pain,

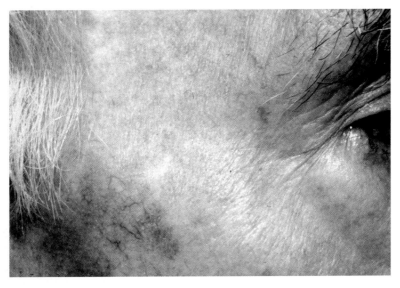

Figure 4
After treatment with low fluence, carbon-assisted, Q-switched Nd:YAG laser.

requiring nonprescription pain medication, (iv) severe pain, requiring prescription pain medication, or (v) extreme pain, requiring a physician call. At the end of the study, each subject assessed their satisfaction with the laser treatment as follows: (i) unsatisfactory results, not worth the time and effort; (ii) fair results, but wishing the results were better; (iii) good results, satisfied with the procedure; and (iv) excellent results, very satisfied. The investigators also evaluated improvement based on a percentile scale: 0% to 25% (poor), 26% to 50% (fair), 51% to 75% (good), and 76% to 100% (excellent).

Independent investigator assessment showed six of eight subjects having at least a fair clinical improvement in rhytides. Two of eight subjects showed a poor outcome. In contrast, subject assessment was fair in five of eight subjects; two subjects reported an unsatisfactory outcome; one subject reported a good overall outcome.

At 24 hours after each treatment, 80% of subjects reported complete absence of pain. Mild pain, not requiring pain medication, was present in 20% of subjects. Only one subject reported pain at seven days, after each treatment.

Petechiae were observed in 75% of subjects immediately after each treatment. Thirty-three percent of subjects had pinpoint bleeding immediately after each treatment (Figs. 5 and 6). No erythema, edema, purpura, pigmentary changes, or scarring was observed at one month after each treatment and at three months following the last treatment.

In a study evaluating the histologic changes seen after Q-switched Nd:YAG nonablative treatment, six female subjects ranging in age from 48 to 63 years received laser treatment (5). Subjects had Fitzpatrick skin types II–IV. Subjects were precluded from using any topical

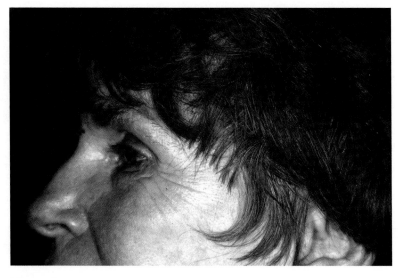

Figure 5
Before treatment with high fluence, Q-switched Nd:YAG laser.

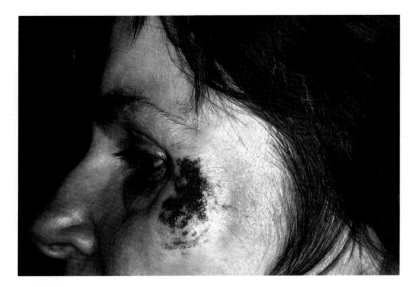

Figure 6
Petechiae and bleeding immediately after treatment with high fluence, Q-switched Nd:YAG laser.

collagen–promoting agents for one month prior to the study and during the entire course of the study. Sun-damaged 4×4 cm areas of infra-auricular skin were exposed to a 1064 nm Q-switched Nd:YAG laser at fluences of 7 J/cm^2 and a 3-mm spot size. Two laser passes, with a 10% to 20% overlap, were used in all subjects in an attempt to promote petechiae as the visible endpoint. Petrolatum dressings were applied for one week after treatment. 3 mm punch biopsies were taken from each subject before treatment. Photographs were taken of the biopsy sites. Again, three months after the last treatment, another biopsy was taken from a different previously treated area. Histologic specimens were evaluated blindly by a board of certified dermatopathologists.

Four of six skin biopsy specimens obtained three months after laser treatment showed mild fibrosis with histologic improvement in pretreatment solar elastosis. There was a mildly thickened upper papillary collagen zone, with an improvement in the organization of collagen fibrils. The remaining two specimens showed no changes. Histologic study of human skin obtained three months after high-energy, short-pulse carbon dioxide laser shows a papillary dermal repair zone, composed of dense, compact collagen bundles in parallel alignment with the epidermal surface. Such findings were seen in kind but not in degree in this study (Figs. 7 and 8).

Friedman et al. (6) recognized the inherent limitations of photographic and clinical evaluation of improvement after nonablative treatment. They analyzed the results in two subjects after five treatments with a low fluence, Q-switched Nd:YAG laser. Clinical results were analyzed using a 30-mm, three-dimensional microtopograhpy imaging system (PRIMOS, GFM, Teltow, Germany). Six-month results, as

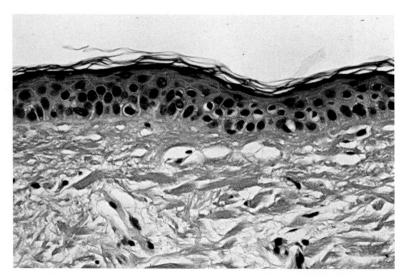

Figure 7
Histologic thinned epidermis and dermis seen with solar elastosis.

measured by this three-dimensional method, showed a decrease in skin roughness of 26%. Such methods provide a more precise measurement of clinical improvement than is seen with clinical and/or photographic evaluation.

Because a thermal effect is sought in the upper papillary dermis, and *millisecond non–Q-switched Nd:YAG lasers* have a greater heating

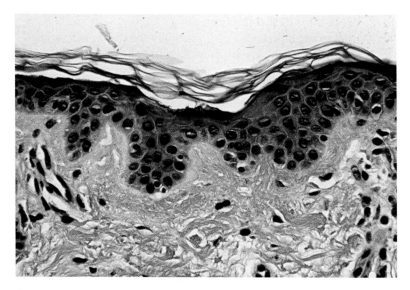

Figure 8
Histologic hyperplastic epidermis and thickened epidermis seen after treatment with the Q-switched Nd:YAG laser.

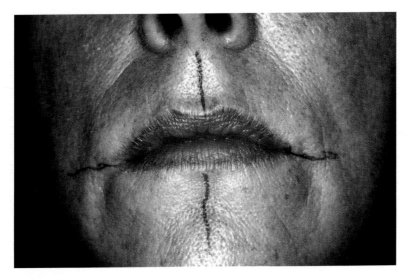

Figure 9
Before treatment with millisecond Nd:YAG laser.

capacity than their nanosecond Q-switched counterparts, such lasers are currently being used for nonablative dermal remodeling (Figs. 9 and 10). There are limited data as to the success of these systems. In theory, because the 1064 nm wavelength is less well absorbed by water, than are the 1320 nm Nd:YAG, 1450 nm diode, and 1540 nm Erbium glass wavelengths, a greater dermal wound can be created. Conversely, it has been anecdotally suggested that the 1064 nm wavelength, because of its greater dermal

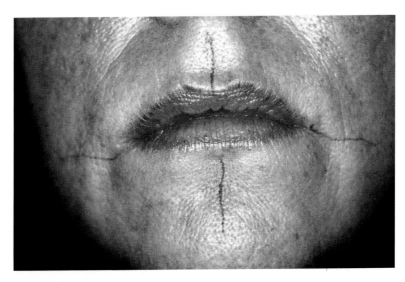

Figure 10
After treatment with millisecond Nd:YAG laser.

penetration, may lead to a increased scarring. There are no scientific data to prove this latter premise.

In one of the first studies performed with a non–Q-switched millisecond Nd:YAG laser, 10 Fitzpatrick type II-III skin subjects were treated at fluences of 100 to 130 J/cm^2, pulse durations of 3 to 8 ms, and up to 5 treatments over an eight-week period (7). They were followed for six months after their final treatment. Side effects were minimal with only one subject showing posttreatment blistering. This healed without scarring. Most patients showed some degree of clinical improvement. It is also possible that combining another wavelength with the use of a 1064 nm near-infrared system can lead to better results. Goldberg (8), in a small study of 10 subjects, and Lee (9), in a large study of 150 subjects found that the clinical improvement following treatment with both a millisecond Nd:YAG laser and a millisecond KTP laser was better than that seen when either the Nd:YAG or KTP laser was used alone.

1064 nm Nd:YAG lasers have been, and will continue to be, used for nonablative dermal remodeling. Future studies are required to compare the results obtained using this wavelength with those obtained using many other currently available wavelengths for this technique.

including sun protection may be used in conjunction to further enhance results.

CoolTouch® Applications

Rhytids

The initial Food and Drug Administration's (FDA) indication for the 1320 nm CoolTouch® laser was for treatment of periocular rhytids. The initial area tested with this device, starting in 1999, was the periorbital region, to reduce lower lid and lateral canthus (crow's feet) rhytids. As our understanding of the concept of dynamic skin lines evolved, it became obvious that use of botulinum toxin in these regions immediately after the first 1320 nm laser treatment greatly enhanced the efficacy of these treatments. We now routinely inject 10 units of Botox® at the lateral canthus and just below it, immediately after the initial treatment is performed. The rationale to restrict movement centers on the fact that the collagen remodeling induced by the 1320 nm laser will no longer be influenced by dynamic movement. Therefore, collagen synthesis will be more effective when Botox® is injected into the rhytids, rather than adjacent to them, leading to improved clinical results. Although the initial patients who were treated from 1999 to 2001 were extremely pleased with the improvement in the appearance of their skin, overall satisfaction rate has improved to over 90% with the addition of botulinum toxin. We typically counsel the patients to expect a 50% improvement and warn them that 20% of patients do not respond to the treatment at all. Advantages for the 1320 nm wavelength for treating rhytids include extremely low morbidity (we have had only one patient in thousands, who developed a blister posttreatment with a slight depression), speed of the CoolTouch® treatments, and the no downtime aspect. As collagen regeneration continues for several months after CoolTouch® treatments, patients are reevaluated six months after their last treatment to determine whether another round of three to five treatments would be beneficial. We explain to our patients that maintenance therapy at least once a year may be necessary, especially in areas of dynamic skin lines owing to underlying muscle movement, and that Botox® may be required again during the next round of treatment.

The perioral region is another target area in which the 1320 nm laser device has been utilized. This is a much more treatment-resistant region, probably related to even more profound effects of dynamic muscle movement. We inform patients that they may only observe a 20% to 30% improvement, and that typically two rounds of three- to five-month treatments sessions spaced six months apart may be necessary. Recently, we have treated patients concomitantly with botulinum toxin along the upper lip, using 4 U of Botox® injected in the middle of the upper lip just below the central nares with 2 U each bilaterally (Fig. 4). We have observed markedly improved results and vastly accelerated improvement. Overall, it is best to underestimate results in this region and patients will be pleased when they observe more than they expected. The perioral region, and the upper lip in particular, is the most difficult area to treat

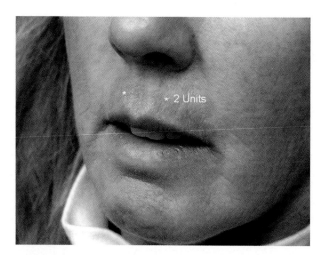

Figure 4
Sites of supplemental botulinum toxin injection. Each site (*asterisk*) receives
2 U of Botox® cosmetic.

with any laser, including ablative devices. Thus, it is not surprising that
1320 nm wavelength has the least effective results in this region. Some
examples of clinical results are shown in Figure 5.

Acne Scarring

The 1320 nm CoolTouch® laser has also been cleared by the FDA for the
treatment of acne scarring and active acne. The mechanism for improvement in active acne is heating, with subsequent shrinkage of sebaceous
glands. Although there are few clinical trials on light-based treatments
for active acne, we have observed some improvement with 1320 nm laser.
Blue light is known to work by activating porphyrins on the surface of
Propionibacterium Acnes (19). We believe that active acne will respond
with about an 80% improvement with three treatments, spaced three
weeks apart, using 1320 nm CoolTouch® laser.

The results using 1320 nm laser for atrophic acne scarring have been
greater than initially predicted by proponents of ablative resurfacing.
Atrophic acne scarring is a common condition that results from inflammation with subsequent collagen degradation, dermal atrophy, and fibrosis
(20). Ablative skin resurfacing has been shown to improve acne scarring
through epidermal vaporization and dermal thermal damage, which lead
to collagen shrinkage and dermal remodeling (21,22). Its use, however, is
limited by a prolonged postoperative recovery period and by complications including scarring, infection, and persistent pigmentary changes.

Previous studies looking at effects of 1320 nm laser on atrophic acne
scarring have included small numbers of patients with limited follow-up
periods; results have generally been encouraging (23–26). In a study on

(A)

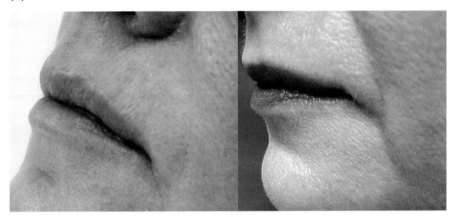

(B)

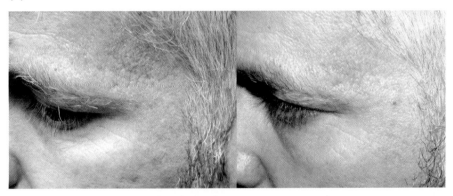

(C)

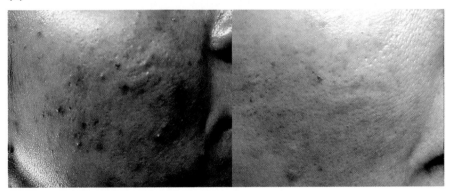

Figure 5
Clinical examples of results with 1320 nm. (**A**) Upper lip after four treatments, one month apart. (**B**) Temporal region with acne scarring after three treatments, one month apart. Image on right taken just before the 4th treatment. (**C**) Right cheek after six treatments, one month apart. Notice reduction in active acne as well as improvement in acne scarring.

Asian patients, there was a patient evaluation of about 40% improvement.(26). Mild to moderate clinical improvement was observed after the series of three treatments in the majority of patients treated in a study comparing 1320 nm laser with 1450 nm laser (24). A study at our site involving 29 patients (skin phototypes I–IV) with facial acne scarring was conducted, in which each patient received a mean of 5.5 (range 2–17) treatments with the 1320 nm Nd:YAG laser (27). Objective physician assessment scores of improvement were determined by side by side comparison of preoperative and postoperative photographs at a range of 1 to 27 months (mean = 10.4 months) postoperation. Subjective patient self-assessment scores of improvement were also obtained. The results obtained by both physician and patient assessment scores, showed that acne scarring was significantly improved. Mean improvement was 2.8 ($P < 0.05$) on a 0 to 4 point scale by physician assessment and 5.4 ($P < 0.05$) on a 0 to 10 point scale by patient assessment. No significant complications were observed. We have not seen the postinflammatory hyperpigmentation reported in a small percentage of Asian patients (26). These improvements in acne scarring parallel the other previously published studies.

Based on our clinical experience and on published studies, we explain to patients that acne scarring may be improved by approximately 50%. We also warn them that about 20% of the patients may not respond at all and may need another method of treatment, including ablative treatments. Results with fractional resurfacing are encouraging and this may turn out to be a valuable alternative. The nonresponders may not be able to synthesize enough collagen or may have no net gain, with as much collagen breakdown as collagen buildup at the treatment sites. As acne scarring results from the inflammatory response to *Propionibacterium acnes* and the subsequent collagen degradation, dermal atrophy, and fibrosis, which is genetically determined, some patients may have collagen degradation when inflammation is induced with the 1320 nm laser.

Although atrophic acne scars tend to respond to laser treatment, the deeper ice pick and boxcar scars tend to be more resistant to 1320 nm and other infrared laser wavelengths. Patients should be aware that a series of (about five or six) treatments spaced one month apart may be necessary. We find that it takes more treatments to remodel acne scars than to remodel fine rhytids. Similar to rhytids, reevaluation occurs six months after an initial series of treatments. At that time, another round of treatment may be necessary. In contrast to dynamic skin lines, acne scar improvement appears to last much longer. Once the scar is remodeled, unless there is further inflammation, it is unlikely that further scarring will occur. We have follow-up records for over six years, and patients who have demonstrated improvement after the initial series of treatments maintain that improvement for many years. Nonablative laser skin resurfacing with a 1320 nm Nd:YAG laser can effectively improve the appearance of facial acne scars with minimal adverse sequelae and with long lasting results.

SUMMARY

Patients have become very interested and aware of minimally invasive therapies for skin rejuvenation. With longer work hours translating to less available time, most patients cannot afford the recuperation time required after more invasive therapies. Nonablative treatments have become the modality of choice for many patients.

The CoolTouch® 1320 nm pulsed Nd:YAG laser provides gradual improvement of skin tone with minimal morbidity, and an answer to many patients who seek to satisfy their desire for less rhytids, improved surface texture, and reduced acne scarring. With aging and the accompanying increase in facial skin laxity, acne scars become more prominent and adult patients often seek treatment for this as part of the rejuvenation process. A noticeable diminution of rhytids around the eyes, mouth, hands, cheeks, or the entire face can be achieved for 80% of patients with a series of CoolTouch® 1320 nm treatments while preserving the epidermis and skin color. Combination treatments with botulinum toxin type A, may lead to improved results.

There are no pigmentary changes with this wavelength as it is only absorbed by water. Thus, it is safe for all ethnic skin types. Risks of scarring or blistering are virtually nonexistent when the procedure is performed properly. Morbidity is extremely low, there is no downtime, and the procedures are quick and simple to perform with minimal parameters to manipulate. The treatment is highly effective for mild rhytids and acne scars, and has replaced much of ablative resurfacing. Combinations treatments with other methods of rejuvenation are commonly employed.

14

1540 and 1450 nm Noninvasive Rejuvenation

Murad Alam
Section of Cutaneous and Aesthetic Surgery, Department of Dermatology, Northwestern University, Chicago, Illinois, U.S.A.

Te-Shao Hsu
SkinCare Physicians, Chestnut Hill, Massachusetts, U.S.A.

Jeffrey S. Dover
Department of Medicine (Dermatology), Dartmouth Medical School, Hanover, New Hampshire, U.S.A.; Section of Dermatologic Surgery and Cutaneous Oncology, Department of Dermatology, Yale University School of Medicine, New Haven, Connecticut, U.S.A.; and SkinCare Physicians, Chestnut Hill, Massachusetts, U.S.A.

Kenneth A. Arndt
SkinCare Physicians, Chestnut Hill, Massachusetts, U.S.A.; Department of Dermatology, Harvard Medical School, Boston, Massachusetts, U.S.A.; Department of Medicine (Dermatology), Dartmouth Medical School, Hanover, New Hampshire, U.S.A.; and Section of Dermatologic Surgery and Cutaneous Oncology, Department of Dermatology, Yale University School of Medicine, New Haven, Connecticut, U.S.A.

Video 16: Noninvasive Rejuvenation

INTRODUCTION

Nonablative laser and light treatments, also known as photorejuvenation, have over the past five years largely co-opted traditional carbon dioxide and erbium (Er):YAG ablative resurfacing. Nonablative procedures purport to provide many of the same benefits as ablative procedures, without the protracted downtime associated with cutaneous re-epithelialization. As such, these minimally invasive therapies have become an accepted modality for reducing the visible signs of photodamage in young and middle-aged adults, and as a result, the number of devices available for this indication has proliferated. In this chapter, two nonablative lasers, the 1450 nm diode laser and the 1540 nm Er:glass laser are discussed. There are some preliminary studies to indicate that these lasers may have efficacy in the nonablative treatment of facial rhytides.

1540 nm ERBIUM:GLASS LASER

Laser Parameters

The 1540 nm Er:glass laser is a flashlamp pumped system that derives its midinfrared emission wavelength from a specific codoped Yb:Er:phosphate glass material. One variant of this device, the Aramis (Quantel Medical, Clermond-Ferrand, France) laser, can deliver up to 5 J in 3 ms. The operation is in either single shot mode or pulse-train configuration, with repetition rate up to 3 Hz (1). Contact cooling is delivered through a sapphire window. Another Er:glass device (Candela Corp, Wayland, Massachusetts), not commercially available in the United States, has been used at pulse energies up to 1.2 J, with a pulse-width of 1 ms; in pulse-train mode, the laser can be fired at 8 Hz (2).

Investigations of Efficacy for Nonablative Indications

Since this is a relatively new device used in dermatology and skin surgery, the number of published studies is limited. Among the earliest studies is one by Ross et al. (2), in which, the authors cite their earlier unpublished work on a farm pig model. When treated with the Er:glass laser, pig skin displayed partial epidermal preservation and significant dermal collagen denaturation and shrinkage. Despite the significant sparing of the dermis, and possibly because of the dermal effects, pitted scarring was observed after healing.

In their human protocol, Ross et al. (2) enrolled eight men and one woman, with an average age of 74. Seven postauricular sites (four on one side and three on the other) were irradiated in each patient, and in each patient, one side was treated with a single laser pass and the other with two passes. A control eighth site was treated with contact cooling alone. At each treatment site, the cooling tip was applied for two seconds at −10°C, followed by a series of laser pulses delivered at 8 Hz. Pulse energies ranged from 400 to 1,200 mJ, and when a second pass was applied, this was initiated three to five seconds after the completion of the first pass. Punch biopsies were obtained in the immediate postoperative period and at two months, and were processed with hematoxylin and eosin (H&E) staining.

Mordon et al. (1) conducted their study on the abdominal skin of male hairless rats, which have a superficial muscular layer 800 μm deep that permits easy analysis of potential thermal denaturation in the deep dermis. Different combinations of fluence and cooling were evaluated. Specifically, with regard to fluence, single 3 ms pulses of 26, 28, and 30 J/cm^2 were used; the fourth setting entailed a pulse train (1.1 J, 3 Hz, 15 and 30 pulses). Each of these fluences was tried separately with cooling of −5°C, 0°C, and +5°C. Biopsy specimens were obtained postoperatively at 24 hours, 3 days, and 7 days, and stained with H&E as well as Masson trichrome (for collagen), orcein (for elastic fibers), periodic acid Schiff (for fibrin), and with Alcian blue (for mucopolysaccharides).

Two more recent human studies have been performed by Fournier et al. (3) and Lupton et al. (4). In the former, Fournier et al. (3) provided a series of four treatments, six weeks apart, to four perioral and periorbital rhytides on each of the 60 patients (58 women), who had a mean age of 47 and Fitzpatrick skin types from I to IV. Perioral rhytides were treated with five passes (40 J/cm²) and periorbital rhytides with three passes, and in both cases, a fluence of (24 J/cm²) was used. All treatments were at 2 Hz. Measurement of results was by photography before, immediately after, seven days after, and six weeks after the first treatment, and before and six weeks after for the next three treatments. Skin biopsies using a 3 mm punch were harvested before, seven days after, three weeks after, and two months after a single treatment on each of the three patients. Pre- and postoperative ultrasound imaging and silicone imprints were also obtained.

Even more recently, Lupton et al. (4) treated 24 women, with mean age 47 and Fitzpatrick skin types I to II, who had mild to moderate periorbital and/or perioral rhytides. The overall approach was very similar to that used earlier by Fournier. Three consecutive monthly treatments were delivered. Each treatment entailed three passes to periorbital areas and five passes to perioral areas using a 2 Hz repetition rate, a 10 J/cm² fluence, a 3.5 ms pulse duration, and a contact cooling temperature of 5°C. Outcome measures included photographic and clinical assessment after each treatment, and at one, three, and six months following the final treatment. Additionally, 3 mm skin biopsies were obtained at baseline, immediately following the first treatment, and one and six months after the final treatment.

Clinical and Technical Outcomes

Mordon et al.'s (1) animal study revealed that single pulses were more likely to induce detectable epidermal damage than the pulse-train irradiation. With the pulse-train approach, epidermis and hair follicles remain intact after treatment, with the dermis showing homogenized changes and fibroblastic proliferation by day 3 to day 7. Typically, the dermal wound was 200 μm thick, and was centered between 250 μm and 300 μm deep in the skin.

On a global satisfaction scale of one to four (four being the optimum), six weeks after the final treatment, patients under the study by Fournier et al. (3) offered an average rating of 3.06, with 62% being satisfied (3) or very satisfied (4). Statistical analysis of the silicone imprints showed a significant decrease in anisotropy, or unevenness, from before treatment to after treatment. Ultrasound imaging performed 18 weeks after the first treatment confirmed a 17% thickening of the dermis. Histologic findings included decrease in dermal elastic fibers, and thickening and improved horizontal orientation of upper dermal collagen two months following treatment. Independent observers usually noted wrinkle improvement after the third procedure or six weeks after the entire treatment series, but none of the wrinkles completely disappeared.

Lupton et al. (4) measured clinical improvement on a different 4-point scale (1 = <25% improvement; 2 = 25–50% improvement; 3 = 51–75%

improvement; $4 = >75\%$ improvement). Six months posttreatment, patients rated their improvement at 1.6 and 1.3, respectively, in the periorbital and perioral areas; the corresponding ratings of a blinded reviewer were 2.1 and 2.0. On histology, mild tissue edema and inflammation were seen immediately after treatment, and six months after treatment, a mild increase in dermal fibroplasia was noted.

Adverse Effects

In general, adverse effects appear mild following the newer treatment approaches of Fournier and Lupton. Fournier et al. (3), incredibly, reported no side effects in any of the 222 patients treated except minimal pain in two of them. Lupton et al. (4) found mild transient erythema and edema in virtually all patients, with about 40% of them experiencing mild pain during treatment. A single patient had reactivation of oral herpes simplex infection.

Earlier investigators, who blazed the way with dose-finding experiments, obviously noted more significant side effects. Specifically, Ross et al. (2) saw not only posttreatment erythema and edema, but also epidermal whitening that occasionally devolved into erosions and ulcers. One to two months later, atrophic scarring and "pits" appeared at these sites. The authors noted that their treatment parameters resulted in peak dermal injury at about 1 mm depth, and this may have been too deep. Mordon et al. (3) support this conclusion by the result seen in their animal model, that deep dermal and muscle necrosis is directly proportional to temperature and fluence.

Significant eye injury is possible to the operator and patient when the 1540 nm laser is used, and therefore appropriate precautions should be taken. On the one hand, the 1540 nm wavelength does not penetrate the cornea well and consequently does not represent a threat to the retina. However, this system is not truly "eye-safe" since 1540 nm light is highly absorbed by the corneal stroma, and this absorption can cause significant damage to corneal tissue (5,6). A recent study, that irradiated rabbit corneas with a 1540 nm device (Laser Sight Technologies, Winter Park, Florida), found deep corneal injuries consistent with energies above $56 \, \text{J/cm}^2$ (7). Grossly, these injuries appear as white opacities, and they may herald permanent visual disability. While fluences used in nonablative applications are lower, caution is prudent as even the compilers of the American National Standards Institute (ANSI) standards appear oblivious of this risk (8).

Conclusions: Theory and Practice

Several general conclusions can be drawn from current research on nonablative treatments with the 1540 nm Er:glass laser.

 1. To optimize the dermal effect and clinical improvement associated with treatment, fluence and cooling parameters must be carefully

selected. Shorter cooling times will result in cooling confined to the superficial dermis, and a peak temperature zone that is shallow in the skin; longer or more intense epidermal cooling will push the peak temperature zone deeper into the dermis. As ablative resurfacing models, including medium-depth chemical peeling, dermabrasion, and carbon dioxide laser ablation, have revealed that dermal remodeling occurs at a depth of 100 to 400 μm from the skin surface, this is the layer that should be targeted for nonablative treatment (2). More recent studies have verified that dermal fibroplasia and collagen thickening in this region are associated with clinical improvement.

2. The Er:glass laser appears to emit light at a wavelength useful for inducing focal dermal injury (1). The human dermis absorption coefficient is such that light energy is predominantly deposited in the dermis when the incident wavelength is between 1.3 and 1.8 μm. This range includes the 1.32 μm Nd:YAG laser, the 1.45 μm diode laser, and the 1.54 μm Er:glass laser, the last one associated with the most dermal absorption and least dermal scatter. The Er:glass laser is also a useful device for nonablative treatment because its emission wavelength corresponds with a trough in the melanin absorption coefficient. Compared to the other midinfrared lasers, the 1540 nm laser is less absorbed by melanin, and thus is less prone to induce pigmentary side effects.

3. The mechanism underlying clinical improvement following nonablative treatment with the Er:glass laser is not well understood. It is possible that collagen in the upper dermis is increased and arrayed more horizontally; fibroblast proliferation has also been observed. These findings are similar to those seen with other nonablative devices, and it is not clear what specific effects, if any, the Er:glass laser has, compared to other lasers. Despite clinical confirmation of postoperative edema, routine mucin stains have not demonstrated this swelling to be associated with increased deposition of glycosaminoglycans (2).

4. This nonablative treatment can provide modest improvements in rhytides in certain patients, with minimal side effects. Wrinkles are not completely removed but may be softened. For most patients, treatment is associated with slight discomfort, and postoperative erythema and edema that resolves within a few hours or in a day or two. Multiple treatments seem necessary for clinical efficacy. In general, intermediate treatments are associated with lesser satisfaction of the patients, and therefore patients should be advised that a noticeable improvement, even if actually obtained, might not be evident until the treatment cycle is completed.

1450 nm DIODE LASER

Laser Parameters

The 1450 nm diode laser is a 14-watt device (Smoothbeam, Candela Corp., Wayland, Massachusetts) that also emits radiations in the midinfrared range. In investigational protocols, pulse widths of 160 to 260 ms have been used with a repetition rate of 0.5 to 1.0 Hz. Cooling is achieved via a dynamic cooling device (DCD), and laser energy is delivered through a 4 mm spot size (9).

Investigation of Efficacy for Nonablative Indications

This laser has been used both for treatment of facial rhytides and for treatment of active acne. Acne treatment can be considered as an extension of the nonablative applications of this laser, as the mechanism of directed dermal injury appears to be the same.

Very little published research is available regarding the nonablative efficacy of this laser, which is marketed as a nonablative device. Goldberg et al. (9), in a recent study involving 19 women and one man, who collectively spanned Fitzpatrick skin types I to IV and ranged in age from 42 to 70, treated Glogau class I and class II rhytides. In 12 subjects, the treated rhytides were periorbital, and in the remainder, they were perioral. Two to four treatment sessions, at one-month intervals, were performed for each patient. Unfortunately, Goldberg et al. (9) do not provide any treatment parameters such as fluence, pulse width, repetition rate, or number of passes. Outcome measures were pre- and postoperative photography, pre- and postoperative optical profilometry, and clinical assessment.

Additional studies are apparently under preparation. Tanzi, Alster, and Lupton (10–13) describe randomized studies in which patients received treatment to either the left or the right sides of their faces, with the contralateral side serving as a control. A study of 20 patients has examined treatment of transverse necklines, and the outcome measures have included a blinded rater assessment as well as in vivo microtopography (PRIMOS Imaging System; GFM, Germany). In this investigation, mean fluences of $11.6 \, \text{J/cm}^2$ were used with a 6 mm spot, and with cooling settings of 10 ms of precooling, 20 ms of intracooling, and 20 ms of postcooling. For the treatment of atrophic facial scars, 1450 nm diode laser has been compared to 1320 nm Nd:YAG laser, according to a pending study of 20 patients in which, the diode-treated side received fluences of 9 to 14 J/cm^2 via nonoverlapping 6 mm spots during a single pass.

Acne treatment with the 1450 nm device has been reported in studies that have targeted back acne. After recruiting 27 male subjects with back acne, Paithankar et al. (14) randomized a $36 \, \text{cm}^2$ area of skin on one side of each subject's back to be the treatment site, with an equivalent-sized area on the other side serving as a control treated with cryogen alone. Four treatments spaced three weeks apart were administered to the entire area of the treatment sites, rather than to just where acne form papules had been marked. The average treatment fluence was 18 J/cm^2. Apart from clinical assessments, outcome measures included lesion counts and skin biopsies immediately after treatment, and at 6-, 12-, and 24-week follow-up visits.

Clinical and Technical Outcomes

Goldberg et al. (9) found that 7 out of the 20 patients showed no obvious improvement after treatment, 10 experienced mild improvement, and three had moderate improvement at the sites of their laser-treated rhytides. Clinical improvement was correlated with optical profilometry findings but not with the number of treatments. Perioral sites showed the least improvement.

According to Tanzi, Alster, and Lupton (10–13), in left–right face studies, the treated sides have indicated clinical and histologic improvement of rhytides, but periorbital rhytides improved more. Three-dimensional in vivo microtopography confirmed this clinical finding. Moreover, the 1450 nm laser may be superior to the 1320 nm Nd:YAG device for nonablative treatment of atrophic facial scars.

Paithankar et al. (14) found a statistically and clinically significant reduction in acne lesion counts after treatment, and the mean reduction was five or more lesions. On completing their 24-week follow-up, 14 of the 15 patients had no residual acne lesions in the treated areas. Histologic findings were epidermal preservation, but rupture of the pilosebaceous unit and thermal coagulation of the sebaceous lobule and follicle. Given the low density of sebaceous glands on the back, these changes were not observed in many biopsy samples. The authors report that long-term follow-up biopsies of similarly treated back and face skin showed no difference from baseline in adnexal structures, including sebaceous glands and follicles. Significantly, research with shorter pulse diode lasers (810 nm) used in combination with indocyanine green (ICG) dye has indicated similar transient necrosis of sebaceous glands followed by long-term improvement of acne (15). The underlying mechanism of epidermal sparing and dermal injury is consistent with the nonablative paradigm, and different from aminolevulinic acid (ALA), photodynamic therapy (PDT) and other laser/light based acne treatments that achieve their effect by depopulating *Propionibacterium acnes*. Further studies of the treatment of facial acne are under way.

Adverse Effects

Immediate erythema usually occurs after nonablative use of the 1450 nm laser for treatment of facial rhytides. This can vary from mild to severe and may be concomitant with the emergence of small edematous papules, lasting one to seven days, which were first noted by Goldberg et al. (9). Postinflammatory hyperpigmentation is rare, and hypopigmentation, persistent erythema, and scarring are not reported.

After the use of this laser for nonablative treatment of acne, the side effects are similar (14). The hallmarks are erythema and edema, with mild to severe hyperpigmentation in about 10% of subjects. Purpura and scarring are absent.

Conclusions: Theory and Practice

There is a paucity of peer-reviewed data regarding the efficacy of the 1450 nm diode laser for nonablative treatment of rhytides. The few presumptive conclusions are as follows:

1. Multiple treatments with the 1450 nm diode laser may soften facial rhytides in some treated patients, but these reductions are typically modest (9).
2. The histologic mechanisms underlying the treatment of rhytides by this modality are not well described (9,14). Based on the action of the 1450 nm laser in the treatment of acne, the mechanism may include selective heating of the dermis and sparing of the epidermis. Acne improvement has been linked to transient sebaceous gland necrosis after laser treatment.

REFERENCES

1. Mordon S, Capon A, Creusy C, Fleurisse L, Buys B, Faucheux M, Servell P. In vivo experimental evaluation of skin remodeling by using an Er:glass laser with contact cooling. Lasers Surg Med 2000; 27:1–9.
2. Ross EV, Sajben FP, Hsia J, Barnette D, Miller CH, McKinlay JR. Nonablative skin remodeling: selective dermal heating with a mid-infrared laser and contact cooling combination. Lasers Surg Med 2000; 26:186–195.
3. Fournier N, Dahan S, Barneon G, Diridollou S, Lagarde JM, Gall Y, Mordon S. Nonablative remodeling: clinical, histologic, ultrasound, imaging, and profilometric evaluation of a 1540 nm Er:glass laser. Dermatol Surg 2001; 27:799–807.
4. Lupton JR, Williams CM, Alster TS. Nonablative laser skin resurfacing using a 1540 nm erbium glass laser. A clinical and histologic analysis. Dermatol Surg 2002; 28:833–835.
5. Allen RG, Polhamus GD. Ocular thermal injury from intense light in laser applications in medicine and biology. New York: Plenum Press, 1989:286.
6. Ham WT, Mueller HA. Ocular effects of laser infrared irradiation. J Laser App 1991; 3:19–21.
7. Clarke TF, Johnson TE, Burton MB, Ketzenberger B, Roach WP. Corneal injury threshold in rabbits for the 1540 nm infrared laser. Aviat Space Environ Med 2002; 73:787–790.
8. ANSI, American National Safety Standard for Safe Use of Lasers (ANSI Z136.1–1993). Orlando, FL: Laser Institute of America, Inc., 1993.
9. Goldberg DJ, Rogachefsky AS, Silapunt S. Non-ablative laser treatment of facial rhytides: a comparison of 1450-nm diode laser treatment with dynamic cooling as opposed to treatment with dynamic cooling alone. Lasers Surg Med 2002; 30:79–81.
10. Alster TS, Lupton JR. Are all infrared lasers equally effective in skin rejuvenation. Sem Cutan Med Surg 2002; 21:274–279.
11. Tanzi EL, Alster TS. Comparison of a 1450-nm diode laser and a 1320-nm Nd:YAG laser in the treatment of atrophic facial scars: a prospective clinical and histological study. Dermatol Surg 2004; 30:152–157.
12. Alster TS, Tanzi EL. Treatment of transverse neck lines with a 1450 nm diode laser. Lasers Surg Med 2002; 14(suppl):33.
13. Tanzi EL, Alster TS. Comparison of a 1450 nm diode laser and a 1320 nm Nd:YAG laser in the treatment of atrophic facial scars. Lasers Surg Med 2000; 27:1–9.
14. Paithankar DY, Ross EV, Saleh BA, Blair MA, Graham BS. Acne treatment with a 1450 nm wavelength laser and cryogen spray cooling. Lasers Surg Med 2002; 31:106–114.
15. Lloyd JR, Mirkov M. Selective photothermolysis of the sebaceous glands for acne treatment. Lasers Surg Med 2002; 31:115–120.

15

Intense Pulsed Light and Nonablative Approaches to Photoaging

Robert A. Weiss and Margaret A. Weiss
Department of Dermatology, The Johns Hopkins University School of Medicine,
Baltimore, Maryland, U.S.A.

Mitchel P. Goldman
Department of Dermatology/Medicine, University of California, San Diego,
California, U.S.A. and La Jolla Spa MD, La Jolla, California, U.S.A.

Video 17: Quantum SR/IPL

INTRODUCTION

One of the most controversial light-based technologies, first introduced for clinical studies in 1994, and cleared by the U.S. Food and Drug Administration (FDA) in late 1995 as the Photoderm™ (ESC/Sharplan, Norwood, Massachusetts, now Lumenis, Santa Clara, California), is the noncoherent filtered flashlamp intense pulsed light (IPL) source. It was initially launched and promoted as a radical improvement over existing methods for the elimination of leg telangiectasia, because of pressure from venture capital groups that funded its development in response to the perceived need for a new leg vein therapy. Another important feature recognized earlier was the IPL's ability, as a specific modality, to minimize the possibility of purpura common to pulsed dye lasers (PDL). In reality, the device turned out to be of far greater utility for indications other than leg telangiectasias. The road to usability, reproducibility, and good results was a long one. Ironically, it is now considered the gold standard for the treatment of many of the signs of photoaging.

The initial claims of IPL causing less purpura formations than short-pulsed PDLs have turned out to be true and have been confirmed by numerous investigators (1–10). Present day indications have expanded far beyond the treatment of leg veins to include hair removal, facial telangiectasias, virtually all skin vascular conditions, scarring, pigmentation, and poikiloderma of Civatte. The most recent addition in the realm of nonablative treatment of photoaging is known as facial rejuvenation or photorejuvenation (1–3,11,12).

The IPL device consists of a flashlamp housed in an optical treatment head with water-cooled reflecting mirrors. An internal filter overlying the flashlamp prevents wavelengths less than 500 nm from being emitted. Optically coated quartz filters of various types (cut-off filters) are placed over the window of the optical treatment head to eliminate wavelengths lower than that of the filter. Available cut-off filters are of 515, 550, 560, 570, 590, 615, 645, 690, and 755 nm. For faster recycling times, certain optical heads have water circulating around the flashlamp. Finally, to allow optimal transmission of light by decreasing the index refraction of light to the skin as well as promoting a "heat-sink" effect, filter crystals are optically coupled to the skin with a water-based gel.

Although Lumenis is the largest and most well known of the IPL device manufacturers, other manufacturers now supply pulsed light devices (Table 1). Because there exists virtually no peer-reviewed published data on these other devices, the subsequent discussion focuses on the Lumenis technology.

Table 1
Manufacturers and Brand Names of Intense Pulsed Light Device

Manufacturer	Brand name	Output	Spot sizes	Fluence (max.)
Lumenis (Santa Clara, California) (www.lumenis. com)	Photoderm^{TM} VL/PL	515–1200 nm	4 × 8 mm, 8 × 35 mm,	90 J/cm^2
	Epilight	590–1200 nm	10 × 45 mm	
	Lumenis One	1 Hz	8×15 mm and 15×35 mm	
	Multilight HR	515–1200 nm	2×6 mm,	
	Vasculight HR®	515–1200 and	2×9 mm	
	Quantum SR	1064 nm laser	560–1200 nm	
	Quantum HR	560–1200 and		
	Vasculight – SR®	1064 nm laser		
Energis Technology (Swansea, U.K.) (www.energiselite. com)	Energis Elite IPL	600–950 nm	10 × 50 mm	19 J/cm^2
Danish Dermatologic Development A/S, (Hørsholm, Denmark)	Elipse	Wavelength 400–950 nm	10 × 48 mm	22 J/cm^2
Medical Bio Care	OmniLight FPL	515–920 nm		45 J
OptoGenesis	EpiCool – Platinum	525–1100 nm		60 J
Primary Tech	SpectraPulse	510–1200 nm		10–20 J
Syneron	Aurora DS	580–980 nm		10–30 J/cm^2
Palomar (Burlington, Massachusetts)	EsteLux Y G	525–1200 nm 500–670/ 870–1400 nm		15 J 30 J
Alderm (Irvine, California)	Prolite	550–900 nm	10 × 20 mm and 20 × 25 mm	10–50 J

WAVELENGTH

The working premise for IPL is that noncoherent light, like many laser wavelengths, can be manipulated with filters to meet the requirements for selective photothermolysis. Thus, for a broad range of wavelengths, the absorption coefficient of blood in the vessel was higher than that of the surrounding bloodless dermis. When filtered, the Lumenis IPL device is capable of emitting a broad bandwidth of light from 515 to approximately 1200 nm. (Other IPLs have different wavelength outputs.) This bandwidth is modified by application of filters, which exclude the lower wavelengths. Although the output is not uniform across this spectrum and has been demonstrated beyond 1000 nm, it has been shown that during a 10 msec pulse, relatively high doses of yellow light at 600 nm are emitted, with far less red and infrared (4) (Fig. 1). The peak emission of the optical treatment head in the 600 nm region and other yellow wavelengths most likely facilitates selective absorption by bright red superficial vessels.

Filters presently applied for vascular lesions are 515, 550, 560, 570, and 590 nm. Longer filters of 615, 645, 695, and 755 nm, which cut-off much more of the yellow wavelengths, are used most commonly for photoepilation and, possibly, fibroblast stimulation. The key factor in using IPL successfully turned out to be not only filtering and eliminating the lowest wavelengths emitted by the flashlamp, but a limitless capacity to manipulate pulse durations and to couple these pulse durations with

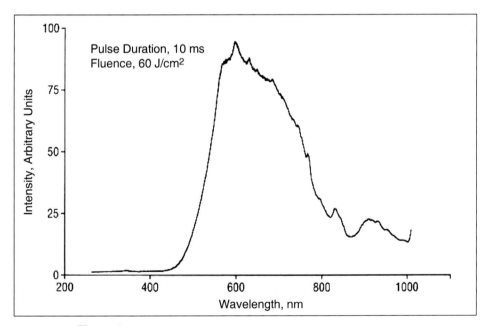

Figure 1
Emission spectrum of an intense pulsed light head with 515-nm filter at 10-msec pulse duration. Peak output shown by line is at 600 nm. *Source*: Courtesy of Laser Zentrum, Hannover, Germany.

precise resting or thermal relaxation times programmable in a Windows[TM] environment using C++. This has been termed as "multiple synchronized pulsing" by the authors.

Selectivity is theoretically obtained for deoxyhemoglobin throughout the 600- to 750-nm range. While oxyhemoglobin is characterized by a very high absorption coefficient up to 630 nm, absorption drops at longer wavelengths but rises again to a broad peak in the near infrared (800–900 nm) range (Fig. 2). The absorption pattern of deoxyhemoglobin is similar to oxyhemoglobin up to 600 nm, but absorption does not drop as fast as that of oxyhemoglobin at 600- to 750-nm. It has been shown that blue telangiectasias of the leg are only slightly more deoxygenated compared with red telangiectasias (13). In addition, by treating a vessel with multiple pulsing, oxygenated hemoglobin is converted to deoxygenated hemoglobin during the first portion of the sequential pulsing. Predictions were thus made that wavelengths in the 600- to 750-nm range were preferable for treating relatively deoxygenated blue leg telangiectasia.

An additional advantage of working at higher wavelengths is that longer wavelengths are absorbed less by melanin. Melanin absorption is greatest in the ultraviolet range (240–360 nm) and decreases steadily as a function of increasing wavelength. As absorption of light by skin is determined primarily by melanin, longer wavelengths not only penetrate more deeply, reaching relatively deeper blood vessels, but also avoid more non-specific melanin absorption with accompanying epidermal damage.

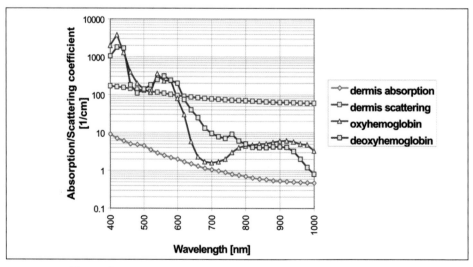

Figure 2

Absorption curve of hemoglobin in different states of oxygenation. Because collagen absorbs very little on its own, the primary components absorbing light are hemoglobin and melanin (melanin not shown). There is a zone from 600- to 750-nm in which deoxyhemoglobin has preferential absorption.

SPOT SIZE

Spot size plays a very important role in treating blood vessels of the legs, because spot size, along with wavelength, affects penetration depth. A small spot size leads to rapid scattering with a rapid decay of fluence by depth (14). Penetration is therefore more efficient with a large spot size. A depth of 4 mm should be attainable with the 8 × 35 mm rectangular spot size of the IPL device, considering an average wavelength of 800 nm (Table 2).

With a large spot size, a tremendous amount of light energy is delivered to the skin. The large planar front of light emitted by the large footprint IPL must be directed using a water-based interface between the crystal and the skin. The water-based gel serves critical functions of enhancing optical coupling, minimizing reflections, and maintaining continuity of the index of refraction of the skin–air interface. Clinical experience has also emphasized the role of gel as a heat sink. Heat is generated by near infrared wavelengths in the epidermis during the programmed 2 to 8 msec of the flashlamp pulse. Water-based gel is efficient at absorbing heat from the epidermis and without its use, the skin quickly overheats and protein denaturation of the epidermis occurs causing subsequent blistering. The gel may also be necessary as a filter for higher wavelengths. As water absorbs some wavelengths beyond 1000 nm, some of the ineffective or potential tissue damaging-near-infrared wavelengths may be removed prior to being absorbed by the target.

For treating deeper, larger vessels requiring a much higher fluence, one may more safely increase fluence, while protecting the overlying skin by chilling the gel. A general rule is that when working with the large footprint of IPL, a 1- to 2-mm layer of gel between the crystal and the skin is highly desirable (Fig. 3). This has been more recently termed "floating" the crystal on the gel and is the technique recommended when not using an integrated chilled crystal. In addition, the use of a refrigerated air cooling system with the topical gel provides even more comfort. The colder the gel, the more efficient it becomes as a heat sink.

Table 2
Spot Size vs. Wavelength

Spot size	Light penetration depth (595 nm)	Light penetration depth (800 nm)
1 mm	0.8 mm	1.5 mm
2 mm	1.1 mm	2.0 mm
5 mm	1.25 mm	2.5 mm

For 800 nm, the penetration appears to be half the diameter of the spot size. Therefore an 8-mm wide crystal should permit penetration down to 4 mm.
Source: Courtesy of ESC/Sharplan, Norwood, MA.

(A)   **(B)**

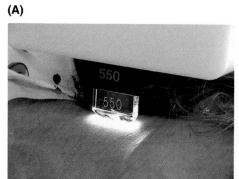 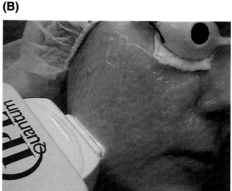

Figure 3
(**A**) Proper spacing of the crystal from the skin with a 2-mm layer of gel or floating the crystal in gel. If the crystal rests directly on the skin, the likelihood of epidermal injury is far greater. (**B**) With a Peltier cooling device incorporated into the crystal, the layer of gel required is much less.

PULSE DURATIONS (TABLES 3, 4, AND 5)

Allowing proper thermal relaxation time between pulses theoretically prevents elevation of epidermal temperatures above 70°C, and is an inherent advantage of "multiple sequential pulsing" of the IPL device. Thermal relaxation time is the amount of time taken for the temperature of a tissue to decrease by a factor of $\varepsilon = 2.72$ as a result of heat conductivity. For a typical epidermis of 100 micron thickness, the thermal relaxation time is about 1 msec. For a typical vessel of 100 (0.1 mm) and 300 (0.3 mm) microns, the thermal relaxation time is approximately 4 and 10 msec, respectively. Therefore vessels greater than 0.3 mm cool more slowly than the epidermis with a single pulse. For larger vessels, however, multiple pulses may be advantageous, with delay times of

Table 3
Suggested IPL Parameters for Leg Veins

Vein size (mm)	Filters (nm)	First pulse (msec)	Delay time (msec)	Second pulse (msec)	Fluence (J/cm^2)
< 0.2	550	2.4	10	2.4	25–35
0.2–0.5	550–570	2.4	15	4–6	25–40
0.6–1	570–590	2.4–3	15	6	30–40
1–1.5	570–590	2.4–3	15–25	7–12	35–45
1.5–2.0	590	8	20–50	8–12	40–60
Unresponsive at > 2 mm	590	Long pulse mode 12 msec	30–40 msec	Long pulse mode 12 msec	60–70

Table 4
Suggested IPL Parameters for Common Facial Vascular Lesions and Photorejuvenation

Vascular lesion	Filters (nm)	First pulse (msec)	Delay time (msec)	Second pulse (msec)	Fluence (J/cm^2)	No. of sequential pulses
Telangiectatic matting	550	2.4	10–15	4.0	22–30	Double
Nasal alae telangiectasia	570	2.4–3.0	10–15	5.0–7.0	32–44	Double
Hemangioma	570	2.4–3.0	10–20	6.0–8	32–42	Double
Poikiloderma	515, 550	1.5–2.4	10–20	2.4–4.0	22–36	Single or double
Photodamage—mild	550–570	2.4	10–20	4.0	25–38	Double
Photodamage—moderate (first treatment)	570–590	2.4	10–20	4.0–6.0	22–40	Double
Photodamage—severe	590 or higher	2.4–4.0	20–40	4.0–6.0	22–45	Double

10 msec or more between pulses for epidermal cooling. This delay time must be increased with larger vessels as thermal diffusion across a larger vessel elongates the thermal relaxation time. Multiple sequential pulsing with delay times permits successive heating of targeted vessel(s) with adequate cooling time for the epidermis and the surrounding structures.

These theoretical considerations imply the following: (1) vessels smaller than 0.3 mm should theoretically only require a single pulse, although a double pulse should have no adverse effect on treatment, (2) double or triple pulses should be spaced 10 msec or longer to accommodate normal epidermal thermal relaxation times, and that even safer might be a 15- to 20-msec thermal relaxation time (which is recommended for patients with skin types that are highly reactive to thermal damage such as Asian skin), (3) bright red lesions (oxyhemoglobulin) are better treated with 515 to 590 nm filters, (4) blue lesions (deoxyhemoglobulin) should be

Table 5
Suggested Parameters for IPL Photoepilation

Fitzpatrick skin type	Filter (nm)	Fluence (J/cm^2)	Pulse durations (msec)	Delay between pulses (msec)
II	615	39–42	3.3–5 (two pulses)	30
III	645	34–36	3.0 (three pulses)	30
IV	695	34–40	3.0 (three pulses)	40
V	695, 755	38–40	5–7 (two pulses)	50–60

treated with 590 nm or higher filters, (5) darker skin (melanin) should always be treated with the highest filter available, with double pulses, and accompanied by increasing delay times between pulses (typically 20–40 msec) to allow for increased skin thermal relaxation times. For example, treatment of melasma in an Asian skin individual would involve use of a 590 or 640 nm filter, double pulsed with 3 to 4 msec pulse durations, and use of fluence just enough to cause a slight pinkness of the treated areas.

The treatment of darker skin individuals (types IV–VI) and/or patients with hyper-reactive melanocytes becomes an increasing concern when performing photoepilation. In these cases, the 755 nm filter is used primarily with delay times between pulses from 50 to 100 msec to give plenty of time for the skin to cool down avoiding thermal damage.

CONCEPTS OF MULTIPLE SEQUENTIAL PULSING

The new concepts for IPL and what has most contributed to the success of the technique, are the ability to elongate pulse durations for larger vessels, to shorten pulse durations for smaller vessels, and to use these in a variety of combinations of synchronized short and long pulse widths. For many laser devices assessed to treat leg veins, a longer pulse duration (up to 50 msec) has led to better clinical results (15). For a small vessel (0.3 mm), heat distribution is assumed to occur instantaneously. For a larger vessel this cannot be assumed, because more time is required to have heat pass from just inside the superficial vessel wall through the vessel to the deeper wall. Additional cooling time is required to release the accumulated heat from the core to the vessel surface. These principles were demonstrated using double pulse experiments with the 585 nm yellow dye laser in which larger vessels of PWS (>0.1 mm) absorbed greater energy fluences before the development of purpura after double pulses spaced 3 to 10 msec apart (16). In another study using pulsed laser irradiation at 585 nm, pulse durations were chosen between short pulse (0.45 msec) and long pulse (10 msec) (17). From the results it was demonstrated that long-duration pulses caused coagulation of the larger diameter vessels, whereas small-caliber vessels and capillaries showed resistance to photothermolysis at these parameters. This concept has been termed *photokinetic selectivity*.

Applying this to IPL, we have found that increasing pulse durations for IPL up to 12 msec causes larger vessels (0.5 mm or greater) to undergo more effective clinical photothermal coagulation while sparing the epidermis (6). Obeying the principles of "thermokinetic selectivity" using IPL, we understand that the smaller overlying vessels in the papillary dermis do not absorb wavelengths efficiently at longer pulse durations, and thus cause less epidermal heating. Longer thermal diffusion times for larger vessels are best served with longer pulse durations for IPL.

The concept of double pulsing for larger telangiectasia is to allow pre-heating of vessels with absorption by smaller vessels with the first pulse. This allows the surrounding structures to cool. In addition oxygenated hemoglobin turns to deoxygenated form, which absorbs longer wavelengths. And, the larger vessel starts to retain heat. The secondcoupled, longer pulse then heats up the larger vessels further in the area under the crystal.

TREATMENT OF PHOTOAGING WITH IPL

Facial Telangiectasias

The treatment of facial telangiectasias is the foundation for treatment of photoaging by IPL. Clinical observations were made following treatment of facial telangiectasias, that is, skin texture became smoother. This observation was made by the authors while treating patients during the period 1995–1997. The authors found it easier to treat facial telangiectasias than leg telangiectasias, as they are generally more uniform in size and depth with a thinner overlying epidermis. Facial telangiectasia have a thinner vessel wall than leg veins making them more susceptible to endothelial thermal damage. Response is more predictable to with our clinical results approaching a 95% resolution rate of facial telangiectasias after one to three treatments. The parameters for IPL of facial telangiectasia include a double pulse of approximately 2.4 to 4 msec duration with a 550-nm filter in light skin and 570-nm filter in darker skin patients. Typical, delay times are 10 to 20 msec between pulses with 10-msec delay in light skin and 20 to 40 msec in dark and/or Asian skin. Fluences required are much less than that used for leg veins, typically between 28 and 35 J/cm². Higher fluences are used when the second pulse duration is greater than 4.0 msec so that a double pulse of 3.0 and 6.0 msec usually requires a fluence of 40 to 45 J/cm² to effectively treat a larger facial vessel (up to 1 mm diameter). The advantage of the IPL over the PDL is that with the large spot size an entire cheek of telangiectatic matting can be treated using less than a dozen pulses in less than five minutes (Fig. 4). In addition, there is little if any development of purpura. For either larger more purple telangiectasias typically seen on the nasal alae, or venous lakes or adult port-wine stains, the same settings as for small vessels of leg may be employed, that is, a short pulse followed by a long pulse.

Poikiloderma

A frequently seen manifestation of photoaging is poikiloderma of Civatte. This photoaging process presents an erythematous, pigmented, and finely wrinkled appearance that occurs in sun-exposed areas, mostly on the neck, forehead, and the upper chest. For areas of poikiloderma on the neck and lower cheeks consisting of pigmentation and capillary matting, the IPL device is ideal with use of a 515-nm filter, which allows absorption both by melanin and hemoglobin simultaneously (Fig. 5). For patients with more dyspigmentation, one begins with higher filters, such as the 550- or 560-nm filter, to prevent too much epidermal absorption, which would result in crusting and swelling of the skin lasting for several days.

(A)   **(B)**

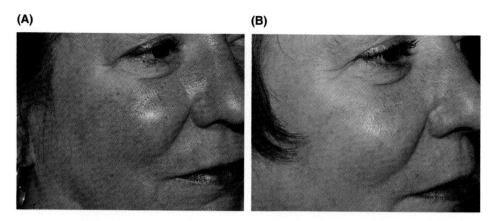

Figure 4
(**A**) Patient with rosacea and the entire cheek is treated with 30 pulses.
(**B**) Results after three treatments spaced one month apart.

Additional treatments with the IPL may be performed with a 550-, 560-, or 570-nm filter to treat the vascular component of poikiloderma. For patients with the most severe form of poikiloderma, one may need to begin with the 590 nm filter and use lower filters on subsequent treatments.

Treatment of poikiloderma is one of the most effective uses of the IPL technology (1). In a recent study, 135 patients randomly selected with typical changes of poikiloderma of Civatte on the neck and/or the upper chest were treated with one to five treatments using IPL. Parameters included the 515- and 550-nm filters with pulse durations of 2 to 4 msec, either single or double, with a 10-msec delay. Fluences were between 20 and 40 J/cm^2. Clearance over 75% was reported in both telangiectasia and hyperpigmentation. The total incidence of side effects was 5% including temporary hyper- and hypopigmentation. In many cases, improved skin texture was noted both by physician and by patient as a consequence of treatment. Possibly because of either the near infrared component of IPL and/or an interaction of blood vessels with release of various endothelial and fibroblastic growth factors, there appears to be a collagen remodeling effect with improved skin texture, reversing the cutaneous atrophy component of poikiloderma of Civatte.

Photorejuvenation

The overall appearance of aging skin is primarily related to the quantitative effects of sun exposure with resultant UV damage of structural components such as collagen and elastic fibers. Appearance, however, is also affected by genetic factors, intrinsic factors, disease processes such as rosacea, and the overall loss of cutaneous elasticity associated with age. With excessive sun exposure in addition to depletion of the ozone layer, visible signs of aging have become more evident in younger individuals. Photorejuvenation has been described as a dynamic nonablative process

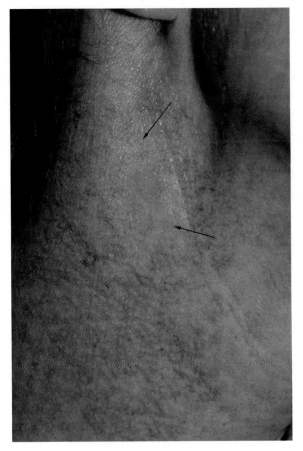

Figure 5
Treatment of poikiloderma of the neck. Initial treatment of a single 3-msec pulse, 25 J/cm^2, 515-nm filter shows clearance in area of two test pulses. Test area outlined in arrows.

involving the use of the IPL to reduce mottled pigmentation and telangiectasias, and to smooth the textural surface of the skin (2). The treatment is generally administered in a series of three to six procedures in three- to four-week intervals. The entire face is treated, rather than a limited affected area, and the patient may return to regular activities immediately. Marketing has made the public and medical community aware of these changes through various unsuccessfully applied service trademarks such as Photofacial, Fotofacial, Facialite, and others. An example of photorejuvenation of photoaging is shown in Figure 6 .

Zelickson and Kist (20,21) have demonstrated that IPL treatment results in an 18% increase in collagen Type-1 transcripts, whereas PDL treatment results in a 23% increase in collagen Type-1 transcripts. This may explain the improvement in fine wrinkling with photorejuvenation. A further investigation demonstrated that collagen I, III, elastin, and

(A)   **(B)**

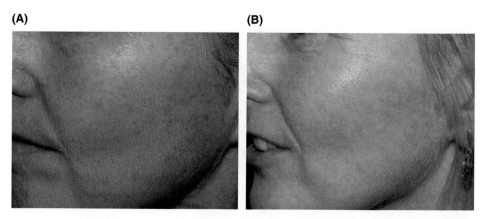

Figure 6
Photorejuvenation (**A**) before and (**B**) after three treatments. Excellent reduction of the photoaging components of mottled pigmentation, telangiectasias,
and smoothing of the textural surface of the skin.

collagenase increased in 85% to 100% of patients and procollagen
increased in 50% to 70% of patients.

Hernandez-Perez and Ibiett (22) evaluated the histologic effects of
five IPL treatments with 570 to 645 nm, 2.4 to 6.0 msec, delay 20 msec,
and 25 to 42 J/cm^2. They showed epidermal thickening of 100 to 300 μm,
better cellular polarity, a decrease in horny plugs, new rete ridge formation, decreased elastosis, and dermal neocollagen formation.

However, Prieto et al. (23) in a histologic study in patients with
rosacea did not see evidence of changes in collagen, elastic, or reticular
fibers, but did note coagulated demodex, which recurred after three
months. They treated patients at the following parameters: 560 nm, 2.4
to 4.2 msec, 15-msec delay, 28 to 36 J/cm^2, and five times every month.

Negishi et al. (24) treated 73 patients in five sessions with the Quantum IPL every three to four weeks at the following settings: 560 nm, 2.8
to 6.0 msec, 20- to 40-msec delay, and 23 to 27 J/cm^2. The authors also
showed that 80% of Japanese patients had greater than 60% improvement
in pigmentation and erythema with smoother skin. The Quantum IPL
has an integrated skin cooling crystal that cools the epidermis to 40°C
during IPL and 65°C without cooling.

With the original IPL, Negishi et al. (25) reported photorejuvenation in 97 Japanese patients using 550- to 570-nm cut-off filters (550
and 570 nm for pigment and telangiectasia, respectively). Patients were
treated three to six times at two- to three-week intervals with IPL at settings of 28 to 32 J/cm^2, 2.5 to 4.0/4.0 to 5.0 msec, 20- to 40-msec delay
without topical anesthesia. The authors noted that 49% had greater than
75% improvement in pigmentation with 33% having greater than 75%
improvement in telangiectasia and 13% having a greater than 75%
improvement in skin texture. Approximately 50% of the other patients
had a greater than 50% improvement in these parameters as well. There

were no episodes of hyperpigmentation including four patients with melasma. Histologic evidence of collagen and elastic fiber proliferation in papillary and subpapillary layer was present in the biopsies taken at the end of the study.

The treatment of freckling is also improved with IPL photorejuvenation. Huang et al. (26) used 550 to 590 nm filters with 25 to 35 J/cm^2, 4 msec single or double pulse, 20- to 40-msec delay time, one to three treatments (mean 1.4) at 4-week intervals. Their endpoint consisted of graying or perilesional erythema. A 91.7% of patients were extremely/very satisfied with treatment. Kawada et al. (27) also treated freckling and lentigos in Asian skin. They utilized a Quantum IPL at the following parameters: 560 nm, 20 to 24 J/cm^2, 2.6 to 5.0 msec, 20-msec delay, three to five treatments at two- to three-week intervals. No adverse effects were seen, and patients reported that small patches and ephelides responded best (48% greater than 50% improvement; 20% greater than 75% improvement).

Weiss et al. (28) evaluated 80 of their initial patients treated for vascular lesions to determine if "photorejuvenation" also occurred. Images from three subsequent visits including one follow-up at four years were graded. There was an 80% improvement in pigmentation, telangiectasia, and skin texture. Hypopigmentation lasting for one year occurred in 2.5%, temporary mild crusting occurred in 19%, erythema for more than four hours in 15%, hypo- or hyperpigmentation in 5%, and rectangular footprinting in 5%.

In a recent study, 49 subjects with varying degrees of photodamage were treated with a series of four or more full-face treatments at three-week intervals using IPL (Vasculight^{TM} IPL, Lumenis, Santa Clara, California). Fluences varied from 30 to 50 J/cm^2 with typical settings of double or triple pulse trains of 2.4 to 4.7 msec with pulse delays of 10 to 60 msec. Cut-off filters of 550 or 570 nm were used for all treatments (2). Photodamage, including wrinkling, skin coarseness, irregular pigmentation, pore size, and telangiectasias, was improved in more than 90% of the patients. Treatments involved IPL of the entire facial skin except in males, who elected to avoid treatment of the beard area because of potential hair loss. In this study, 72% of subjects reported a 50% or greater improvement in skin smoothness, and 44% reported a 75% or greater improvement. Minimal side effects were reported with temporary discoloration consisting of a darkening of lentigines, which resolved completely within seven days. Two subjects reported a "downtime" of one and three days because of moderate to severe swelling.

The use of IPL with a thermoelectrically chilled crystal delivery system (Quantum SR) on 20 patients for photorejuvenation has also been evaluated (29). These patients underwent three monthly IPL treatments on the face, neck, and/or anterior chest. A 560-nm cut-off filter was used with a double pulse of 2.4 and 6.0 msec separated by a 15-msec delay time. Fluences ranged from 26 to 30 J/cm^2. Telangiectasia improved in 84% of patients, dyspigmentation in 78%, and skin texture in 78%. Side effects were minimal and consisted of localized edema in 50% for less than eight hours and erythema lasting from 2 to 24 hours.

The dual-mode filtering IPL system, Elipse Flex DDD was evaluated in 20 women for facial photorejuvenation (30). First, areas of telangiectasia were treated with a pulse duration of 14 to 30 msec. A second pass was then made with a double pulse of 2.5 msec with a 10-msec delay. Two types of filters were used, 530 to 750 nm at an energy of 11 to 17 J/cm^2 and 555 to 950 nm at a fluence of 13 to 19 J/cm^2. Both groups reported significant improvement in both telangiectasia and pigmentation without adverse sequelae.

Combination IPL Photorejuvenation

Photorejuvenation may also be enhanced with combination procedures, such as the use of IPL with 1064- and 1320-nm Nd:YAG laser treatments (31,32), microdermabrasion (33), and the use of botulinum toxin A (Botox®, Allergan, Irvine, California) (34). Muscle relaxation with botulinum A allows for parallel collagen formation over a static dermis. The use of 1064-, 1320-, and 1450-nm wavelengths causes significant structural change in the dermis, which can enhance new collagen formation, further reducing wrinkling.

Miscellaneous Pigmentation

In addition to hyperpigmentation from photodamage as described in the preceding section, other forms of pigmentation have been successfully treated with IPL. Nineteen Chinese patients ranging in age from 8 to 51 years with postburn hyperpigmentation were treated in three to seven sessions with 550, 570, and 590 nm filters at the following parameters:1.7 to 4 msec, 15- to 40-msec delay, 28 to 46 J/cm^2 (35). A 7 greater than 50% improvement was seen in 78 % of the patients 32% greater than 75% improvement, and 2/19 had no improvement. There was no recurrence during the 11 to 32 months of follow-up.

PSR

The combination of IPL and photodynamic therapy sensitizers, such as 5-amino levulinic acid (ALA) (Levulan, DUSA Pharmaceuticals, Wilmington, Massachusetts), allow for new options in the treatment of severely photodamaged skin (36), and may offer a significant cosmetically beneficial alternative to photodynamic treatments with blue light for such conditions as actinic keratoses (37), early skin cancers (38), and cystic acne (39).

We have termed this advanced technique as photodynamic skin rejuvenation (PSR). The PSR application of PDT involves activation of a specific photosensitizing agent, ALA, by the conventional intense pulsed light provided by the VascuLight or Quantum system. This process produces activated oxygen species within cells, thus resulting in their elimination or destruction. The topically active agent, ALA, is the precursor in the heme biosynthesis pathway of protoporphyrin-9, which facilitates cellular destruction. Exogenous administration of ALA, along with 410-nm continuous blue light, has been FDA cleared for the treatment of actinic keratosis and appears to have significant long-term efficiency (40). However, in clinical practice, a variety of light sources has been used in photodynamic therapy in an effort to reduce downtime and discomfort for patients and to enhance the clinical and cosmetic outcome of the procedure. Alexiades-Armenakas and co-workers (41) were the first to describe the use of 595-nm pulsed light with ALA to treat actinic keratoses. Advantages over blue light therapy were a decrease in pain during treatment as well as post-treatment erythema and crusting.

As 595 nm is not an optimal peak of absorption for ALA, a broader wavelength such as that found with the IPL should be even more efficacious in activating ALA. IPL treatments are under study for such enhanced benefits of photodynamic therapy (42). Short duration PDT, using Levulan for 15 to 60 minutes, coupled with IPL has shown significant benefit in the treatment of precancerous conditions such as actinic keratoses as well as actinically damaged skin. Additionally, early evidence shows a significant degree of cosmetic enhancement (Fig. 7).

Other variations of the procedure under study involve single IPL treatments with higher fluences and longer application times, resulting in dramatic decreases in actinic damage with a relatively short duration of healing. Additionally, initial studies show promise in application of topical ALA and IPL skin treatments using photorejuvenation, in conditions such as moderate to severe acne and rosacea. The mechanism for improvement in acne and rosacea is because of the enhanced absorption of ALA by sebaceous glands. This enhanced absorption followed by photoactivation with IPL, damages the sebaceous gland causing its involution. A decrease in the size and/or activity of the sebaceous gland then leads to an improvement in acne.

(A)　　　　　　　　　　　　　　　　　　**(B)**

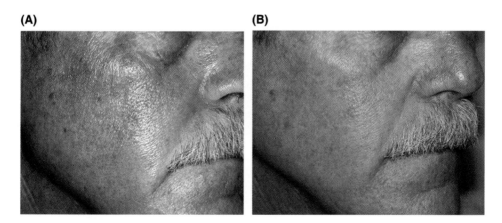

Figure 7
(**A**) Extensive photodamage and actinic keratosis in a 55-year-old man.
(**B**) Six months after treatment with ALA applied to the entire face and left on for 1 hour followed by IPL to the entire face with a 560-nm filter, 32 J/cm^2, double pulse of 3.0 and 6.0 with a 10-msec delay time.

In addition, combination of the IPL procedure with pharmacologic treatments, such as metronidazole topical cream (Metro Cream®, Galderma Laboratories), has resulted in significant overall levels of success in the treatment of rosacea (43). The combination of IPL treatment with a variety of depigmenting agents such as Trilumena®, (Galderma Laboratories) has also resulted in a greater resolution of melasma (44).

TREATMENT TECHNIQUE

Photorejuvenation

Floating Technique

For nonchilled crystals, a thick layer of gel must be placed onto the crystal and absolutely no pressure applied as the crystal is placed over the target area, floating the crystal in gel. Compressing this 2- to 3-mm layer of gel against the skin will result in crystal placement too close to the skin, thus, greatly increasing the risks of epidermal injury. Plastic spacers are available to increase the uniformity of distance of crystal and thickness of gel, although most users simply float the crystal by holding the weight of the IPL head in their hands.

To minimize rectangular footprinting, a 10% overlap of pulse placement is used or, alternatively, a second pass may be performed with the direction 90° from the original direction.

Close Contact Technique

To minimize pain and to facilitate uniform treatment from operator to operator, contact cooling or epidermal anesthetic creams were utilized. Attaching a cooling device, which surrounds the crystal, has been shown to produce better results with fewer side effects (12). Cooling is maintained by circulating water at 1°C through the metal collar around the crystal. The newest devices incorporate a chilled crystal, which is kept in close contact with the skin, while only a small layer of chilled water-based gel is placed between the crystal and the skin. Fluence must be lowered. With absolutely minimal pressure, the cooling device with the crystal is placed directly onto the skin overlying the targeted area. No pressure is applied as the target vessels may shut with compression. EMLA anesthetic cream is not used before treatment as there is a high incidence of vasoconstriction produced by the prilocaine component of EMLA. LMX 5% lidocaine (Ferndale Labs, Ferndale, Michigan) is a better choice, but is usually requested by 50% of the patients when using lower fluences and the direct contact method of the chilled crystal.

ADVERSE REACTIONS

During our initial clinical trials with IPL, three patients with tanned legs developed immediate desquamation of the epidermis resulting in hypopigmentation (2.5%), lasting for four to six months in two patients and one year in the third with no permanent pigment change. This occurred at $40 \, J/cm^2$ with a single pulse of 3 msec. No reaction like this has been observed on the face. No long-term sequelae were noted.

In our subsequent experience with thousands of treatment sessions, there has been about a 2% incidence of scattered areas of crusting in areas of increased pigmentation. This typically heals within seven days by peeling off. We accelerate this process by having the patients apply a moisturizer twice a day and/or undergo a treatment with microdermabrasion one to two days after IPL treatment. When there is no underlying pigmentation, crusting occurs primarily on curved body areas such as the neck over the sternocleidomastoid muscle curvature. Purpura occurs in scattered, isolated pulses in about 4% of treatments. Purpura is more likely when the 515-nm filter is used or when the pulse durations are too short, such as coupling a 2.4-msec pulse duration, with another 2.4-msec pulse duration. The purpura from IPL is different than typical short pulse PDL purpura in that resolution occurs within two to five days as opposed to the one to two week purpura seen with PDL treatment.

Other adverse effects of IPL include a stinging pain described as a brief grease splatter, electric shock, or rubber band snapping on the skin during treatment. Typically patients tolerate over 150 pulses per session. Treatment pain can be minimized by a number of topical anesthetic creams such as LMX (lidocaine 4%) (Ferndale Labs, Ferndale, Michigan); EMLA is not used. Occasionally a thin nontreated stripe between reticular footprints can be seen (Fig. 8). This is easily corrected with subsequent treatment applying the crystal over the nontreated sites or proceeding with treatment using the crystal rotated 90° from the original direction. In the past eight years, we have observed very few patients in whom small rectangular spots of hypopigmentation at the

(A) **(B)**

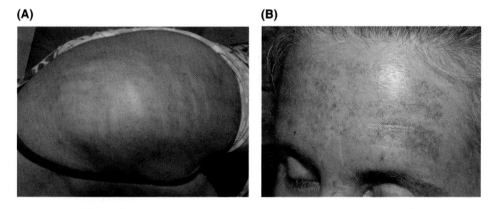

Figure 8
(**A**) Rectangular footprints because of fluence too high for the pulse duration selected. (**B**) Crusting, a side effect which clears within several days to a week. This only occurs when an erythematous rectangular footprint is observed immediately posttreatment.

lateral neck margins have persisted at the end of two years. This was preceded by epidermal desquamation.

With the newest progressive set of parameters, the incidence of acute side effects has been markedly reduced. Side effects include a mild burning sensation, lasting less than 10 minutes noted in 45%, and erythema, which typically lasts several hours to three days. Mild cheek swelling or edema occurs 25% of the time with full-face treatments primarily after the initial treatment, and lasts from 24 to 72 hours. Short-term hyper- or hypopigmentation (greater than two months) has been noted in approximately 8% to 15% of sites treated.

REFERENCES

1. Weiss RA, Goldman MP, Weiss MA. Treatment of poikiloderma of Civatte with an intense pulsed light source. Dermatol Surg 2000; 26(9):823–827.
2. Bitter PH. Noninvasive rejuvenation of photodamaged skin using serial, full-face intense pulsed light treatments. Dermatol Surg 2000; 26(9):835–842.
3. Goldberg DJ, Cutler KB. Nonablative treatment of rhytids with intense pulsed light. Lasers Surg Med 2000; 26(2):196–200.
4. Raulin C, Schroeter CA, Weiss RA, Keiner M, Werner S. Treatment of port-wine stains with a noncoherent pulsed light source: a retrospective study. Arch Dermatol 1999; 135(6):679–683.
5. Jay H, Borek C. Treatment of a venous-lake angioma with intense pulsed light [letter]. Lancet 1998; 351(9096):112.
6. Weiss RA, Weiss MA, Marwaha S, Harrington AC. Hair removal with a non-coherent filtered flashlamp intense pulsed light source. Lasers Surg Med 1999; 24(2):128–132.
7. Raulin C, Schroeter C, Maushagen-Schnaas E. Treatment possibilities with a high-energy pulsed light source (PhotoDerm VL). Hautarzt 1997; 48(12):886–893.
8. Raulin C, Weiss RA, Schonermark MP. Treatment of essential telangiectasias with an intense pulsed light source (PhotoDerm VL). Dermatol Surg 1997; 23(10):941–945.
9. Raulin C, Goldman MP, Weiss MA, Weiss RA. Treatment of adult port-wine stains using intense pulsed light therapy (PhotoDerm VL): brief initial clinical report [letter]. Dermatol Surg 1997; 23(7):594–597.
10. Schroeter C, Wilder D, et al. Clinical significance of an intense, pulsed light source on leg telangiectasias of up to 1 mm diameter. Eur J Dermatol 1997; 7:38–42.
11. Sadick NS, Weiss RA, Shea CR, Nagel H, Nicholson J, Prieto VG. Long-term photo-epilation using a broad-spectrum intense pulsed light source [In Process Citation]. Arch Dermatol 2000; 136(11):1336–1340.
12. Weiss RA, Sadick NS. Epidermal cooling crystal collar device for improved results and reduced side effects on leg telangiectasias using intense pulsed light. Dermatol Surg 2000; 26(11):1015–1018.
13. Sommer A, Van MP, Neumann HA, Kessels AG. Red and blue telangiectasias. Differences in oxygenation? Dermatol Surg 1997; 23(1):55–59
14. Keijzer M, Jacques SL, Prahl SA, Welch AJ. Light distributions in artery tissue: Monte Carlo simulations for finite-diameter laser beams. Lasers Surg Med 1989; 9(2):148–154.
15. Adrian RM. Treatment of leg telangiectasias using a long-pulse frequency-doubled neodymium:YAG laser at 532 nm. Dermatol Surg 1998; 24(1):19–23.
16. Dierickx CC, Casparian JM, Venugopalan V, Farinelli WA, Anderson RR. Thermal relaxation of port-wine stain vessels probed in vivo: the need for 1–10 millisecond laser pulse treatment. J Invest Dermatol 1995; 105:709–714.
17. Kimel S, Svaasand LO, et al. Differential vascular response to laser photothermolysis. J Invest Dermatol 1994; 103(5):693–700.
18. Goldman MP, Eckhouse S. Photothermal sclerosis of leg veins. ESC Medical Systems, LTD Photoderm VL Cooperative Study Group [see comments]. Dermatol Surg 1996; 22(4):323–330.
19. Green D. Photothermal sclerosis of leg veins [letter; comment]. Dermatol Surg 1997; 23(4):303–305.
20. Zelickson B, Kist D. Pulsed dye laser and photoderm treatment stimulates production of type-I collagen and collagenase transcripts in papillary dermis fibroblasts [Abstract]. Lasers Surg Med 2001; 13(suppl):33.
21. Zelickson B, Kist D. Effect of pulse dye laser and intense pulsed light source on the dermal extracellular matrix remodeling [Abstract]. Lasers Surg Med Abstract 2000; 12(suppl):17.

22. Hernandez-Perez E, Ibiett EV. Gross and Microscopic Findings in Patients submitted to nonablative full face resurfacing using intense pulsed light. Dermatol Surg 2002; 28: 651–655.

23. Prieto VG, Sadick NS, et al. Effects of intense pulsed light on sun-damaged human skin, routine, and ultrastructural analysis. Lasers Med Surg 2002; 30:82–85.

24. Negishi K, Wakamatsu S, et al. Full-face photorejuvenation of photodamaged skin by intense pulsed light with integrated contact cooling. Lasers Surg Med 2002; 30:298–305.

25. Negishi K, Tezuka Y, Kushikata N, Wakamatsu S. Photorejuvenation for Asian skin by intense pulsed light. Dermatol Surg 2001; 27:627–632.

26. Huang, et al. Intense pulsed light for the treatment of facial freckles in Asian skin. Dermatol Surg 2002; 28:1007.

27. Kawada A, Shiraishi H, et al. Clinical improvement of solar lentigines and ephelides with an intense pulsed light source. Dermatol Surg 2002; 28:504–508.

28. Weiss RA, et al. Rejuvenation of photoaged skin: 5 yr results with IPL. Dermatol Surg 2002; 28:1115.

29. Beasley KL, Weiss RA, Weiss MA. New parameters for intense pulsed light rejuvenation with a thermoelectrically chilled crystal delivery system. Cosmet Dermatol 2002; 15: 14–16.

30. Troilius A, Bjerring P, Dierickx C, Christiansen K. Photorejuvenation with a double exposure procedure using a new IPL system. Laser Surg Med 2002; 14(suppl):29.

31. Goldberg DJ, Whitworth J. Laser skin resurfacing with the Q-switched Nd:YAG laser. Dermatol Surg 1997; 23:903–907.

32. Fatemi A, Weiss MA, Weiss RA. Short-term histologic effects of nonablative surfacing: results with a dynamically cooled millisecond-domain 1320 nm Nd:YAG laser. Dermatol Surg 2002; 28:172–176.

33. Tan MH, Spencer JM, Pires LM, Ajmeri J, Skover G. The evaluation of aluminum oxide crystal microdermabrasion for photodamage. Dermatol Surg 2001; 27(11):943–949.

34. Fagien S, Brandt F. Primary and adjunctive use of botulinum toxin type A in facial aesthetic surgery. Clin Plast Surg 2001; 28:127–148.

35. Sun Ho, et al. Prospective study on the treatment of postburn hyperpigmentation by IPL. Lasers Surg Med 2003; 32:42.

36. Ruiz-Rodriguez R, San-Sanchez T, Cordoba S. Photodynamic photorejuvenation. Dermatol Surg 2002; 28:742–744.

37. Fritsch C, Goerz G, Ruzicka T. Photodynamic therapy in dermatology. Arch Dermatol 1998; 134:207–214.

38. Kalla K, Merk H, Mukhtar H. Photodynamic therapy in dermatology. J Am Acad Dermatol 2000; 42:389–413.

39. Hongcharu W, Taylor CR, Chang Y, Aghassi D, Suthamjariya K, Anderson RR. Topical ALA-photodynamic therapy for the treatment of acne vulgaris. J Invest Dermatol 2000; 115(2):183–192 (PMID: 10951234).

40. Fowler JF, Zax RH. Aminolevulinc acid hydrohloride with photodynamic therapy: efficacy outcomes and recurrence 4 years after treatment. Cutis 2002; 69:6S.

41. Alexiades-Armenakas M, Kauvar ANB, et al. Laser-assisted photodynamic therapy of actinic keratoses. Lasers Surg Med 2002; 14(suppl):24.

42. Gold MH. The evolving role of aminolevulinic acid hydrochloride with photodynamic therapy in photoaging. Cutis 2002; 69:6S.

43. Dahl MV, et al. Topical Metronidazole maintains remission of rosacea. Arch Dermatol 1998; 143:679–683.

44. Taylor SC, Torok HM, et al. Efficacy and safety of a new triple combination agent for the treatment of facial melasma. Cutis. In press.

45. Raulin C, Werner S, Hartschuh W, Schonermark MP. Effective treatment of hypertrichosis with pulsed light: a report of two cases. Ann Plast Surg 1997; 39(2):169–173.

46. Gold MH, Bell MW, Foster TD, Street S. Long-term epilation using the EpiLight broad band, intense pulsed light hair removal system. Dermatol Surg 1997; 23(10):909–913.
47. Schumults CD, Goldberg DJ. Blinded comparison of two intense pulsed light (IPL) systems for hair removal: clinical efficacy and complication rate. Lasers Surg Med 2003; 15(suppl):31.
48. Weiss RA, Weiss MA. Early clinical results with a multiple synchronized pulse 1064 nm laser for leg telangiectasias and reticular veins. Dermatol Surg 1999; 25(5):399–402.

16

Advanced Sclerotherapy: The Sclerosing Foam

Alessandro Frullini

Studio Flebologico, Incisa Valdarno, Florence, Italy

Video 18: Sclerosing Foam

What is important the most is the concentration inside the vein, not in the syringe.
　　—R. Tournay (1949)

INTRODUCTION

This famous axiom from Raymond Tournay (1), the French father of sclerotherapy, continues to be valid even a fifty years after its first enunciation, and the recent advance of foam sclerotherapy, puts these words in a new light. With the sclerosing foam (SF), it is possible for the first time, to achieve full control on drug concentration inside the vein and on the time of contact between the sclerosing agent and the endothelium (2).

The idea of using air and drug in combination is quite old; Egon Orbach (3) from Berlin, later from New Haven (U.S.A.), in 1944 employed this in his "air block" technique which used sodium tetradecyl sulphate (STS). The method has been extensively used in the following years only in the treatment of telangiectasias, because it was found that in larger veins, the air present in the upper part of the vessel impeded full contact between STS and the vein inner wall.

The idea was to create an air meniscus, which could separate blood and the injected bolus. In his early reports, Orbach stated that "the method improved the rate of success of sclerotherapy by 10%" without significant complications, if the amount injected was below 3 cc (4).

Subsequently, it was determined that the method worked well only in smaller veins, and is still in use for the treatment of telangiectasias.

In 1993, Juan Cabrera, a Spanish vascular surgeon from Granada, proposed the use of CO_2 mixed with STS or polidocanol (POL) in order to form a therapeutic foam (2). This represented a true revolution in the stagnant world of sclerotherapy: from the time of Orbach, only three major achievements (injection–compression technique according to Fegan, use of

317

POL as a sclerosing agent by Henschel, and echo-guided sclerotherapy) (5–7) represented a true step forward in the treatment of superficial venous insufficiency. Even though many doctors were capable of treating saphenous insufficiency with sclerotherapy, until then surgery was considered the gold standard of treatment for superficial varicosities in most medical institutions, sclerotherapy played a role only in the management of minor varicosities (8).

The possibility of permanently eliminating the saphenous trunk and its collaterals with a single injection, with low costs, no hospitalization, no anesthesia, and a virtually painless treatment, has completely changed the perspective of varicose vein treatment.

Many authors subsequently reported different methods for foam production.

In 1997, Alain Monfreux (9) reported a technique utilizing a glass syringe and a sterile plug to produce a weak foam. Two years later, Patrick Benigni and Symon Sadoun (10–12) presented their personal technique to produce POL foam with a disposable syringe.

In 1999, Mingo-Garcia (13,14) reported on the "Foam medical system," a specially designed device that he had utilized to prepare a good quality foam.

The year 2000 represented a turning point in foam sclerotherapy: Lorenzo Tessari (15) presented his three-way tap technique which was capable of extemporarily preparing a very good foam with extremely reduced cost. The clinical trials immediately gave very encouraging results, and the foam gained popularity among doctors and patients (16–20).

In the same year, I presented my personal method (Frullini method) (21) which was capable of generating foam with characteristics similar to the Tessari's one; later G. Gachet (22) reported another technique.

In the meantime, the pharmaceutical companies started to show interest in foam and at present, a British company is developing a well-standardized "industrial grade" microfoam which could represent the ultimate foam for varicose vein treatment.

FOAM AND SF

Sclerotherapy is a therapeutic process triggered by the injection of drugs capable of transforming the wall of a varicose vein into a fibrotic cord. The typical end point of sclerotherapy should be permanent occlusion, but this does not always occur with liquid sclerosants. The main factors for insufficient sclerotherapy are the size of the vein and the impossibility to control blood flow inside it, during injection.

With classical liquid sclerosants, the injection of a volume of drug inside a vein segment raises the inner drug concentration to a peak, then there is a plateau, and finally a lowering of the drug/blood ratio. The shape of the curve is ruled by the speed of injection, the ratio of injected volume/size of the vessel, and by the blood flow. Sclerosis will be triggered only if the level of drug concentration decreases below a threshold or what I call "minimal effective concentration," for a sufficient period of time.

In a telangiectasia, we can expect a linear rise and then a relatively long plateau; at this stage only the drug will be present inside the telangiectasia.

In a 10 mm great saphenous vein (GSV) segment with a significant ostial reflux and large reentry perforators, even with the use of echo-guided sclerotherapy and large needles (e.g., 20 gauge), the peak will be reached slower than in the previous example. The concentration of the sclerosant in that vein segment will be related to the drug dilution and to all hemodynamic phenomena that occur during the sclerosing time (e.g., respiration, leg movements, etc.).

This can explain why sclerotherapy has never been a problem of drug power for telangiectasia and why saphenous sclerosis has always been difficult.

The introduction of SF has completely changed this perspective: when foam is injected, it forms a coherent bolus inside the vein. Due to its properties, this bolus has a controlled and uniform concentration, and can be controlled in site for a definite time. This will lead to optimal and, for the first time, controlled sclerosis.

Foam is a nonequilibrium dispersion of gas bubbles in a relatively small volume of liquid which contains surface-active macromolecules (surfactants). These preferentially adsorb at the gas/liquid interfaces and are responsible for the tendency of a liquid to convert into foam and for the stability of the produced dispersion (23–26).

The SF is a mixture of gas and a liquid solution with tensioactive properties; the gas must be well tolerated or physiologic, and the bubble size should be preferably below 100 microns. The behavior of a SF is different when injected, if compared to the action of a liquid solution (19).

The most common mistake made with regard to foam is to consider it as a single entity. In fact, according to the method chosen, it is possible to produce very different foams, with different characteristics, complication rate, and therapeutic indications.

We can classify foams by the bubble's diameter

1. Froth more than or equal to 1 mm
2. Foam more than 100 microns
3. Minifoam less than 100 and more than 50 microns
4. Microfoam less than 50 microns

or by the relative quantity of liquid (the shape is the result of the competition between surface tension and interfacial forces)

1. Wet foam (nearly spherical bubbles – wetness or the volume fraction of liquid is over 5%)
2. Dry foam (polyhedral bubbles – the volume fraction of liquid is below 5%).

Wet foam has the maximum stability because when the bubble is polyhedral there is a increased competition between surface tension and interfacial forces. Uniform diameters also mean more stability because smaller bubbles empty in to larger ones according to Laplace law. Extemporary SF, like Monfreux's one, often have a bimodal expression: it acts as dry foam with polyhedral bubbles in the very first moments after generation, then when dissolution of bubbles creates a wetter environment, the foam assumes characteristics of a wet foam with spherical bubbles. More standardized SF (e.g., Tessari's foam) appears to be wet even in the initial stage. This gives more stability and uniformity (Figs. 1 and 2).

According to the range of variation of diameter, we can also classify foams as:

1. High standardization (industrial grade)
2. Medium standardization
3. Poor standardization.

The foam is always in evolution, even when it seems very stable. Several factors introduce disorder in nonequilibrium systems where drainage (draining of liquid from foam), disproportionation (change in bubble size distribution), and coalescence (fusion of bubbles) will lead to dissolution. This can be slowed in several ways but, for medical use, therapeutical properties are more important than lasting time.

Another important aspect of foam is its response to forces or rheology: in fact, the SF exhibits striking mechanical properties because it elastically resists to pushing if this is made gently (as inside a vein) or reacts

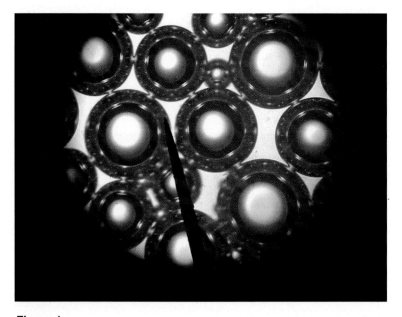

Figure 1
Optical microscope appearance of a wet foam produced with STS 3% Monfreux method (later stage) (120×).

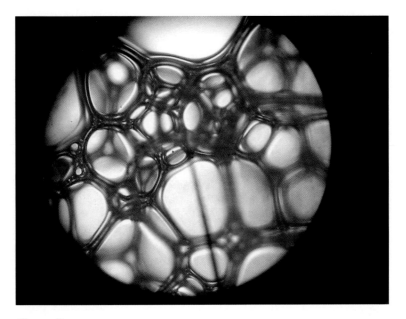

Figure 2
Optical microscope appearance of a dry foam produced with STS 3% Monfreux method (earlier stage) (120×).

as a liquid if pushed forcefully in a syringe (syringeability); so a foam can exhibit features of different basic states of matter.

SF shows peculiar properties: adhesiveness and compactness (with the possibility of manipulating the foam after injection and displacing effect on blood), syringeability (or possibility of being injected with a small needle without losing its characteristics), greater volume for the same quantity of liquid agent (possibility to treat longer vein segment), long duration (long enough for therapeutical action), enhanced spasm generation (less risk of blood collection inside the sclerosed vein), echovisibility, enanhcement of sclerosing power with reduced drug dose and concentration, and selectivity of action on endothelium (lesser risk in case of extravasation).

Again, it must be stressed that each property has a different expression according to the type of foam, where only industrial grade highly standardized foam shows the best properties, safety, and results.

TECHNIQUES FOR SF PREPARATION

Apart from Orbach technique that we do not consider to produce true foam, the very first report of a foam was from the Spanish vascular surgeon Juan Cabrera in 1997 (27,28). He never exactly explained the method for preparation because he patented it and sold it to a company that has developed his technique (Varisolve®, Provensis, U.K.). We only know that it was produced with a specially designed device which was capable of forming extemporarily a sterile, high-standard microfoam with CO_2. Large quantities of foam were injected under Duplex control with immediate deambulation.

Cabrera's foam has been perfected by Provensis and its launch in the market is estimated in the near future.

Later in 1997, Alain Monfreux from Toulouse (France) described his technique (MUS technique): A 3-cc glass syringe with a small quantity of POL or STS was closed with a sterile plug and the piston was gently pulled and held in tension for one to two minutes. The air slowly entered through the interface between the piston and the body of the syringe generating the foam (9). This had a relatively large size of bubbles and was quite dry; the resulting shape of bubbles in the very first seconds after the injection was polyhedral, and the mechanical properties were poor. Notwithstanding this, several positive reports appeared in literature, with encouraging results in treatment of telangiectasia and large veins (29–33). No severe complications were reported, but the system was not for single use; therefore in 1999, Sica and Benigni (34) presented a new method of injection using a disposable syringe. Unfortunately, their foam had a very short lifetime and so this method of injection was not very practical.

In 1999, Garcia Mingo (14) presented the results of the "Foam medical system," a special device where 1% to 1.5% POL and helium (1:10 ratio) were employed to produce microfoam, which was then probably cooled.

Dr. Garcia cannulated the saphenous trunk and collaterals first, elevated the leg to empty the superficial network, and then started foam infusion.

Garcia Mingo reported good results, but at this moment, I am not aware of any other doctor utilizing a similar device.

In December 1999, Dr.Lorenzo Tessari demonstrated his three-way tap method to Dr. Attilio Cavezzi and me. We suddenly realized that this method was superior to all extemporary foam methods used till then moment. We started a pilot-study in February 2000 and then a larger trial in order to evaluate its safety and outcome (17).

To produce Tessari's foam with STS, a three-way stopcock is needed, coupled with 2.5 and 5 mL syringes. The first is filled with 0.5 cc of drug, the second with 2 to 2.5 mL of atmospheric air. Taking care not to detach the syringes (I the keep the third unutilized way of the tap in firm contact with a solid surface in order to avoid any detachment), 20 quick passages of the solution are made. After the first 10 passages, the tap is narrowed to the maximum level possible. This will form foam of a high quality and consistence, especially when STS is utilized and if the silicone contents of the syringes are low. Even if Dr. Tessari has popularized the method using a long catheter for injection, I don't advice this way of foam administration. When using foam the site of delivery is not important because foam forms a coherent bolus which migrates inside the vein, under total echographic control, even for long segments. Moreover, the exposure to the relatively wide inner

Table 1
Different Characteristics of Sclerosing Foams

Author	Type	Wetness	Standard	Compactness	Duration time
Cabrera	Microfoam	Wet	Very high	High	Long
Monfreux	Foam	Dryer	Very low	Low	Long
Sadoun	Foam	Wet	Low	Low	Very short
Tessari	Minifoam	Wet	High	High	Long
Frullini	Minifoam	Wet	High	High	Long
Gachet	Foam	Dryer	Low	Low	Very short

surface of the catheter, will interfere with the structure of the SF altering its characteristics.

In 2000, I presented a different method; I generated the foam in a vial of sclerosing solution, providing that the vial had a rubber cap (21). A small connector was used in the original description to couple the syringe and vial, but it is easily possible to perforate the rubber cap with the syringe prefilled with air. A minimum of five passages is generally necessary to create a good foam (similar to Tessari's one). It is necessary to choose the size of the vial and the syringe properly (a 50 mL vial cannot be coupled with a 1 mL syringe!).

Foam generation is due to the Venturi effect that occurs when a fluid (liquid detergent) is forcefully passed through a narrow passage.

A precise definition of the physical properties and characteristics of different foams has not been published, but for practical purpose, it is possible to summarize as in Table 1.

CLINICAL APPLICATIONS OF FOAM SCLEROSANTS

Foam has been already employed in almost every field of phlebology (19). Moreover, new and exciting indications have been tried with success. I will try to make an analysis of the reported data for the most common indications.

SF in Telangiectasias and Reticular Veins

J.P. Henriet (30), in 1997, first reported about the utilization of foam of POL in telangiectasias. He started using it in 1995 and reported more than 22,000 injections in 3200 patients utilizing Monfreux's method.

POL concentration was in the range of 0.1% to 0.2% and the foam amount produced was 3 mL. Good results were reported in a nonobjective manner stressing the low complication rate and the advantages of the technique.

Two years later, the same author published another report on more than 10,263 patients (about 70,000 injections) (30–33).

POL concentration was in the range of 0.3% to 0.4 % for reticular veins and 0.1% to 0.2% for telangiectasias. No serious side effects were reported.

In 1999, Sadoun and Benigni published the result of a pilot-study in a small group of patients with lateral thigh telangiectasia, comparing liquid 0.25% POL with the same drug in a foamy form. Again, the Monfreux method was employed to prepare the SF . In this group, an enhanced power was observed for SF even with a higher rate of minor local complications.

In 2001, Frullini et al. (17) and Tessari et al. (18), published a pilot-study on Tessari's foam produced with STS. A subgroup was represented by small varicosities. Good results were reported, but again with an unexpected rate of minor local complications.

From my experience, it is clear that telangiectasia is the worst indication for Tessari's SF at this moment; this type of treatment is too powerful to be employed in every telangiectasia. Moreover, the adhesiveness and compactness of SF. produce a longer contact with endothelium keeping the foam for a very long time in situ. I generally prefer to use liquid sclerosants, i.e., POL for standard telangiectasias. POL foam (or very seldom STS one) is reserved for resistant cases of telangiectatic matting that, on the contrary, is a very good indication for SF made with POL foam 0.1% to 0.25%. Reticular veins can be treated quite safely with POL foam 0.2% to 0.3% and spasm generation is always very satisfactory.

Due to its lower compactness, Monfreux foam is the most appropriate for use in telangiectasias. Thicker foams such as Tessari's or Frullini's are difficult to push into these small vessels. On the contrary, dry foam such as as Monfreux's can be injected easily in telangiectasia; and as it has a lower power, can be handled more safely. The treatment is performed as usual, but larger quantity of product can be used in a single injection, because the foam has the same activity at the site of injection as well as away from it. There is no risk of having a diluted and then inactive drug as when liquids are employed.

When using smaller needles (e.g., 30 gauge), the treatment is sometimes disturbed by a flow of foam that covers the tip of the needle (this phenomenon is more frequent when a disposable syringe technique is adopted). To avoid this, care has to be taken to push the piston very gently progressing with little steps. In this way, blanching of the vessel without the quick backflow of blood will be observed.

This spasm generation is then controlled and when the contact time between the foam and the endothelium is sufficient, I promptly massage the field in order to push away the foam.

This means that in treating telangiectasia with foam, the *time factor* is essential in avoiding complications; with liquid sclerosants time of exposure rarely has a definite role (only in prolonged injections that should anyway be avoided in case of liquid sclerosants). With foam, it is possible to control this time and generate a perfect spasm in the treated area. Obviously, this also means that with improper time of exposure, local complications will be more frequent than with liquids.

SF for Saphenous Trunks and Collaterals

The first series on Cabrera's microfoam was published in 1997, and was the report of 261 GSVs treated with echo-guided injection of standardized microfoam (2). The method has been already described in a Spanish publication in 1993 (35).

In 1999, the first paper in English literature on foam sclerotherapy was published (31) and in 2000, Frullini and Cavezzi (32) presented their results on 167 large veins treated with echosclerosis-utilizing foam. In the same year, Cabrera et al. (36) presented the first report on the long-term result of foam sclerotherapy. In a retrospective analysis, 500 insufficient GSVs were treated with POL 1% to 3% microfoam. Refluxing GSV was detected at five years in only 14% and disappearance of all superficial branches was reported in 96.5%.

Apart from Cabrera's technique that is currently developed by Provensis (U.K.) with the name of Varisolve® and that will be available in the near future, the treatment with STS or POL foam is generally performed in saphenous trunk with echo-color-Doppler (ECD) guide.

The ideal patient for the treatment is over 60 years old, preferably with an inguinal recurrence or a GSV smaller than 10 mm (measured in the standing position) who does not wish to have the leg operated on. In my opinion, younger patients can be treated with surgery, but in case they refuse it is ideal to treat them with sclerotherapy.

For case of inguinal cavernoma or GSV insufficiency, I perform a thorough ECD, examination with the patient in standing position. Then I ask the patient to lie down and I reexamine the injection site echograpically.

I prefer to inject the GSV at the upper third of the thigh with a plain 20 gauge needle or a small cannula, but the injection can be given more distally. When using foam there is no need for a long catheter as that would worsen the quality of the foam and would transform a simple procedure into a cumbersome and expensive one.

When the saphenic reflux is to be directed into a large thigh collateral from a short, insufficient segment of GSV, I often use a small cannula positioned in the collateral and inject after elevating the leg. This helps in emptying the vein segment to be treated.

A compression is never made at the groin on the sapheno-femoral-junction (SFJ) during the injection, because the blood must flow freely from the area I want to treat and that is to be filled with foam. A lace positioned in this site would hamper the emptying of GSV leaving some blood at the junction. On the contrary, on echograpic visualization, the compression is applied just when the foam is visualized at the SFJ or immediately after injection and spasm generation.

STS 1% to 1.5% and 2% to 3% POL are usually chosen to prepare a thick foam with the Tessari's or Frullini's method. To my knowledge, 8 mL of this foam is not associated with serious complications and is enough in most cases of GSV insufficiency less than 9 mm. Larger veins could occasionally need more concentrated liquid or greater quantity of foam. Anyway, I recommend that no more than 10 mL of foam be used.

This is a safety warning that must be kept in mind when using extemporary foam. Industrial-grade foam can be used safely in larger volumes, but the coalescence rate of even the best extemporary foam is a definite risk in injections of more than 10 mL of foam.

Eccentric compression is then applied to the entire limb with proper pads fixed with non-wowen-adhesive bandage, and a 30- to 40-mm stocking. I instruct the patient to walk immediately after the procedure and then to walk frequently during the following week (at least two hours on day 1). Stocking and pads are kept for 48 hours and subsequently, only the stockings (but not pads) are removed during the night.

SF for Recurrences

The definition of recurrent varicose veins includes three distinct situations: (i) the true recurrence where at duplex examination neovascolarization is observed in the site of a previous ligature and division, (ii) the untreated segments in a limb where proper treatment has been administered in a different superficial venous network, and (iii) the progression of the disease with development of new varices.

In any case, this is the best indication for SF. Patients with recurrences are often older than patients asking treatment for the first time, and those who are sometimes disappointed by previous surgery.

Surgery for recurrent varicose veins has a higher incidence of complications and recovery is generally longer than for primary cases (29).

Injection of SF in neovascularization (e.g., inguinal cavernoma) has a high rate of success due to higher endothelial sensitivity and to the lower thickness of the venous wall (37). Moreover, tortuosity of these vessels makes control on foam manipulation easier.

My preferred method of treatment for inguinal neovascularization includes echo-guided injection right in the cavernoma at the groin or at the upper thigh (the rule is easiest access for best safety). I am not really concerned about the amount of foam that passes into the deep system at the neo-junction, because if for a standard size cavernoma, 3 mL of foam is used due to tortuosity and high compliance vessels with their typically tiny wall, only an insignificant amount of sclerosing material will pass during the injection in femoral vein. Moreover, just after removal of the needle, I apply a gentle pressure on the inguinal crease pushing the foam downward into the collateral branches.

Sometimes the "starry sky" picture can be seen in the femoral vein or the echographic imaging of sclerosing product in the deep vein. This has never been associated with complications and is to be considered, in my opinion, only the visualization of something common for every sclerosant injection, but not commonly seen when foam is not used.

The preferred drug for recurrences is STS 1% to 2%. The drug is injected immediately after foam production, and therefore everything must be ready at that moment. Surprisingly, the simple injection of a cavernoma usually suffices to treat all the limb collaterals. This is due to the mono-reflux system that often is present in surgical recurrences.

The compression protocol is the same for saphenous trunks and patients are reviewed after seven days. A second injection is generally given at that time only in case of failure to demonstrate occlusion, but this occurs very rarely. Additional injections on collaterals are generally given later if still necessary.

The necessity for long-term compression in these limbs has to be stressed. Up to six months of treatment with a a 30- to 40-mm stockings are necessary to improve skin condition and to help sclerosis to become optimal.

SF for Miscellaneous Indications

Foam has been already used in the treatment of vascular malformations with excellent results by Cabrera and by others (28–38).

Foam injections have also been tried in the treatment of pelvic varicocele (39). Further field of applications will be certainly suggested in the near future as SF could be injected in virtually every vessel through a vascular catheter. Considering that SF has a specific selectivity and its action can be confined to small segments, it will be interesting to determine a potential role for foam in occlusion of bleeding vessels or in cases where ischemic necrosis is sought for (e.g., metastatic liver).

COMPLICATIONS WITH SF

When we consider the complications of the treatment with foam, it is necessary to be precise which kind of foam has been used.

It is most important to understand that it is not possible to list all the complications of foam, but we can only report the complications seen with the use of different foam.

Obviously, the standard will be the SF which has a lower rate of complications. On the contrary, low quality foam will be associated with higher risk of complications, even if the indication and the technique of administration are correct.

The first concern of foam users was the effect of injected gas inside the vein. Much experimental work has been done in the past on animals in defining the extrapolated lethal dose of air (40,41).

The main observations from these works were that air can be injected safely in small amounts. Larger doses need a longer time for administration. It was postulated that the lethal dose of injected air for a 60-kg human was 480 mL injected in 20 to 30 seconds.

SFs made with atmospheric air are generally administered with a total volume below 8 mL. Rarely a 10 mL injection is necessary, and I never advice the use of this volume for a medium or low standard foam (e.g., Monfreux foam). The coalescence rate in those foams is so high that significant air embolism could occur.

Minor complications have often been reported with foam. These are similar to those seen with liquid sclerosants, with the exception of telangiectasias treatment, where pigmentation and skin necrosis have been reported even from experienced doctors. This is due to the higher sclerosing power of foam (19–32).

Among major complications, partial deep vein thrombosis (DVT) has been reported. In every case, DVT was asymptomatic and without sequelae at three months (31). A similar rate of DVT has been reported in the surgery of varicose veins (42). Unfortunately, varicose veins patients treated with classical sclerotherapy are rarely studied with duplex immediately after the treatment as the patients treated with echo-guided injection. Therefore, it is difficult to have similar data on the incidence of DVT after classical sclerotherapy.

Anyway, lowering the concentration of the sclerosing drug used for foam generation and generally avoiding large volume injections in the short saphenous vein (SSV) (less than 2 mL) will be extremely important in lessening the chance of a DVT. This has to be considered a rare and generally limited complication, but the need for routine ECD controls after treatment has to be stressed.

CONCLUSIONS

Lower limbs varicose veins are not to be simply considered as defects that have to be removed. Instead venous insufficiency is a disease, genetically inherited and jeopardized from improper lifestyle.

To cure this disease in a permanent way is a utopia, but control on the clinical situation can be simply obtained with the therapeutic tools we have today.

The choice between the best treatments in every clinical situation is always debatable. SF only adds a new extraordinary therapeutical tool. The near future will tell us if industrial foam will be the best and the least invasive treatment for superficial venous insufficiency.

Notwithstanding this, I still believe that the best treatment will be only able to control venous insufficiency in a given moment. The maintenance of this control has a key role in keeping the patient free of the so-called *recurrences* or, in my opinion, what is best called the *uncontrolled progression of the disease.*

REFERENCES

1. Stemmer R. Studio fisico dell'iniezione sclerosante. In: Tournay R, ed. Terapia Sclerosante delle varici. Raffaello Cortina Editore, Milano: 1984:65–72.
2. Cabrera Garrido JR, Cabrera Garcia-Olmedo JR, Garcia-Olmedo Dominguez MA. Elargissement des limites de la schlérothérapie: noveaux produits sclérosants. Phlébologie 1997; 50(2):181–188.
3. Orbach EJ. Sclerotherapy of varicose veins: utilization of intravenous air block. Am J Surg 1994:362–366.
4. Orbach E. Vene Varicose. In: Samuels S, ed. "Le Malattie Vascolari" Società Editrice Universo 1958.
5. Fegan WG. Continous compression technique of injecting varicose veins. Lancet 1963; 20:108–112.
6. Hofer AE Sklerosierungstherapie bei varizen Arztl Prax 1967; 19/99:2–3.
7. Knight RM, Vin F, Zygmunt JA. Ultrasonic guidance of injections into the superficial system. In: Davy A, Stemmer R, ed. Phlébologie. John Libbey Eurotext Ltd, 1989: 339–341.
8. Neglen P. Long saphenous stripping is favored in treating varicose veins. Dermatol Surg 2001; 27:901–902.
9. Monfreux A. Traitement sclérosant des troncs saphènies et leurs collatérales de gros calibre par la méthode MUS Phlébologie. 1997; 50(3):351–353.
10. Benigni JP, Sadoun S, Thirion V, Sica M, Demagny A, Chahim M. Télangiectasies et varices réticulaires. Traitement par la mousse d'Aetoxisclérol a 0.25%. Présentation d'une étude pilote. Phlébologie 1999; 3(52):283–290.
11. Benigni JP, Sadoun S. Teleangiectases and foam sclerosing agent. In: Henriet JP, ed. Foam Sclerotherapy—State of the Art. Paris: Editions Phlébologique Francaises, 2002:57–60.
12. Sadoun S. Description de deux techniques pour fabriquer de la mousse sclérosant. Phlébologie 2001; 54(4):357–360.
13. Mingo Garcia J. Esclerosis venosa con espuma: foam medical system. Revista Espanola de Medicina y Cirugia Cosmética 1999; 7:29–31.
14. Garcia Mingo J. "Foam medical system" a new technique to treat varicose veins with foam. In: Henriet JP, ed. Foam Sclerotherapy—State of the Art. Paris: Editions Phlébologique Francaises, 2002:45–50.
15. Tessari L. Nouvelle technique d'obtention de la sclero-mousse. Phlébologie 2000; 53(1):129.
16. Cavezzi A. Duplex guided sclerotherapy of long and short saphenous vein with sclerosing foam. In: Henriet JP, ed. Foam Sclerotherapy—State of the Art. Paris: Editions Phlébologique Francaises, 2002: 61–71.
17. Frullini A, Cavezzi A, Tessari L. Scleroterapia delle varici degli arti inferiori mediante schiuma sclerosante di Fibro-vein® con il metodo Tessari: esperienza preliminare. Acta Phlebologica 2000; 1:43–48.
18. Tessari L, Cavezzi A, Frullini A. Preliminary experience with a new sclerosing foam in the treatment of varicose veins. Dermatol Surg 2001; 27:58–60; 1:55–72.
19. Frullini A, Cavezzi A. Sclerosing foam in the treatment of varicose veins and teleangiectases: history and analysis of safety and complications. Dermatol Surg 2002; 28:11–15.
20. Cavezzi A. Sclérotherapie à la Mousse (méthode Tessari): étude multicentrique. Phlébologie 2002; 55(2):149–154.
21. Frullini A. New technique in producing a sclerosing foam in a disposable syringe: the Frullini method. Derm Surg 2000; 26:705–706.
22. Gachet G. Une nouvelle méthode simple et économique pour confectionner de la mousse pour sclérose échoguidée. Phlébologie 2001; 54(1):63–65.

23. Durian DJ. Foam mechanics at the bubble scale. Phys Rev Lett 1995; 75:4780–4783.
24. Durian DJ. Bubble scale model of foam mechanics: melting, nonlinear behavior and avalanches. Phys Rev 1997(E55):1739–1751.
25. Durian DJ. Relaxation in aqueous foams. Bull Material Res Soc 1994; 19:20–23.
26. Cipelletti L, Ramos L. Slow dynamics in glasses, gels and foams. Curr Opin Coll Interface Sci 2002; 7:228–234.
27. Cabrera J Jr, Garcia Olmedo MA, Dominguez JM, Mitasol JA. Microfoam: a novel pharmaceutical dosage form for sclerosants. In: Henriet JP, ed. Foam Sclerotherapy—State of the Art. Paris: Editions Phlébologique Francaises, 2002: 17–20.
28. Cabrera J. Application techniques for sclerosant in microfoam form. In: Henriet JP, ed. Foam Sclerotherapy—State of the Art. Paris: Editions Phlébologique Francaises, 2002:39–44.
29. Frullini A. Sclerosing foam in the treatment of recurrent varicose veins. In: Henriet JP, ed. Foam Sclerotherapy—State of the Art. Paris: Editions Phlébologique Francaises, 2002:73–78.
30. Henriet JP. Un an de pratique quotidienne de la sclérothérapie (veines reticulaires et téleangiectasies) par mousse de polidocanol: faisabilité, résultats, complications. Phlébologie 1997; 50(3):355–360.
31. Cavezzi A, Frullini A. The role of sclerosing foam in ultrasound guided sclerotherapy of the saphenous veins and of recurrent varicose veins: our personal experience. Australian and New Zealand J Phlebology 1999; 3(2).
32. Frullini A, Cavezzi A. Echosclérose par mousse de tétradécylsulfate de sodium et de polidocanol: deux années d'espérience. Phlébologie 2000; 53(4):431–435.
33. Henriet JP. Expérience durant trois années de la mousse de polidocanol dans le traitement des varices réticulaires et des varicosités. Phlébologie 1999; 52(3):277–282.
34. Sica M, Benigni JP. Echosclérose à la mousse: trois ans d'expérience sur les axes saphéniens. Phlébologie 2000; 53(3):339–342.
35. Cabrera Garrido JR, Cabrera Garcia Olmedo JR, Garcia Olmedo Dominguez. Nuevo metodo de esclerosis en las varices tronculares. Pathol Vasc 1993; 1:55–72.
36. Cabrera J, Cabrera J Jr, Garcia-Olmedo MA. Treatment of varicose long saphenous veins with sclerosant in microfoam form: long term outcomes. Phlebology 2000; 15: 19–23.
37. Vin F. La sclérotherapie écho-guidée dans les récidives variqueuses post-opératoires. Phlébologie 1995; 48:25–29.
38. Takashi Yamaki, Motohiro Nozaki, Osamu Fujiwara, Eika Yoshida. Duplex guided foam sclerotherapy for the treatment of the symptomatic venous malformations of the face. Dermatol Surg 2002; 28:619–622.
39. Leal-Monedero J, Zubicoa Ezpeleta S. The role of sclerosing foam in the treatment of pelvic congestion syndrome. In: Henriet JP, ed. Foam Sclerotherapy—State of the Art. Paris: Editions Phlébologique Francaises 2002:79–84.
40. Harkins HN, Harmon PN. Embolism by air and oxygen: comparative studies. Proc Soc Exp Biol Med 1934; 32:178.
41. Richardson HF, Coles BC, Hall GE. Experimental gas embolism: intravenous air embolism. Toronto Can Med Assoc J 1937; 36:584–588.
42. Puttaswamy V, Fisher M, Neale M, Appleberg M. Venous thromboembolism following varicose vein surgery: a prospective analysis. Abstract of The Australian and New Zealand Society of Phlebology Annual Scientific Meeting, May 5–6 2001. J Vasc Surg (Accepted for publication).

17

Principles and Technique of Ambulatory Phlebectomy

Albert-Adrien Ramelet
Spécialiste FMH en Dermatologie et en Angiologie, Lausanne, Switzerland

Robert A. Weiss
Department of Dermatology, The Johns Hopkins University School of Medicine, Baltimore, Maryland, U.S.A.

Video 19: Phlebectomy

INTRODUCTION

Phlebectomy, first described by Cornelius Celsus (25 BC–45 AD), was performed in ancient Rome until it was stopped during the Middle Ages. Not until the 1500s, did phlebectomy resume, with phlebectomy hooks illustrated in the Textbook of Surgery of W.H. Ryff, published in 1545 (1). Lost again, this technique was rediscovered in 1956 by Dr Robert Muller, a Swiss dermatologic surgeon in private practice in Neuchâtel (Switzerland). Dr Muller developed his method (2,3), modestly calling it Celsus' phlebectomy, and eagerly taught this technique to over 300 physicians who visited his office (4–6). This technique is commonly referred to as "Muller's phlebectomy" or "ambulatory phlebectomy (AP)," and is now performed by dermatologic surgeons, vascular surgeons, phlebologists, and others who have had hands-on training with experts in the technique.

This cosmetically refined, safe, effective, and low cost entry technique allows the physician to remove incompetent saphenous veins (except incompetence arising from the sapheno-femoral and sapheno-popliteal junctions), major tributaries, perforators or reticular veins, including veins connected with telangiectasias. Specially designed phlebectomy hooks enable venous extraction through minimal skin incisions (1–3 mm) or needle puncture, assuring complete eradication in most cases. Visual evidence of the vein being extracted typically confirms its eradication.

In contrast to traditional venous ligation, the small size of the skin incision or puncture usually results in little or no scar. Performed under local anesthesia, AP leads to greatly reduced surgical risks compared to traditional surgery for truncal (axial) and reticular varicose veins, and incompetent perforators. In contrast, for these larger veins, sclerotherapy

331

Table 1
Comparative Analysis of Phlebectomy and Sclerotherapy

	Phlebectomy	Sclerotherapy
Pudendal veins	Excellent	Excellent
GSV[a]	Excellent	Fair
GSV primary branch	Excellent	Fair (good with foam)
Reticular varicosities	Good	Excellent
Subdermic lateral venous system	Good	Excellent
Prepatellar	Excellent	Poor-fair
Popliteal fold veins	Excellent	Good
LSV[a]	Excellent	Good
LSV branch	Excellent	Good
Dorsal venous network of the foot	Good	Fair
Feeding veins of telangiectasias	Good	Excellent
Telangiectatic webs	Fair	Excellent
Postsurgical residual varicosities	Good	Excellent

[a]Accompanying treatment of GSV or LSV reflux by endovenous ablation or obliteration techniques such as RF or laser.
Abbreviations: GSV, greater saphenous vein; LSV, lesser saphenous vein; RF, radiofrequency.

involves risks including intra-arterial injection, iatrogenic phlebitis, deep vein thrombosis and pulmonary embolism, skin necrosis, but most of all, residual hyperpigmentation. Unlike sclerotherapy, AP prohibits venous recanalization with recurrence. A comparison of advantages and disadvantages of both techniques is listed in Table 1.

INDICATIONS

This technique provides excellent and definitive results for treating truncal and reticular varicose veins, as long as junctional reflux has been treated and eliminated by an endovenous obliteration technique (chap. 18). When proximal reflux is ignored, only short-term improvement may be obtained, with recurrence seen within 4–12 months after surgery. AP may sometimes be deliberately performed to address an acute problem. Examples include avulsion of a single painful varicose vein in a young mother post-partum who is unwilling or unable to consider more extensive surgery and eradication of a single symptomatic varicose segment or a feeding vein causing a leg ulcer in an elderly individual (4–8).

All types of primary or secondary varicose veins (truncal, reticular, telangiectatic, perforators) may be removed by Muller's phlebectomy. Most of the procedures are ambulatory, but the technique may also be used in conjunction with other surgical procedures such as endovenous laser on radiofrequency (RF) saphenous obliteration.

Regions particularly appropriate for AP include accessory saphenous veins of the thigh, groin pudendal veins, reticular varices (popliteal fold, lateral thigh and leg), and veins of the ankles. Although the dorsal venous network of the foot may be treated, some caution is advised due to the higher incidence of nerve injury. Superficial phlebitis may also be effectively and easily treated by Muller's phlebectomy. Following the incision, the clot is expressed and the vein wall may be removed by the hook, assuring definitive treatment and immediate relief of pain.

PREOPERATIVE EVALUATION OF THE PATIENT

A detailed general and phlebological examination is mandatory before any varicose vein treatment. Minimal evaluation includes a medical history with general health assessment. Contraindications to local anesthesia or the surgical procedure itself must be elicited. Clinical observation and Duplex ultrasound mapping of the varicosities with determination of the origin of reflux is performed. Correction of insufficient perforator reflux, reflux of the sapheno-femoral or sapheno-popliteal junctions, must either precede or accompany any attempt to avulse superficial varicose veins. In addition, evaluation of the integrity of the deep venous system and calf muscle pump must also be performed. Hematologic or other laboratory investigations are not typically normally required, unless indicated by previous disorders revealed by patient history.

INSTRUMENTATION AND OPERATING ENVIRONMENT

This ambulatory procedure is usually performed in an outpatient clinical setting either in an office surgical facility or in the hospital outpatient operating room. An operating table permitting Trendelenburg positioning and the availability of good lighting is required. Direct intraoperative support is seldom necessary, but the presence of a nurse or an assistant in the procedure room is helpful to aid with unexpected bleeding or a vaso–vagal patient response. As the procedure is performed with tumescent anesthesia at very low concentrations of lidocaine, typically 0.1%, the procedure may be easily performed in an office outpatient setting.

Very few surgical instruments are required to perform AP. These include a number 11 scalpel or 18 gauge Nokor™ needle (BD, Franklin Lakes, New Jersey, U.S.) to perform either incisions or simple punctures, mosquito forceps to grasp and avulse the veins and several sets of phlebectomy hooks with different tip designs. The Nokor™ needle is constructed of a scalpel-like point which eliminates skin coring, requires less force, and creates a smoother puncture which results in better healing.

The ideal hook to begin the procedure should have a sharp harpoon to grip the adventitia of the vein, allowing its extraction through a minimal incision and a comfortable grip to prevent fatigue. Blunt hooks (boot hook type) are to be avoided, needing a larger incision and a more aggressive venous dissection possibly causing excessive tissue damage.

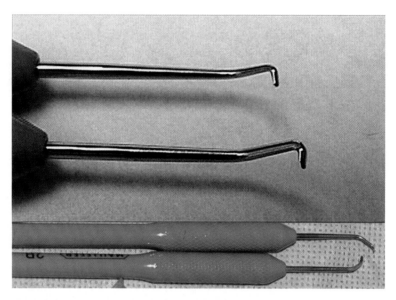

Figure 1
The basic Ramelet phlebectomy hooks with close up of tip.

Two sizes of hook are minimal requirements for most types of phle-
bectomies (Fig. 1). A large hook with a thicker stem is indicated in extraction of larger truncal varicosities and perforators. A thinner hook is
necessary to remove a reticular venous network. There are many type
of hooks presently available to assist with this technique. The Ramelet
hook is used to initially harpoon the adventitia from above, the Oesch
hook, with a short barb, can used to grasp the vein from the side, and
the "original" hook, the Muller, is designed with a large curve to allow
grasping the vein from below (Fig. 2).

The Muller hook, available in four sizes, was the first device to be
developed and was modeled after a crochet hook. The Oesch hook, available in three sizes, is characterized by a massive grip, although one cannot
roll it between the fingers. The "barb" or spike end can be used for lateral
"harpooning" of the vein. The Oesch hook, like the Muller hook, is very
effective for removing larger veins, but less efficacious for reticular veins.
The Oesch hook is best to grasp a vein from the side between a finger and
the skin. The Varady hook is a hook that has a short loop on one end and
a tissue dissector on the other. Thus, Varady's phlebextractor combines
two devices on one stem. The vein is first dissected with the spatula end,
then grasped with the hook end of the phlebextractor. The device must
be frequently reversed in the operator's hand. Because the hook end is
blunt, harpooning is not possible, but is used to lift the entire vein. The
spatula-dissector portion is convenient but no specific advantage over
using any hook itself as a dissector. One exception is in dense fibrous areas
such as overlying the knee in which a blunt dissector may be useful.

The Ramelet hook is relatively inexpensive and is produced in two sizes
which are easily distinguishable by different handle colors (9). A smaller, fine

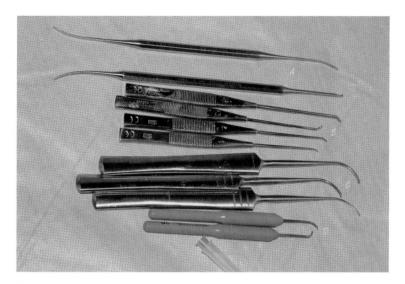

Figure 2
From top to bottom: Varady hooks, Müller hooks, Oesch hooks, and Ramelet hooks.

hook is designed to remove reticular or medium-sized varicose veins. The other has a thicker stem which is useful for large truncal and perforating veins. The grip is easy to grasp allowing finger placement near the tip for leverage and precise touch. Because the stem is short, exacting accurate movement is permitted. It is well adapted to operator's hand, and does not slip minimizing the risks of tearing surgical gloves. The cylindrical shape of the grip permits a gentle rolling of the hook between the fingers, diminishing the amount of rotation of the wrists, thereby minimizing wrist thereby hand stress during the procedure. The shape of the handle minimizes fatigue during removal of long segments. The hook angulation facilitates vein dissection and anchoring. Allowing individual adjustment of the hook angulation permits customization to individual surgeon preferences.

PATIENT MARKING AND ANESTHESIA

Premedication is rarely required and it should be avoided as it may hinder immediate postoperative walking. Immediate ambulation is the best means of prevention of potential vascular complications. To begin with, varicose veins are carefully outlined with a permanent or surgical marking pen when the patient is made to assume a standing position. The patient is then made to assume a supine position for further marking. Cutaneous transillumination may be helpful as veins shift from the standing to supine position relative to the skin surface (Fig. 3) (10). The vein has been shown to shift up to 6 mm from the standing position to the supine position (10). Local anesthesia is given to lift the vein to be avulsed closer to the skin surface.

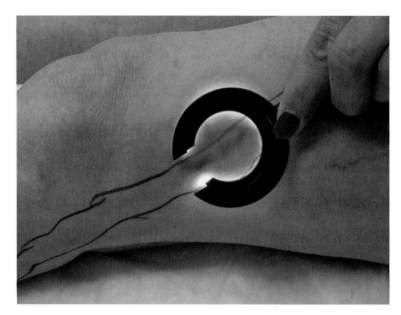

Figure 3
Transillumination assists accurate marking prior to ambulatory phlebectomy—
the varicose vein is seen transilluminated.

While several modalities of local anesthesia have been developed for
this procedure, we find the Klein tumescent technique the most efficacious and advantageous for the procedure. The lidocaine–epinephrine
solution can be buffered to a near neutral pH with 8.4% sodium bicarbonate (add 10% bicarbonate to the anesthetic: 5 mL in 50 mL). This
diminishes the pain resulting from the use of an acidic solution. This preparation may be stored up to two weeks when properly refrigerated (11).

Using the tumescent technique, we routinely inject up to 800 mL of
0.1% to 0.2% lidocaine with epinephrine. Infusion of lidocaine, by using
the tumescent formula of 0.1% lidocaine with 1:1,000,000 epinephrine in
the concentration of 35 mg/kg into the subcutaneous tissues is safe. The
maximum plasma levels reached at 11 to 15 hours postoperatively are
well below the toxic level of 5 mg/mL. Tumescent anesthetic produces
a delay in achieving the peak serum–lidocaine level and does not produce
as high a level as compared with conventional local anesthetic. This
allows coverage for removal of long vein segments. It is possible to inject
large areas of varicose veins quickly by using the Klein tumescent infiltration pump (HK Surgical, San Clemente, California, U.S.) (Fig. 4). Solution is pumped into subcutaneous area of the leg in order to elevate the
veins closer to the skin surface (12,13). This use of tumescent anesthesia,
in which lidocaine is highly diluted in saline or in Ringer solution (1/10),
offers several major advantages (14,15). These include (i) decreased pain
with injection (ii) low toxicity (iii) predissection of the vein from

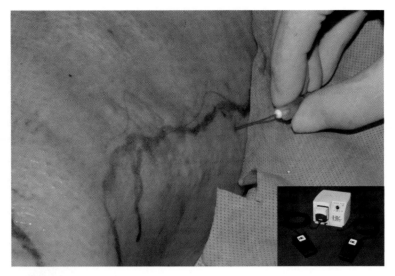

Figure 4
The Klein tumescent peristaltic pump is used to infiltrate large amounts of tumescent fluid. The fluid pressure is seen giving the skin a peau d'orange appearance as the veins are pushed closer to the skin.

surrounding tissue (iv) perioperative compression effect for improved hemostasis and less postoperative bruising, (v) postoperative rinsing and cleansing effect as the solution slowly drains from the punctures, and (vi) long lasting anesthetic properties which reduce patient discomfort well into the next day.

TECHNIQUE

Cutaneous incisions or punctures performed with a No. 11 scalpel blade or 18 gauge needle should be vertical along the vein in the region of the thigh and lower leg. Incisions should only follow the skin lines in flexural areas such as the knees or ankles. The distance between the incisions varies from 2 to 15 cm, according to the size of the vein, presence of perforators, and previous episodes of phlebitis or previous sclerotherapy.

The varicose vein is gently dissected by undermining with the stem of the phlebectomy hook, mainly along its course, slightly perpendicularly to its axis. When freed of its fibroadipose attachments, the liberated vein can be grasped by the harpoon of the hook and easily removed with the help of a mosquito forceps held in the nondominant hand (Fig. 5). The nondominant hand also grips one sterile gauze and assures hemostasis by local compression of the already removed venous network. The whole varicose vein is then extracted progressively from one incision to the other (Fig. 6). Associated perforators are carefully dissected and eliminated by gentle traction or torsion.

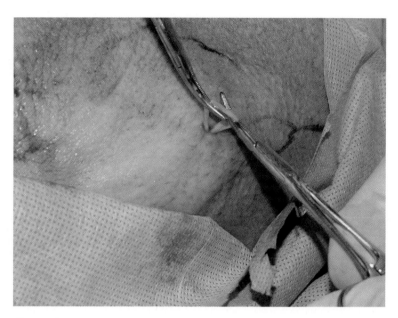

Figure 5
Gentle dissection by undermining with the stem of the hook leads to exteriorization of a vein loop grasped by hemostats.

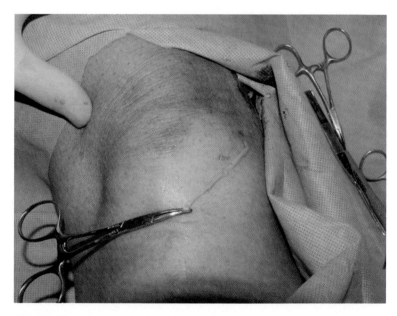

Figure 6
The varicose vein is removed and exposed.

Some areas may be more surgically difficult than others and require more persistence. These include popliteal fold, dorsum of the foot, prepatellar or pretibial, and recurrent varicose veins after phlebitis or sclerotherapy. Hemostasis is achieved with intra- and postoperative local compression. Venous ligation is absolutely not necessary and runs the risk of inflammation and drainage. As vein segments are avulsed the remaining connections sustain slight endothelial disruption which initiates a relatively immediate sealing reaction. As the vein is stretched prior to avulsion, the lumen becomes narrower as well reduces the area to be sealed. No skin sutures or Steri-Strips are required if the operator respects the basic principle of minimal incisions (1–3 mm) and good postoperative compression.

Although extensive varicosities may be operated upon in a single session (60–90 minutes), it is best to operate on each leg in a separate session to allow the patient to return to normal activity immediately. Areas in which hemostasis is more difficult to achieve (popliteal fossa, thighs, groin, major perforators) are surgically removed first, allowing intravascular clotting while the patient remains supine. Gentle local compression for several minutes, by an assistant, may be required.

Sclerotherapy of telangiectasias can be performed immediately before or after the avulsion of the connecting points to reticular veins (16,17). Larger telangiectasias may also be destroyed by gentle subcutaneous curettage (scratching technique) with the harpoon of the hook. Debris of these venules that have been shredded by the hook can be removed through tiny incisions.

Once all targeted veins are avulsed, the leg is thoroughly cleansed with hydrogen peroxide. Persistent bleeding of one incision is easily controlled by additional local compression for several minutes. Drainage of tumescent solution is often blood tinged and can be mistaken for bleeding. Application of antiseptic powder, as described in older literature, is ineffective and must be avoided as it has been reported to induce granulomas even years later (18).

POSTOPERATIVE MEDICATION AND PROPHYLACTIC ANTICOAGULATION

Postoperative pain seldom occurs. Nonprescription acetaminophen is usually adequate for the possible slight discomfort during the initial postoperative evening. Prophylactic anticoagulation is not indicated as the patient moves during the operation and is immediately ambulatory after the phlebectomy with a compression bandage.

POSTOPERATIVE CARE AND BANDAGING

The compression dressing is an essential and critical step to conclude the procedure. The bandage should be applied by the surgeon or a well-trained assistant. The incisions may be covered with a protective film but punctures require no covering. Punctures should remain open to allow tumescent anesthetic to drain. Overlapping sterile gauzes or absorbent pads firmly attached by adhesive tape or nonflexible strips are then placed over the operative sites. The initial compression wrap to hold the absorbant gauze in place consists of a short-stretch material to achieve a low resting pressure but a high working pressure.

A second dressing is typically placed over the first with the second consisting of a high elasticity (long-stretch) bandage or gradient compression stocking. This achieves compression along operating zones minimizing postoperative hemorrhage, pain, and complications. This second dressing covers the entire leg uniformly to prevent isolated edema, constriction or pinching between gauze pads.

The patient is required to walk regularly over the first few days post operatively. The patient is also allowed to work but driving an automobile should be avoided in the ensuing few hours postoperatively, since the motor nerves may be not be functioning properly due to local anesthesia effects. This is of greatest concern for local anesthesia delivered in the popliteal fold in which a temporary foot drop may be observed.

Dressings are changed after 24 or 48 hours, the puncture sites are cleansed with an antiseptic solution and sometimes sprayed with a protective film. No further dressings are needed at this point if the incisions size is minimal, but compression therapy (elastic bandages or compression stockings) is mandatory for 7 to 21 days more, depending on the size of the removed veins, degree of treated reflux, and amount of hematoma. Short showers are allowed four days postoperatively or sooner if the compression is protected by a waterproof covering.

Sclerotherapy of any residual varicosities may be undertaken at three to six weeks postoperatively. Telangiectasias may progressively and spontaneously disappear following varicose vein removal by AP; hence, performing sclerotherapy soon may be unnecessary. Sun exposure should be avoided until the fine erythematous marks have faded else they may become hyperpigmented.

RESULTS

Surgical puncture sites usually clear within several months, but may persist much longer in younger patients with tighter skin, or in ethnic skin patients. These patients should be warned about this possibility. Hematomas rapidly disappear and pigmentation usually fades in a few weeks. Meticulous application of the postoperative compressive dressing diminishes the incidence of bleeding, pain, hematoma, and residual pigmentation. Preoperative and one year postoperative results are shown in Figure 7, which is the result of AP performed in conjunction with endovenous RF ablation. At one year, the results of reduction of venous hypertension in the greater saphenous vein (GSV) is appreciated with excellent medical and cosmetic results. This patient experienced tremendous reduction of pain.

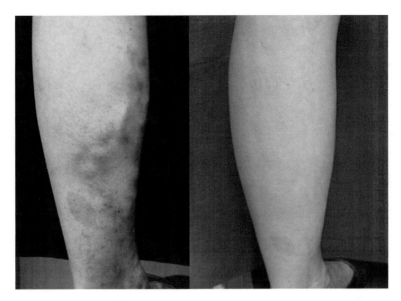

Figure 7
Before and after ambulatory phlebectomy.

AP OF BODY AREAS OTHER THAN THE LEGS

This procedure may also be utilized for removing cosmetically unacceptable dilated periorbital, temporal or frontal forehead venous networks (19),
and venous dilatation of the abdomen, arms or dorsum of the hands.
However, removal of functional veins for purely aesthetic reasons should
be performed extremely cautiously. Other techniques that can be successfully employed are Nd:YAG 1064 nm lasers treatment of facial dilated
veins and foam sclerotherapy on trunk and hand veins.

COMPLICATIONS AND THEIR TREATMENT

Most complications, such as bruising, are benign and resolve spontaneously. The complication rate after AP is relatively low compared to
other methods of surgical vein removal. Some publications have only
in part mentioned complication rates after AP (8,19,20), although two
study summarizes them accurately and completely (20,21).

Poor results may be the consequence of inappropriate patient selection, inaccurate initial diagnosis, or suboptimal technique. Patients with
rapid postoperative recurrence of varicose veins or new onset of purplish
matting indicate insufficient correction of venous reflux. Complications
such as edema, hemorrhage, hematomas, or blisters may be attributed
to incomplete coverage or insufficient time of postoperative compression.
Some complications are relatively unavoidable, no matter what the extent

Table 2
Postoperative AP Complications

Cutaneous
Frequent
  Skin blisters (from friction of compressive dressing)
Less common
  Transient pigmentation
  Keloids
Rare
  Infection
  Contact dermatitis
  Tattooing with marking pen
  Silicotic (foreign body) granuloma
Vascular
Frequent
  Hematomas at 1–2 wks
Less common
  Telangiectatic matting
  Edema (frequent after phlebectomy of dorsum of the foot)
  Lymphatic pseudocyst
Rare
  Postoperative hemorrhage
  Superficial phlebitis
Neurological—all very rare
  Transitory or long-term sensory defect (primarily foot dorsum)
  Carpo-tarsal syndrome after improper compression of the dorsum of the foot
  Neuroma

Abbreviation: AP, ambulatory phlebectomy.

of experience of the operator is (4,21). Complications may be classified as cutaneous, vascular, neurological, or general (Table 2).

Cutaneous Complications

Transitory hyperpigmentation usually fades in few months without any treatment. Hyperpigmentation incidence is much lower for AP than for sclerotherapy. Vesicles secondary to skin shearing from adhesive tape may induce postbullous depigmentation or transitory hyperpigmentation. Contact dermatitis secondary to antiseptic solutions or adhesives is rare, and it heals quickly with topical steroid application.

Infection is highly unusual [4 out of 8000 procedures (0.05%) in our experience] and can be controlled by local application of a topical antibiotic without concomitant systemic antibiotics. Keloids almost never occur, even in predisposed patients, due to the minimal size of the incisions or punctures. Hypertrophic scars may rarely be seen on the dorsum of the foot and respond to typical treatment by intralesional triamcinolone injection, cryotherapy, or pulsed dye lasers.

Tattooing with marking pen ink is unusual. We have observed it only on two occasions with no treatment required since the tattoos were barely visible. If antiseptic powder is used on puncture sites, foreign body granulomas may form which require excision (18). In one case, an association of a foreign body granuloma with necrobiosis lipoidica at each incision site was noted (22).

Vascular Complications

Hematomas are frequent and depend on skin fragility. Immediate postoperative hemorrhage may occur, although is highly unlikely with use of tumescent anesthesia. We routinely reevaluate the postoperative dressing after making the patient to walk in or near the office for 10 to 30 minutes, to check whether tightening or readjustment is required. This is particularly important for patients who may have a long journey home. Postoperative compression plays an important preventative role, but individual variations in coagulation can oppose the action of compression. Some patients rarely complain of persistent (months) subcutaneous nodules, corresponding to deep hematomas in the "tunnel" of the removed vein.

Superficial phlebitis or fibrosis of incompletely removed varicose veins or along neighboring veins may occur. These do not pose a health threat and are best treated conservatively with compression and nonsteroidal anti-inflammatory agents. These "hard areas" as felt by the patients rarely require incision and phlebectomy of the inflamed vein. Deep vein thrombosis has not yet been reported after AP and underscores the safety of the procedure.

Lymphatic pseudocyst may complicate phlebectomy of the ankle, pretibial or popliteal areas. When a soft subcutaneous nodule develops within a few days postoperatively, this lymph collection may be punctured and drained. The best treatment is compression along with gentle circular massage and, in resistant cases, lymphatic drainage. This will usually resolve spontaneously within a few weeks.

Neo-telangiectasias ("telangiectatic matting") are the most annoying complication of phlebectomy, but also an unwanted and frequent complication of sclerotherapy. It is seen much more commonly after "classical ligation" surgery of varicose veins. Its etiology is multiple and poorly understood. In some cases, it depends on a sudden change of venous pressure or persistent reflux. In others, it may be an abnormal "angiogenic" response to the tissue injury. A hypothetical correlation with hormones is controversial and we have not seen this correlation in our patients (23). Matting may spontaneously fade after several months. It may be effectively treated with sclerotherapy using a less inflammatory solution such as glycerin or by various lasers and light sources used to treat bright red (0.1–0.2 mm) vessels.

Neurological Complications

Local anesthesia may diffuse deeply causing temporary anesthesia of larger nerves, particularly in the lateral, popliteal fold which may induce

Table 3
Common Indications for AP

Adjunctive therapy to branch varicosities after endovenous RF and laser ablation
Adjunctive therapy in combination with foam sclerotherapy
Branch varicosities of the greater and lesser saphenous veins
Greater and lesser saphenous vein segments above the fascia (with or without
  concomitant endovenous RF and laser ablation of segments below the fascia)
Short segments of varicose vein causing venous ulcers
Varicose vein segments overlying the patella
Dorsal foot veins remaining after reflux eliminated from above

---

Abbreviations: AP, ambulatory phlebectomy; RF, radiofrequency.

a transitory paralysis of the foot. The mobility of the foot must therefore be evaluated before the patient ambulates. Tumescent anesthesia minimizes this possibility.

Intraoperative manipulation of a sensory nerve is painful since it typically remains functional immediately beyond the region of local anesthesia. It is important for a patient to not be sedated and be able to vocalize pain sensations. For example, the complaints of a shooting pain distal to the phlebectomy indicate the disruption of a perivenular nerve. An astute surgeon will stop the avulsion immediately after the pain reports at a puncture site and thus dramatically reduce the risks of nerve injury. General anesthesia eliminates the patient feedback and therefore incurs greater risks of nerve injury since small nerves adhering to veins may not be visible. Small nerve injury is more frequent in patients previously treated with sclerotherapy. Hyper-, hypo- or total anesthesia secondary to nerve injury usually resolves in some weeks or months. Neuroma has been reported but is very unlikely (24).

LONG-TERM RESULTS

Long-term reflux abolition, varicose vein ablation, and cosmetic results are excellent with AP. Patients can expect that for many years or even decades, there will be few visible veins in the treated area, as long as proximal venous reflux has been definitively treated or new source of proximal reflux has not developed in the interval. In a genetically susceptible individual, new varicose veins may develop and the patient has to be warned about the evolution and progressive nature of venous insufficiency. It is wise for very susceptible patients to see their physicians every three to five years to maintain cosmesis after any venous procedure, since venous hypertension is easier to treat when the spread of pressure has been limited to a smaller anatomic region. This can be done by treating shortly after its initial occurrence. The indications for successful AP are listed in Table 3.

REFERENCES

1. Scholz A. Historical aspects. In: Westerhof W, ed. Leg ulcers. Amsterdam: Elsevier, 1993.
2. Muller R. Traitement des varices par la phlébectomie ambulatoire. Bull Soc Fr Phléb 1966; 19:277–279.
3. Muller R. Mise au point sur la phlébectomie ambulatoire selon Muller. Phlébologie 1996; 49:335–344.
4. Ramelet AA, Monti M. Phlébologie, the Guide. Paris: Elsevier, 1999.
5. Ramelet AA. La phlébectomie selon Muller, description de la technique sous sa forme actuelle. Phlébologie 2004; 57:309–317.
6. Fratila A, Rabe E, Kreysei HW. Percutaneous minisurgical phlebectomy. Seminars in Dermatology 1993; 12:117–122.
7. Muller R, Bacci PA. La flebectomia ambulatoriale. Roma, Salus editrice internazionale, 1987.
8. Muller R, Joubert B. La phlébectomie ambulatoire: de l'anatomie au geste. Paris: Editions médicales Innothera, 1994.
9. Ramelet AA. Muller Phlebectomy, a new phlebectomy hook. J Dermatol Surg Oncol 1991; 17:814–816.
10. Weiss RA, Goldmann MP. Transillumination mapping prior to ambulatory phlebectomy. Dermatol Surg 1998; 24:447–450.
11. Larson PO, Ragi G, Swandby M, Darcey B, Polzin G, Carey P. Stability of buffered lidocaine and epinephrine used for local anesthesia. J Dermatol Surg Oncol 1991; 17:411–414.
12. Vidal-Michel JP, Arditi J, Bourbon JH, Bonerandi JJ. L'anesthésie locale au cours de la phlébectomie ambulatoire selon la methode de R. Muller. Phlébologie 1990; 43:305–315.
13. Krusche PP, Lauven PM, Frings N. Infiltrationsanästhesie bei Varizenstripping. Phlebol 1995; 24:48–51.
14. Sommer B, Sattler G. Tumeszenzlokal Anästhesie. Hautarzt 1998; 49:351–360.
15. Smith SR, Goldman MP. Tumescent anesthesia in ambulatory phlebectomy. Dermatol Surg 1998; 24:453–456.
16. Ramelet AA. Die Behandlung der Besenreiservarizen: Inidikationen der Phlebektomie nach Muller. Phlebol 1993; 22:163–167.
17. Ramelet AA. Le traitement des télangiectasies: indications de la phlébectomie selon Muller. Phlébologie 1994; 47:377–381.
18. Ramelet AA. Une complication rare de la phlébectomie ambulatoire, le granulome silicotique. Phlébologie 1991; 44:865–871.
19. Weiss RA, Ramelet AA. Removal of Blue Periocular Lower Eyelid Veins by Ambulatory Phlebectomy. Dermatol Surg 2002; 28:43–45.
20. Ramelet AA. Complications of ambulatory phlebectomy. Dermatol Surg 1997; 23: 947–954.
21. Olivencia JA. Complications of ambulatory phebectomy: a review of 4000 consecutive cases. Am J Cosmetic Surg 2000; 17:161–165.
22. Vion B, Buri G, Ramelet AA. Necrobiosis lipoidica and silicotic granuloma on Muller's phlebectomy scars. Dermatology 1997; 194:55–58.
23. Davis LT, Duffy DM. Determination of incidence and risk factors for postsclerotherapy telangiectatic matting of the lower extremity: a retrospective analysis. J Dermatol Surg Onc 1990; 16:327–330.
24. De Roos KP, Neumann HAM. Traumatic neuroma a rare complication following Muller's phlebectomy. J Dermatol Surg Onc 1994; 20:681–682.

18

Endovenous Elimination of the Great Saphenous Vein with Radiofrequency or Laser

Robert A. Weiss
Department of Dermatology, The Johns Hopkins University School of Medicine, Baltimore, Maryland, U.S.A.

Mitchel P. Goldman
Department of Dermatology/Medicine, University of California, San Diego, California, U.S.A. and La Jolla Spa MD, La Jolla, California, U.S.A.

Video 20: Closure[TM] *of Great Saphenous Vein: Via Radiofrequency*
Video 21: CTEV[TM] *of Small Saphenous Vein: Via 1320 nm Laser*

INTRODUCTION

Like many other fields of medicine, varicose vein treatment in the 21st century has evolved and adopted more minimally invasive methods. Procedures once performed under general anesthesia in which patients were surgically opened to allow extirpation of organs or structures are being rapidly replaced by techniques that allow the treatment of damaged organ systems with the patient awake and "sealed" from the outside. This revolution has infused the specialty of phlebology with some marvelous new techniques. This chapter will discuss primary concepts and methods in which a patient's damaged and improperly functioning axial vein is treated without requiring its physical removal.

The first attempt at minimizing the extent of surgery for varicose vein disease was to ligate the terminal valve thereby eliminating the source of reflux from the saphenofemoral junction (SFJ) into the great saphenous vein (GSV). Unfortunately treatment of the GSV with incompetence through the SFJ has been demonstrated to result in a high degree of recurrence. When the SFJ is merely ligated and the distal varicose veins are treated with either sclerotherapy or ambulatory phlebectomy long term success rates are very low (1–5). This is secondary to re-anastomosis through hemodynamically significant perforator veins present extending from the knee to the groin which are often not eliminated during the surgical procedure. Therefore, to provide the maximal degree of improvement in abnormal venous hemodynamics, complete surgical removal of the GSV from the

SFJ to the knee has been recommended after ligating the SFJ. This surgical procedure is most-often performed under general anesthesia with patients usually taking several weeks to get back to normal activities.

The first procedure that was developed to replace stripping was the use of a specially designed bipolar radiofrequency (RF) catheter. Radiofrequency energy can be delivered through a specially designed endovenous electrode to accomplish controlled heating of the vessel wall, causing vein shrinkage or occlusion by contraction of venous wall collagen. With worldwide clinical experience on over 60,000 procedures since 1999, this technique has been a valuable addition to treating large varicose veins resulting from saphenous reflux. Shortly after the development of radiofrequency Closure™ (VNUS Medical Technologies, San Jose, California), endoluminal lasers have also been demonstrated to effectively close axial veins through thermal damage to endothelium with subsequent thrombosis and resorption of the damaged vein. These endovenous occlusion techniques are less invasive alternatives to saphenofemoral ligation and/or stripping. They are typically performed under local anesthesia with patients returning to normal activities within 1–2 days.

Although the concept of endovenous elimination of reflux is not new, previous approaches have relied on electrocoagulation of blood causing the resulting thrombus to occlude the vein. The potential for recanalization of the thrombus is high. Within cardiology, application of radiofrequency directly to tissue, not blood, has been effectively applied for ablation of abnormal conduction pathways for arrhythmias (7). Venous occlusion with RF by the mechanism of venous blood coagulation has been previously reported, but is different than the modern approach (8). Another term in the medical literature is endovascular diathermic vessel occlusion, a technique in which a spider-shaped intravascular electrode produces venous occlusion by electrocoagulation with minimal perivascular damage (9).

RF ENDOLUMINAL OBLITERATION (CLOSURE™)

Directing RF energy into tissue to cause its destruction is potentially safer and more controllable than other mechanisms. Delivered in continuous or sinusoidal wave mode, there is no stimulation of neuromuscular cells when using a frequency between 200 and 3000 kHz. The mechanism by which RF current heats tissue is resistive (or ohmic) heating of a narrow rim (<1 mm) of tissue that is in direct contact with the electrode. Deeper tissue planes may be slowly heated by conduction from the small volume region of heating. This is part of the process whereby heat is dissipated by conduction into surrounding normothermic tissue (10). By carefully regulating the degree of heating with microprocessor control, subtle gradations of either controlled collagen contraction or total thermocoagulation of the vein wall can be achieved.

When the RF catheter is pulled through the vein while feedback-controlled with a thermocouple, the surgeon can heat the section of vein wall to a specified temperature. This is a relatively safe process since the temperature increase remains localized around the active electrode provided that close, stable contact between the active electrode and the vessel wall is maintained. By limiting temperature to 85–90°C boiling, vaporization and carbonization of the tissues is avoided (11). In addition, thermography experiments have shown that heating the endothelial wall to 85°C results in heating the vein media to approximately 65°C which has been demonstrated to contract collagen (data on file, VNUS Medical, San Jose, California).

Electrode mediated RF vessel wall ablation is a self-limiting process. As coagulation of tissue occurs, there is a marked decrease in impedance that limits heat generation (12). Alternatively if clot builds up on the electrodes, blood is heated instead of tissue, and there is a marked rise in impedance (resistance to RF). The RF generator can be programmed to rapidly shutdown when impedance rises, thus ensuring minimal heating of blood but efficient heating of the vein wall.

Thus recent technological advances including introduction of specific application electrodes and accompanying microprocessor controlled systems to precisely monitor the electrical and thermal effects has allowed the safe application of this technology. One such system is the Closure^{TM} catheter. This device produces precise tissue destruction with a reduction in the occurrence of undesirable effects such as the formation of coagulum. With the Closure^{TM} catheter system, bipolar electrodes are placed in contact with the vein wall. Unlike the laser systems discussed next, RF requires direct vein wall contact. When the vein wall contracts, the electrodes fold up within the vein allowing maximal physical contraction. Selective insulation of the electrodes results in a preferential delivery of the RF energy to the vein wall and minimal heating of the blood within the vessel.

The catheter design includes collapsible catheter electrodes around which the vein may shrink and a central lumen to allow a guidewire and/or fluid delivery structured within the 5 F (1.7 mm) catheter (Fig. 1). This permits treatment of veins as small as 2 mm and as large as 8 mm. A larger 8 F catheter allows treatment of saphenous veins up to 1.2 mm in diameter. Both catheters have thermocouples on the electrodes embedded in the vein wall, which measure temperature and provide feedback to the RF generator for temperature stabilization. The control unit (Fig. 2) displays power, impedance, temperature, and elapsed time so that precise control may be obtained. The second generation RF generator delivers an audio tone to indicate withdrawal speed. If the pullback is too quick, then the frequency and pitch increase to warn the physician. The unit delivers the minimum power necessary to maintain the desired electrode temperature. For safety, if a coagulum forms on the electrodes, the impedance rises rapidly and the programmed RF generator automatically cuts off. Animal experiments demonstrate endothelial denudation along with denaturation of media and intramural collagen with a subsequent fibrotic seal of vein lumen (Fig. 3). This cannot be accomplished in the goat by sclerotherapy. The goat saphenous vein is a high flow vessel, sclerotherapy would not be very effective as sclerosing solutions require time to interact with the vessel wall but are washed away quickly in these situations.

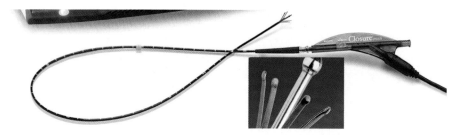

Figure 1
The Closure Plus™ catheter. Inset shows details of electrode tip. (Courtesy of VNUS Medical Technologies, San Jose, CA.)

RF CLOSURE™ USING DUPLEX GUIDED CANNULATION

Over five years of clinical experience suggest that the Closure™ procedure is effective at occluding saphenous veins and abolishing reflux with an 85–90% long-term success rate. Two separate studies evaluated patients treated either with a percutaneous approach or with a vein cut-down allowing access of the Closure™ catheter to treat the proximal GSV with phlebectomy of the distal GS and tributaries.

Enrollment criteria for the first group of patients were symptomatic saphenous reflux with a saphenous vein diameter of 2 to 12 mm. The

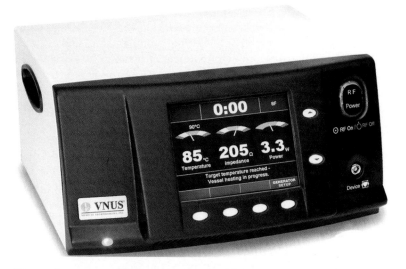

Figure 2
Radiofrequency generator, version 2. Note clear displays of time, temperature, impedance and watts.

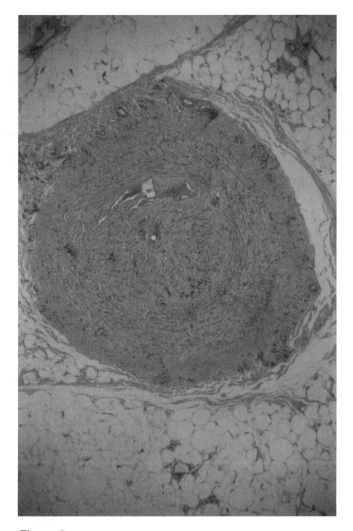

Figure 3
Fibrotic seal of the vein lumen in a sheep model using RF endovenous at 6 weeks.

genders of treated patients was 24% male and 76% female; mean age was 47.2 ±12.6 with a mean vein diameter of 7.4 mm.

Most of the veins treated were above-knee great saphenous (73%), some entire great saphenous (21%) with the remaining including below knee great saphenous, small saphenous, and accessory saphenous (13–15). Adjunctive procedures performed at the time of treatment were phlebectomy on more distal branches in 61% and high ligation in 21%, but the adjunctive procedures did not affect outcome.

Vein occlusion at 1 week has been documented by Duplex ultrasound in 300 out of 308 legs or a success rate of 97%. Occlusion persisted at 6 weeks in 95% and 6 months in 92%. To date all of the patients followed for 6 months to 12 months have remained occluded; in other words, if the saphenous vein is closed at 6 months, this will persist to 12 months and beyond. In our patients, we typically see closure of all the major tributaries at the SFJ except for the superficial epigastric that continues to empty superiorly into the common femoral vein. We believe that there is a high margin of safety by maintaining flow through this tributary. The high flow rate appears to diminish the possibility of extension of any thrombus (in the unlikely event that this would occur) from the GSV. In our personal experience, thrombus has not been observed (5).

For clinical symptoms, the RF endovenous occlusion procedure rapidly reduces patient pain, fatigue, and aching correlating with a reduction in CEAP clinical class for symptoms and clinical severity of disease. When patients have had surgical stripping on the opposite leg, the degree of pain, tenderness and bruising have been far greater on the leg treated by stripping. Side effects of the Closure™ technique have included thrombus extension from the proximal greater saphenous vein in 0.8%, with one case of pulmonary embolus; skin burn (prior to the tumescent anesthesia technique) in 2.5%; clinical phlebitis at 6 weeks in 5.7%; temporary quarter-sized areas of paresthesia in 18%, with most of these occurring immediately above the knee and resolving within 6 months to a year. Thus, compared to most techniques but in particular to traditional surgery of ligation and stripping of similar size saphenous veins, the effectiveness of endovenous RF occlusion is quite high.

RF CLOSURE™ WITH AMBULATORY PHLEBECTOMY

Closure™ with ambulatory phlebectomy was equally as effective as closure of the GSV described above. The first 47 sequential, non-randomized patients who presented to the clinic of one of the authors (MPG) having incompetent GSV from an incompetent SFJ and painful varicosities in 50 legs were treated with the VNUS Closure™ procedure after appropriate informed consent. The varicose veins were marked with the patient standing and again with the patient lying down in the operative position with a Venoscope™ as previously described (16,17). Details of the operative procedure were previously reported (18). In short, after appropriate marking, the area surrounding the GSV and distal tributaries to be treated was infiltrated with 0.1% lidocaine tumescent anesthesia. The amount of tumescent fluid averaged 800 ml with a lidocaine dose of 8 mg/kg. The GSV was then accessed through a 2–3 mm incision in the medial mid thigh usually 20 cm inferior to the SFJ. The proximal portion of the GSV was then treated with VNUS Closure™ and the distal portion including all varicose tributaries were removed with a standard ambulatory phlebectomy technique.

Thirty-nine patients with 41 treated legs were available for evaluation at the longest follow-up period; six patients (nine treated legs) could not be located for re-evaluation after 6 months because of change in residence (often out of state).

The average time to access the GSV in the medial thigh was 7 min (1–30 min). Twenty-seven patients had the GSV accessed in approximately 1 min. The average catheter pullback rate was 2.76 cm/min over an average length of treated GSV of 19 cm (6–42 cm). Complete surgical time including the phlebectomy portion of the procedure was approximately 20 min (range 13–35 min).

Ninety-five percent of all patients could resume all pre-operative activities within 24 hours; the other 2 patients could resume all activities within 48 hours. Every patient had complete elimination of leg pain and fatigue and 21 of 22 patients who presented with ankle edema had resolution of this problem. All patients said that they would recommend this procedure to a friend.

Adverse sequelae were minimal with four patients complaining of heat distal to the SFJ during the procedure that resolved with additional tumescent anesthesia. Twenty-eight of 50 treated legs had some degree of purpura lasting 1–2 weeks. Five patient legs developed mild erythema over the GSV Closure[TM] site that lasted 2–3 days. Eight legs had an indurated fibrous cord over sites of ambulatory phlebectomy that lasted up to 6 months. No new varicose veins were noted in three patients with recurrent reflux in the GSV. One patient who developed reflux had the development of new veins at 1 year post-treatment (6).

Three separate papers detail a similar cohort of patients treated in a multicenter study ranging from 16–31 clinics, with 210–324 patients, with 6–12 month follow-up (15,19,20). The vein occlusion rate at 1 year examination was 91.6% from 9 centers and 81.9% from 14 centers. Forty-nine patients were followed at 2 years with Duplex scans and showed a 89.8% closure rate. There was a 3% incidence of paresthesia as well as a 1.6% rate when treatment was confined to the thigh. Two limbs (0.8%) developed scaring from skin burns and 3 patients developed a DVT with 1 embolism. The reason for the increase in adverse effects appears to be the use of general anesthesia without tumescent anesthesia.

Sybrandy and Wittens from Rotterdam reported 1 year follow-up of 26 patients treated with VNUS Closure[TM] (21). They reported 5 patients with postoperative paresthesia of the saphenous nerve and one with a cutaneous burn for an overall complication rate of 23%. One patient (3.8%) had total recurrence of the GSV; one patient (3.8%) could not be treated due to a technical failure; eight patients (30.8%) had closure of the GSV but with persistent reflux of the SFJ; 50% of patients had closure of both the GSV and SFJ. They reported a total of 88% of patients with a totally occluded GSV.

The probable reason for the increase in adverse effects was their use of a spinal anesthesia instead of the recommended tumescent anesthesia. In addition they treated all patients from the ankle proximally, which exposed the GSV within the calf to heat from the RF catheter. Their mean operating time was 67 minutes (range, 25–120 minutes).

Another report describes 2 episodes of DVT in 29 patients treated with the RF Closure[TM] (22). Patients were treated with a groin incision and passage of the catheter from the groin downward. The authors do not report the type of anesthesia used or the length of vein treated; it is presumed that patients were not ambulatory and were treated under general anesthesia. The important information to come out of a review of various treatments of the GSV is that the use of tumescent anesthesia in awake patients who can ambulate immediately after the procedure is important in preventing skin burns and DVT. Treatment when limited to the GSV segment above the knee is also important in preventing paresthesia to the saphenous nerve.

TUMESCENT ANESTHESIA FOR ENDOVENOUS PROCEDURES

The development of the RF closure technique for treating the incompetent GSV was completed by multiple specialties with dermatology taking a significant role. Dermatologic surgeons are experts in the use of liposculpture surgery with the tumescent anesthesia technique, and were the first to apply tumescence to ambulatory phlebectomy and/or ligation of the GSV and its tributaries.

A patent was filed on March 10, 1999 for a technique for using tumescent anesthesia with radio-frequency or other energies for endoluminal closure. Our patent #6,258,084 was granted on July 10, 2001. Tumescent anesthesia or the placement of large volumes of dilute anesthesia in a peri-vascular position serves several purposes:

1. to protect perivascular tissues from the thermal effects of intravascular energy such as RF,
2. to decrease the diameter of the treated vein to allow for better contact of the RF electrodes with the vein wall, and thus secondarily reduce intravascular blood for non-specific coagulation,
3. provide better and safer anesthesia for patients, and
4. for laser procedures, tumescence helps to shrink the vein and lumen to prevent the fiber tip from contacting the vein wall directly. This allows the laser energy to flow proximally into the lumen, minimizing the risk of perforating holes in the vein wall.

Our initial results revealed that, using this method, the GSV could be sealed with endovenous techniques as a totally painless procedure with little down-time and immediate ambulation of the patient. Our combined clinical experience with endovenous techniques spans 5.5 years with well over 1000 endovenous patient treatments including RF and various lasers. Post-treatment Duplex evaluation data at regular time intervals exists on the vast majority of these patients. Our experience with tumescent anesthesia utilized in every one of our patients is complete lack of DVT. The incidence as measured by Duplex ultrasound follow-up at 3–14 days is 0%. We firmly believe that the use of tumescent anesthesia in unsedated conscious patients followed by immediate ambulation at the conclusion of the procedure is the reason for our lack of serious adverse sequelae such as DVT.

In our experience using tumescent anesthesia, only two patients have developed focal numbness 4 cm in diameter on the lower medial leg. These resolved within 6 months. No skin injury or deep vein thrombosis has been observed in any of our patients using RF Closure™.

CLINICAL TECHNIQUE FOR RF CLOSURE™

The patient undergoes a Duplex ultrasound to determine venous anatomy and the presence of reflux at the SFJ and the size of the GSV at the terminal valve. Presently, patients with reflux in the greater or lesser saphenous vein are candidates if the vein size does not exceed 1.2 mm. Reflux may originate at the junction itself as this region may be safely treated.

The procedure begins with the vein to be treated marked on the skin using Duplex ultrasound. (Fig. 4). An appropriate entry point is selected. This is usually just below where reflux is no longer seen in the greater saphenous vein or where the vein becomes too small to cannulate with a 16-gauge introducer set. For the majority of patients in our series, this is at a point just above or below the knee along the course of the GSV. Before proceeding the patient's feet are wrapped in warm material or socks to minimize vasoconstriction, a heating pad is placed under the thigh and a small amount of 2% nitrol paste is rubbed onto the intended entry point to minimize vasoconstriction during the initial cannulation process.

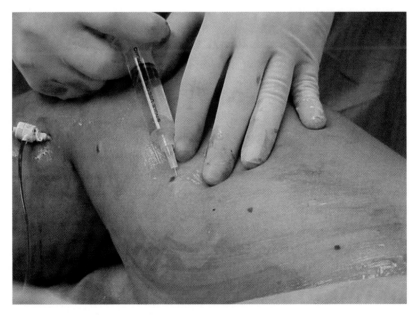

Figure 4
Local anesthesia is being placed along the previously marked GSV.

The patient is then prepped and draped, after which 0.1 cc of 1% lidocaine without epinephrine is injected at the pre-marked site. With Duplex guidance, a 16-gauge needle is inserted through the skin and guided into the saphenous vein. When venous return is noted through the attached syringe, the Closure™ catheter may at this point be placed directly through the needle into the vein. Because this permits some slow leakage of blood around the Closure™ catheter during the procedure, we prefer to insert a sheath with a flapper valve through which the Closure™ catheter is then advanced. Others prefer gaining entry via a venous cut-down or pulling of the vein close to the surface with an ambulatory phlebectomy hook. Our technique requires one needle puncture only and is more likely to result in better cosmesis.

In order to place the sheath a guidewire must be first inserted through the 16 gauge needle initially inserted into the skin. The guidewire is passed approximately 5 cm into the GSV. The sheath is then threaded along the guidewire, piercing the skin; its progress is followed by Duplex until it is seen firmly placed within the lumen of the GSV. After establishing the intraluminal placement of the sheath, the guidewire is carefully withdrawn.

The Closure™ catheter, with a diluted heparin solution or plain normal saline dripping at one drip per second through a central lumen, is now inserted through the sheath. Its progress up the GSV is monitored by Duplex. If the catheter gets hung-up on a valve or slight bend of the GSV, the catheter is twisted or external pressure is applied to the leg to change the shape of the GSV. Sometimes the patient must rotate the leg.

Once the Closure™ catheter is in place, tumescent anesthesia (consisting of 0.1% lidocaine neutralized to pH 7 with sodium bicarbonate) is injected between the skin and the cannulated GSV. Tumescent anesthesia volume is typically 300–600 cc for the course of the vein along the thigh. Duplex monitoring of the anesthesia injection at the SFJ is recommended as the shape of the SFJ is changed from the round "hook" to a straighter path.

After the tumescent anesthesia is completed, the final check of the position of the catheter is made with Duplex. The tip is positioned with the electrodes deployed. The tips of the electrodes are placed so that they align with the base of the terminal valve cusps, usually at least 1 cm below the terminal valve. It is important to deploy the electrodes below the entry point of the superior epigastric tributary. Impedance and temperature is continuously monitored once the RF electrode is plugged into the RF generator. Prior to commencing treatment, the normal impedance of the vein wall should be between 200 and 350 ohms and the thermocouple should transmit a baseline temperature with full tumescence of 28–32°C.

The RF is then applied; the physician monitors the temperature and impedance. Within 15 sec the target temperature of 85°C should be reached. With full tumescent anesthesia, it is possible to set the target temperature of 90°C to allow for a 5- to 7-min pullback as the surrounding structures are pushed away from the treated vein and there is a very large capacity heat sink around the targeted saphenous vein.

When the catheter has been pulled back to the introducer sheath site, impedance will suddenly rise and the RF generator cut off. Duplex ultrasound of the SFJ should reveal no flow except the superficial epigastric emptying into the common femoral vein. The GSV should be more echogenic with thicker appearing walls. If flow is seen in the GSV, the procedure may be repeated assuming that the Closure™ catheter can be advanced past the treated distal segment. If one cannot pass the catheter easily no repeat treatment is performed, as vein perforation would be the most likely outcome of such an attempt.

FOLLOW-UP CARE

Class 2 compression hosiery is worn for 3 days with the percutaneous Closure™ technique and 7 days if one is perfoming an adjunctive ambulatory phhlebectomy technique. Patients will note some bruising from the tumescent anesthesia. Anesthesia of the treated portion of the leg may persist for 8–24 hours. To gain experience, we recommend that for the initial cases, one re-evaluate the treated veins at 3 days by Duplex ultrasound. This will allow correlation of results with the pullback rate or any difficulty encountered during the procedure. Once comfortable with the procedure, the physician may want to see the patient for a Duplex ultrasound follow-up study at 6 weeks. At that time, any open segments can be treated by foamed sclerosant Duplex guided sclerotherapy. It has been our experience that when closed at 6 weeks, the GSV will remain closed, fibrosed and almost indistinguishable from surrounding tissue at 6 months. Symptom reduction is rapid with many patients experiencing relief at three days but some not until 6 weeks. Clinical improvement in appearance of varicosities is typically seen within 6 weeks as well.

ENDOVENOUS OBLITERATION OF THE GSV WITH ENDOLUMINAL LASER ABLATION (810 NM, 940 NM, AND 980 NM)

Endovenous laser treatment allows delivery of laser energy directly into the blood vessel lumen in order to produce endothelial and vein wall damage with subsequent fibrosis. It is presumed that destruction of the GSV with laser is a function of thermal destruction. The presumed target for lasers with 810, 940, and 980 nm wavelengths is intravascular red blood cell absorption of laser energy. Unlike RF, it is important for the laser fibers not to be in direct contact with the vein wall. Blood must always be between the fiber and the vein wall as heating of blood with transmission to the wall is the mechanism. Steam bubbles have been shown to occur within blood within the lumen as the primary mechanism for laser effects. Direct thermal effects on the vein wall without the presence of blood probably do not occur. The extent of thermal injury to tissue is strongly dependent on the amount and duration of heat to which the tissue is exposed; for these lasers, this is dependent on multiple factors include blood in the lumen, rate of pullback, and amount of tumescent anesthesia placed around the vein. A uniform layer of blood circumferentially around the fiber will yield the best results with the hemoglobin targeting wavelengths.

One in vitro study model has predicted that thermal gas production by laser heating of blood in a 6 mm tube results in 6 mm of thermal damage (23,24). These authors used a 940 nm diode laser with multiple 15-J, 1 sec pulses to treat the GSV. An median of 80 pulses (range, 22–116) were applied along the treated vein every 5–7 mm. Histologic examination of one excised vein demonstrated thermal damage along the entire treated vein with evidence of perforations at the point of laser application described as "explosive-like" photo-disruption of the vein wall. This produced the homogeneous thrombotic occlusion of the vessel. Since optical properties of a 940 nm laser beam within circulating blood is that it can only penetrate 0.3 mm, the formation of steam bubbles is the mechanism of action of heating surrounding tissue (24).

Initial reports have shown this technique with an 810 nm diode laser to have good short-term efficacy in the treatment of the incompetent GSV, with 96% or higher occlusion at 9 months with a less than 1% incidence of transient paresthsia (25,26). Most patients, however, experience major degrees of post-operative ecchymosis and discomfort. Skin burns have observed by one of the authors (RAW). Deep venous thrombosis extending into the femoral vein have also been recently reported with endovenous laser treatment (27).

Our patients treated with an 810 nm diode laser have shown an increase in post-treatment purpura and tenderness. Most of our patients do not return to complete functional normality for 2–7 days as opposed to the 1 day "downtime" with RF Closure[TM] of the GSV. There is even less downtime with CTEV[TM], discussed in the next section. Recent studies suggest that pulsed 810 nm diode laser treatment with its increased risk for perforation of the vein (as opposed to continuous treatment which does not have intermittent vein perforations but may have irregular areas of perforation) may be responsible for the increase symptoms with 810 nm laser vs. RF treatment (28). Our experience with trying to vary the fluence and treating with a continuous laser pull back vs. pulsed pull back has not resulted in an elimination of vein perforation using an 810 nm diode laser.

A longer wavelength such as 940 nm has been hypothesized to penetrate deeper into the vein wall with resulting increased efficacy. A report of 280 patients with 350 treated limbs with 18 month follow-up demonstrated complete closure in 96% (29). Twenty vein segments were examined histologically. Veins were treated with 1 sec duration pulses at 12 J. Perforations were not present. When the fluence was increased to 15 J with 1.2- and 1.3-sec pulses, microperforations did occur and were said to be self-sealing. The author suggests that his use of tumescent anesthesia as well as the above mentioned laser parameters are responsible for the lack of significant perforations and enhanced efficacy.

A clinical study using an endoluminal 1064 nm Nd:YAG laser in the treatment of incompetent GSV in 151 men and women with 252 treated limbs was reported (30). Unfortunately, the surgeons also ligated the SFJ, which did not allow for a determination of the efficacy of SFJ ablation. Spinal anesthesia was used and the laser was used at 10–15 W of energy with 10 sec pulses with manual retraction of the laser fiber at a rate of 10 sec/cm. Skin overlying the treated vein was cooled with cold water. Unfortunately, this resulted in superficial burns in 4.8% of patients, paresthesia in 36.5%, superficial phlebitis in 1.6%, and localized hematomas in 0.8%.

COOLTOUCH CTEV™ ENDOVENOUS TREATMENT

In an attempt to bypass the problems associated with laser wavelength absorption of hemoglobin, we have developed a 1320 nm endolumenal laser. At this wavelength, tissue water is the target and the presence or absence of red blood cells within the vessels is unimportant. The CoolTouch CTEV™ treatment is an endovenous ablation method using a special laser fiber coupled to the intraluminal use of an infrared 1320 nm wavelength with an automatic pullback device pre-set to pullback at 1 mm/sec (Fig. 5). This 1.32 micron wavelength is unique among endovenous ablation lasers in that this wavelength is absorbed only by water and not by hemoglobin. This makes it significantly different from the other (hemoglobin targeting) wavelengths used for endovenous laser treatments. In our opinion and experience, the CoolTouch CTEV™ at 1320 nm is significantly superior to the other endovenous laser methods both by virtue of the water absorption and the automatic pullback device (31).

When using a wavelength strongly absorbed by hemoglobin, such as 810 nm, there is a lot of intraluminal blood heating with transmission of heat to the surrounding tissue through long heating times. Temperatures in animal models have been reported as high as 1200°C (28). When we have tried ex vivo vein treatment without blood with the fiber in contact with the vein wall, the 810 nm wavelength simply chars the inside of the vein. When blood is added to exvivo veins and is then treated with 810 nm, numerous vein explosions are observed (personal communication, Dr. M. Hirokawa, Tokyo, Japan, 2005).

Minimizing direct contact with the vein wall for hemoglobin-dependent methods minimizes the charring of the vein wall and probably lowers the post-operative pain levels. Ideally for a hemoglobin absorbed wavelength to work, it would be best to have a well-defined layer of hemoglobin between the fiber and the vein wall. In the real world, however, varicose veins are saccular and irregular pockets of hemoglobin are frequently encountered leading to sharp rises in temperature and vein perforations when using hemoglobin absorbing wavelengths such as 810 nm.

Using tumescent anesthesia with a hemoglobin targeting wavelength, it can be very difficult to gauge the correct amount to compress the vein since some hemoglobin is necessary for the mechanism of action. If too much tumescence is used, there can be charring of the inner wall of the vein without heating of the vein wall, with resulting pain and failure to close the vein. For all these potential obstacles to ideal treatment conditions for 810 nm, 940 nm, or 980 nm, it makes far more sense to use a water absorbing

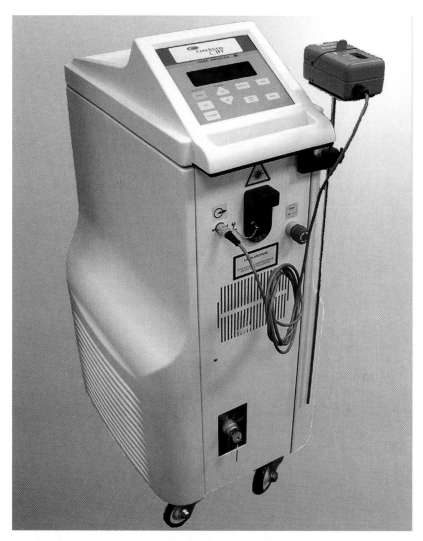

Figure 5
CoolTouch CTEV™ 1320 nm laser and automatic pullback device.

wavelength once cannulated within the vein. Therefore, the 1320 nm wavelength for use in endovenous ablation was explored and clinical trials performed resulting in FDA clearance in September 2004 for treatment of the greater saphenous vein. By August 2005, sufficient data for approval for obliteration of reflux in the lesser saphenous vein were cleared by the FDA.

Percutaneous approaches to smaller leg telangiectasias indicate that deeply penetrating laser wavelengths with significant deoxyhemoglobin absorption, such as 1064 nm Nd:YAG, have the most utility. When veins are targeted through the skin, one exploits the concept of selective photothermolysis. By targeting deoxyhemoglobin, cutaneous leg vessels absorb preferentially to surrounding water, collagen, and other structures. This allows selective destruction of tiny blood vessels without heating surrounding structures. The mechanism of this destruction by 1064 nm laser must be clearly understood by the user. The clinical observation is immediate photodarkening and coagulation. Histologically this is represented by perivascular hemorrhage and thrombi with vessels fragmentation (32). This ultimately leads to vessel clearance in about 75% of targeted areas over a 3-month time frame (33). For the cutaneous approach, this is clearly state-of-the-art but this is not the best approach for endovenous laser ablation in which selective photothermolysis is not a factor.

Endovenous ablation requires maximizing vein shrinkage and closure with the least amount of blood coagulation and the maximum amount of vein wall contraction. We know from earlier methods involving electrosurgical blood coagulation that the long-term success rates based on coagulation of blood are very low (34,35). On the contrary, success rates for radiofrequency vein shrinkage specifically avoiding coagulation of blood are very high (5,13,36). Recently, Proebstle and colleagues designed a study that answers the question of whether endovenous ablation is best accomplished by hemoglobin heating or the approach of using water around the collagen in the vein wall as a target (37). He has had extensive experience with the 940 nm wavelength for endovenous ablation (38). As shown by Proebstle et al., there is a clear advantage of targeting water over hemoglobin when performing endovenous laser. There is a statistically reduced rate of pain post-operatively with a higher rate of success while at the same time applying lower energy. This results in greater safety and efficacy for the patient, our own experience reflects this, with a reduction in pain and bruising of 80% when switching from 810 nm endovenous to 1320 nm endovenous. Having treated over 200 greater saphenous veins with 1320 nm, our incidence of mild pain is 5%. No significant pain interfering with walking has been observed. A typical clinical result is shown in (Fig. 6).

Based on our experience we believe that there is reduced pain reported with 1320 nm vs 940 nm probably due to less vein perforations and more uniform heating by 1320 nm targeting water in the vein wall. Rarely, patients experience mild pain after 1320 nm, but this is probably related to heat dissipated into surrounding tissue, not vein perforations. This might be minimized by using the minimal effective energy to shrink the vein. In our own unpublished studies we have found that emitting 5 W of 1320 nm through a 600-μ fiber moving at 1 mm/sec in a 2-mm thick vein wall, the highest temperature recorded on the exterior of the vein wall was 48°C. Unfortunately in a saphenous vein, for effective sealing and shrinkage, higher energies must sometimes be utilized. In the Proebste et al. (37) study, 8 W of 1320 nm were employed to have the highest intraluminal occlusion and shrinkage but probably accounted for the post-operative pain incidence. We believe that effective energy for vein sealing in our practice is mostly between 5 and 6, thus minimizing post-operative pain to less than 5%. In summary, our experience

(A)   **(B)**

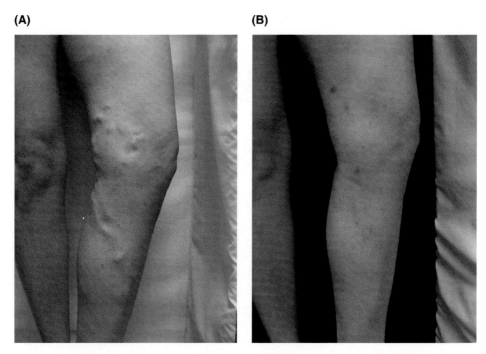

Figure 6
Clinical result seen with CoolTouch CTEV™ 1320 nm laser. (**A**) Before treatment. (**B**) After 6 weeks. There is marked improvement of a varicosity associated with reflux of the greater saphenous vein.

and those of others indicate that 1320 nm water targeting vs. 810 nm,
940 nm, or 980 nm hemoglobin targeting endovenous occlusion is gentler,
leading to far less bruising and post-operative pain.

TECHNIQUE OF COOLTOUCH CTEV™ ENDOVENOUS TREATMENT

The patient is evaluated and marked in an identical manner as with RF
Closure™ of the GSV. An appropriate entry point is selected similar to
RF. This is usually just below where reflux is no longer seen in the greater
saphenous vein. For the majority of patients in our series this is at a point
just above or below the knee along the course of the GSV. A sheath is
placed in the entire length of the vein to be treated up to the sapheno-
femoral junction. Tumescent anesthesia is then injected along the vein
and injected subfacially to separate and dissect the targeted vein, and
to provide a layer of thermal protection around the vein. Some blood
is always in the vein and that gets gently heated from its water content.
Direct fiber contact with the vein wall is not important as the energy
for heating water is propelled in an arcing field from the distal end of

the fiber facing into the lumen proximally. Once tumescent anesthesia is achieved and totally surrounds the targeted vein, a 600 um laser fiber is inserted with CTEV^{TM}. A helium neon aiming beam that is continuously illuminated when the laser is on ensures that the laser fiber is in the superficial venous system and can be used to monitor automatic pullback visually. The sheath acts to protect the vein during the insertion of the optical fiber. However, the sheath must be completely removed from the vein prior to application of laser energy. This is performed so that the automatic pullback device may pullback the fiber unimpeded. If the laser fiber retracts within the sheath thermal destruction of the sheath occurs with no energy transmission to the vein wall.

Correct placement of the laser fiber tip 2 cm distal to the SFJ is confirmed through Duplex visualization of the fiberoptic in the tumescent anesthesia compressed saphenous vein combined with viewing the aiming beam through the skin. Pullback is set for 1 mm/sec and the laser is set for 5–6 W at 50 Hz. The laser is fired for 2–3 sec to visualize sealing of the targeted vein on Duplex. The laser is then stopped for a moment while the pullback device is turned on. Once the laser fiber is seen to be getting pulled back on Duplex, the laser is immediately switched on. Vein shrinkage can be monitored visually by Duplex ultrasound as the water is heated circumferentially. Having the fiber pointed directly at a vein wall should be avoided. The progress can be monitored by Duplex or visually by the aiming beam reaching the skin surface from within the vein. As the fiber approaches the entry site, the laser is stopped.

SUMMARY

The latest techniques for endovenous occlusion using radiofrequency ablation catheters or endoluminal laser targeting water are our preferred methods to treat saphenous related varicose veins. These methods are well proven to offer a less invasive alternative to ligation and stripping and can be supplemented by sclerotherapy, particularly foamed sclerosant sclerotherapy. Clinical experience with endovenous techniques in over 1000 patients shows a high degree of success with minimal side effects, most of which can be prevented or minimized with use of tumescent anesthesia. Tumescent anesthesia is critical to the safety of endovenous techniques. Within the next 5 years, these minimally invasive endovenous ablative procedures involving saphenous trunks should have virtually replaced open surgical strippings. Already over 100,000 patients have been treated worldwide.

REFERENCES

1. Munn SR, Morton JB, MacBeth WAAG, McLeish AR. To strip or not to strip the long saphenous vein? A varicose vein trial. Br J Surg 1981; 68:426–428.
2. McMullin GM, Coleridge Smith PD, Scurr JH. Objective assessment of high ligation without stripping the long saphenous vein. Br J Surg 1991; 78:1139–1142.
3. Rutherford RB, Sawyer JD, Jones DN. The fate of residual saphenous vein after partial removal or ligation. J Vasc Surg 1990; 12:422–428.
4. Sarin S, Scurr JH, Coleridge Smith PD. Assessment of stripping the long saphenous vein in the treatment of primary varicose veins. Br J Surg 1992; 79:889–893.
5. Weiss RA, Weiss MA. Controlled radiofrequency endovenous occlusion using a unique radiofrequency catheter under duplex guidance to eliminate saphenous varicose vein reflux: a 2-year follow-up. Dermatol Surg 2002 Jan; 28(1):38–42.
6. Goldman MP, Amiry S. Closure of the greater saphenous vein with endoluminal radio-frequency thermal heating of the vein wall in combination with ambulatory phlebectomy: 50 patients with more than 6-month follow-up. Dermatol Surg 2002 Jan; 28(1):29–31.
7. Olgin JE, Kalman JM, Chin M, Stillson C, Maguire M, Ursel P, et al. Electrophysiolo-gical effects of long, linear atrial lesions placed under intracardiac ultrasound guidance. Circulation 1997 Oct 21; 96(8):2715–2721.
8. Gradman WS. Venoscopic obliteration of variceal tributaries using monopolar electro-cautery. J Dermatol Surg Onc 1994; 20(7):482–485.
9. Cragg AH, Galliani CA, Rysavy JA, Castaneda-Zuniga WR, Amplatz K. Endovascular diathermic vessel occlusion. Radiology 1982 Jul; 144(2):303–308.
10. Haines DE. The biophysics of radiofrequency catheter ablation in the heart: the impor-tance of temperature monitoring. Pacing Clin Electrophysiol 1993 Mar; 16(3 Pt 2):586–591.
11. Haines DE, Verow AF. Observations on electrode-tissue interface temperature and effect on electrical impedance during radiofrequency ablation of ventricular myocardium. Cir-culation 1990 Sep; 82(3):1034–1038.
12. Lavergne T, Sebag C, Ollitrault J, Chouari S, Copie X, Le HJ, et al. [Radiofrequency ablation: physical bases and principles]. Arch Mal Coeur Vaiss 1996 Feb; 89 Spec No 1:57–63:57–63.
13. Pichot O, Kabnick LS, Creton D, Merchant RF, Schuller-Petroviae S, Chandler JG. Duplex ultrasound scan findings two years after great saphenous vein radiofrequency endovenous obliteration. J Vasc Surg 2004 Jan; 39(1):189–195.
14. Lurie F, Creton D, Eklof B, Kabnick LS, Kistner RL, Pichot O, et al. Prospective ran-domized study of endovenous radiofrequency obliteration (closure procedure) versus ligation and stripping in a selected patient population (EVOLVeS Study). J Vasc Surg 2003 Aug; 38(2):207–214.
15. Merchant RF, Depalma RG, Kabnick LS. Endovascular obliteration of saphenous reflux: a multicenter study. J Vasc Surg 2002 Jun; 35(6):1190–1196.
16. Weiss RA, Goldman MP. Transillumination mapping prior to ambulatory phlebectomy. Dermatol Surg 1998; 24:447–450.
17. Smith SR, Goldman MP. Tumescent anesthesia in ambulatory phlebectomy. Dermatol Surg 1998 Apr; 24(4):453–456.
18. Goldman MP. Closure of the greater saphenous vein with endoluminal radiofrequency thermal heating of the vein wall in combination with ambulatory phlebectomy: prelimin-ary 6-month follow-up. Dermatol Surg 2000 May; 26(5):452–456.
19. Chandler JG, Pichot O, Sessa C, Schuller-Petrovic S, Osse FJ, Bergan JJ. Defining the role of extended saphenofemoral junction ligation: a prospective comparative study. J Vasc Surg 2000 Nov; 32(5):941–953.

20. Manfrini S, Gasbarro V, Danielsson G, Norgren L, Chandler JG, Lennox AF, et al. Endovenous management of saphenous vein reflux. Endovenous Reflux Management Study Group. J Vasc Surg 2000 Aug; 32(2):330–342.
21. Sybrandy JE, Wittens CH. Initial experiences in endovenous treatment of saphenous vein reflux. J Vasc Surg 2002 Dec; 36(6):1207–1212.
22. Komenaka IK, Nguyen ET. Is there an increased risk for DVT with the VNUS closure procedure? J Vasc Surg 2002 Dec; 36(6):1311.
23. Proebstle TM, Sandhofer M, Kargl A, Gul D, Rother W, Knop J, et al. Thermal damage of the inner vein wall during endovenous laser treatment: key role of energy absorption by intravascular blood. Dermatol Surg 2002 Jul; 28(7):596–600.
24. Proebstle TM, Lehr HA, Kargl A, Espinola-Klein C, Rother W, Bethge S, et al. Endovenous treatment of the greater saphenous vein with a 940-nm diode laser: thrombotic occlusion after endoluminal thermal damage by laser-generated steam bubbles. J Vasc Surg 2002 Apr; 35(4):729–736.
25. Min RJ, Zimmet SE, Isaacs MN, Forrestal MD. Endovenous laser treatment of the incompetent greater saphenous vein. J Vasc Interv Radiol 2001 Oct; 12(10):1167–1171.
26. Navarro L, Min RJ, Bone C. Endovenous laser: a new minimally invasive method of treatment for varicose veins–preliminary observations using an 810 nm diode laser. Dermatol Surg 2001 Feb; 27(2):117–122.
27. Mozes G, Kalra M, Carmo M, Swenson L, Gloviczki P. Extension of saphenous thrombus into the femoral vein: a potential complication of new endovenous ablation techniques. J Vasc Surg 2005 Jan; 41(1):130–135.
28. Weiss RA. Comparison of endovenous radiofrequency versus 810 nm diode laser occlusion of large veins in an animal model. Dermatol Surg 2002 Jan; 28(1):56–61.
29. Bush RG. Regarding "Endovenous treatment of the greater saphenous vein with a 940-nm diode laser: thrombolytic occlusion after endoluminal thermal damage by laser-generated steam bubbles". J Vasc Surg 2003 Jan; 37(1):242.
30. Chang CJ, Chua JJ. Endovenous laser photocoagulation (EVLP) for varicose veins. Lasers Surg Med 2002; 31(4):257–262.
31. Goldman MP, Mauricio M, Rao J. Intravascular 1320-nm Laser Closure of the Great Saphenous Vein: A 6- to 12-Month Follow-up Study. Dermatol Surg 2004 Nov; 30(11):1380–1385.
32. Goldberg SN, Hahn PF, Tanabe KK, Mueller PR, Schima W, Athanasoulis CA, et al. Percutaneous radiofrequency tissue ablation: does perfusion-mediated tissue cooling limit coagulation necrosis? J Vasc Interv Radiol 1998 Jan; 9(1 Pt 1):101–111.
33. Weiss RA, Weiss MA. Early clinical results with a multiple synchronized pulse 1064 nm laser for leg telangiectasias and reticular veins. Dermatol Surg. In press 1998.
34. Lewin JS, Connell CF, Duerk JL, Chung YC, Clampitt ME, Spisak J, et al. Interactive MRI-guided radiofrequency interstitial thermal ablation of abdominal tumors: clinical trial for evaluation of safety and feasibility. J Magn Reson Imaging 1998 Jan; 8(1):40–47.
35. Otsu A, Mori N. Therapy of varicose veins of the lower limbs by light coagulator. Angiology 1971 Mar; 22(3):107–113.
36. Sofka CM. Duplex ultrasound scan findings two years after great saphenous vein radiofrequency endovenous obliteration. Ultrasound Q 2004 Jun; 20(2):66.
37. Proebstle TM. Comparison of 940 nm and 1320 nm endovenous ablation. Dermatol Surg. In press 2005.
38. Proebstle TM, Gul D, Kargl A, Knop J. Endovenous laser treatment of the lesser saphenous vein with a 940-nm diode laser: early results. Dermatol Surg 2003 Apr; 29(4):357–361.

19

Radiofrequency Tissue Tightening: Thermage

Carolyn I. Jacob
Northwestern Medical School, Department of Dermatology, Chicago Cosmetic Surgery and Dermatology, Chicago, Illinois, U.S.A.

Michael S. Kaminer
Department of Dermatology, Yale Medical School, Yale University, New Haven, Connecticut, U.S.A.; Department of Medicine (Dermatology), Dartmouth Medical School, Dartmouth College, Hanover, New Hampshire, U.S.A.; and SkinCare Physicians of Chestnut Hill, Chestnut Hill, Massachusetts, U.S.A.

Video 22: Thermage

INTRODUCTION

Rapid advances in skin rejuvenation treatments have been seen in the new millennium, with patient demand and improved technology driving the development of treatments that require little or no recovery time. A new nonlaser procedure for tightening the skin uses radiofrequency to heat the dermis and potentially the subdermal tissues. The ThermaCool TC™ by Thermage has been recently cleared by the FDA for the non-invasive tightening of periorbital rhytides using this proven mechanism of tissue tightening. In this chapter we will outline the new radio-frequency technology and explore its place among the armamentarium of facial rejuvenation. We will also briefly discuss early stage work that uses this technology for acne treatment and body skin tightening.

To meet the demands of aging baby boomers, who desire an ever-youthful appearance, many devices and drugs have been developed. Previously, carbon dioxide and Erbium:YAG lasers were developed to produce skin rejuvenation through epidermal ablation and dermal heating. Although effective, these ablative lasers require 5 to 10 days of epidermal healing and may cause erythema that lasted for weeks to months. Recently, nonablative lasers have been researched, tested, and proved to provide dermal neocollagenesis while protecting the epidermis. These less invasive lasers improve facial rhytides from 0% to 75%, by subjective evaluation (1). Unfortunately, these technologies often require multiple, time-consuming treatment sessions, use highly delicate optics, and can be quite costly to acquire and maintain. In addition, results from nonablative lasers can be quite subtle, and they can vary significantly from patient to patient in both magnitude and duration of effect.

Radiofrequency tissue tightening is a recently introduced complement to and, in some applications, alternative to nonablative laser technologies. Earlier radiofrequency technologies were low-energy modifications of traditional ablative radiofrequency electrosurgery units that were used with limited success for cosmetic purposes to improve the surface of the skin (2,3). Recently, a new nonlaser radiofrequency device delivering much higher energy was developed to both remodel and tighten collagen in the deeper dermis and subcutaneous tissue to improve lax or aging skin. The ThermaCool TC^{TM} (Thermage, Hayward, California, U.S.A.) device uses a novel form of radiofrequency energy to create a uniform field of dermal and even subdermal heating, while contact cooling protects the epidermis. This device can safely deliver higher energy fluences to a greater tissue volume than nonablative lasers. In November 2002, the ThermaCool TC^{TM} received FDA approval for the reduction of periorbital rhytides (4).

MECHANISM OF ACTION

The ThermaCool TC^{TM} radiofrequency device has four key components: a radiofrequency generator, a handpiece, a cooling module, and disposable treatment tips. Radiofrequency energy production follows the principle of Ohm's law, which states that the impedance Z (Ω) to the movement of electrons creates heat relative to the amount of current I (A) and time t (sec) (Fig. 1).

The radiofrequency generator supplies a 6 MHz alternating current across a specially modified monopolar electrode to deliver volumetric heat to tissue in a targeted manner. A disposable return pad that is connected to the patient's flank creates a path of travel for the radiofrequency signal. The generator is regulated by a Pentium^{TM} chip–based internal computer that processes feedback, including temperature of the tip interface with the skin, application force, amount of tissue surface area contact, and real time impedance of the skin. This information is gathered by a microprocessor in the handpiece and relayed to the generator via high-speed fiber optic link.

A unique capacitively coupled electrode disperses energy uniformly across the very thin (1/1000 of an inch) dielectric material on the treatment tip, thereby creating a uniform electric field (Fig. 2). The radiofrequency generator operates at 6 MHz, which changes the polarity of

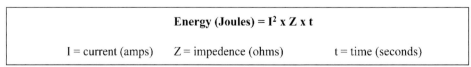

Energy (Joules) = I² x Z x t

I = current (amps)   Z = impedence (ohms)   t = time (seconds)

Figure 1
Ohm's law.

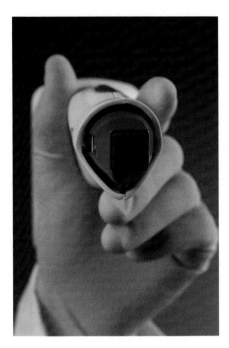

Figure 2
The unique capacitively coupled electrode treatment tip. *Source*: Courtesy of Thermage.

an electrical field in biological tissue six million times per second. The charged particles of the tissue within the electric field change orientation at the same frequency, and the dermal tissue's natural resistance (expressed in Ohms law as Z) to the movement of electrons generates heat. This friction from electron movement creates volumetrically distributed deep dermal heating (Table 1). Before, during, and after delivery of the radiofrequency energy, a cryogen spray delivered onto the inner surface of the treatment tip membrane provides cooling to protect the dermis from overheating and subsequent damage. The treatment tip continually monitors heat transmission from the skin via thermisters mounted on the inside of the dielectric membrane. The cryogen spray also

Table 1
Unique Properties of Radiofrequency Dermal Heating with the ThermaCool TC™

Energy used	6 MHz alternating current radiofrequency
Treatment tip	Capacitive coupling creating a uniform electric field
Distribution of heat	Volumetric heating with no edge effect

provides cooling of the upper portion of the dermis. This creates a reverse thermal gradient through the dermis and results in volumetric heating and tightening of deep dermal and even subdermal tissues (Fig. 3). The depth of this heating is dependent on the geometry of the treatment tip and the duration of cooling. Newer sizes and speeds of treatment tips are under investigation. New designs will allow for variations in treatment parameters, target even deeper heating delivery, and provide more vigorous epidermal protection.

Each treatment cycle consists of three phases: precooling, cooling and treatment, and postcooling. A treatment cycle is about six seconds with the initial generation of treatment tips and about two seconds with recently developed "fast" treatment tips. Also, with the new "fast" treatment tips, the handpiece microprocessor aborts the treatment pulse to protect against burning if all four corners of the tip are not in complete contact with the skin.

The initial feasibility study of this radiofrequency device coupled with a concurrent epidermal cooling system utilized a three-dimensional Monte Carlo simulation mathematical model to gauge the theoretical temperature distribution within human skin (5). The results showed that this treatment tip design produces volumetric heating deep within the dermis and yet protects the superficial skin layers from thermal injury. This creates a much greater temperature rise below the surface than in the epidermis. The depth of the radiofrequency field in tissue varies with the surface area of the treatment tip electrode design. The larger the tip electrode surface area, the deeper the heat produced. The amount of heat generated depends on the impedance of the tissue being treated with each

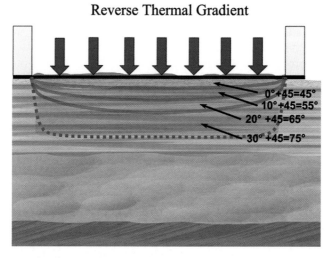

Figure 3
The reverse thermal gradient created via simultaneous cooling of the epidermis and heating of the dermis. *Source*: Courtesy of Thermage.

pulse and on the selected treatment setting. The depth of the protected tissue zone at the surface is controlled by the cooling time and intensity. Therefore, the degree and depth of heat generated in the tissue can be customized by changing the size and geometry of the tip electrode, the amount of energy delivered (which is directly correlated to tissue impedance), and the cooling parameters designated for a given energy setting. These heating, cooling, and energy parameters are programmed into a small eprom chip located within each disposable treatment tip, with manufacturer-optimized parameters that are automatically upgraded without active user intervention or generator software upgrade.

In vivo studies have shown that this volumetric radiofrequency tissue heating creates a dual effect. Primary changes to collagen occur as heat disrupts hydrogen bonds, thereby altering the molecular structure of the triple helix collagen molecule and resulting in collagen contraction (6,7). Secondary to the immediate thermal contraction of collagen, a more gradual contraction that is caused by of wound healing is predicted to occur over time as collagen regenerates, leading to a thicker remodeled dermis. Animal studies have documented that the Thermacool TC[TM] device can achieve dermal collagen heating as shallow as the papillary dermis or as deep as the subcutaneous fat (8). Additional animal studies examined $1\,cm^2$ treatment tips with 2- and 6-second cycle times, described as "fast" and "standard" treatment tips, respectively. Lactate dehydrogenase (LDH) and heat shock protein (HSP) stainings were used to determine the depth of action for these two treatment tips. Results showed that the depth of treatment was the same for both the "fast" and the "standard" treatment tips. This was observed histochemically when the enzyme (LDH) or protein (HSP) was inactivated. It was noted from this experiment was that the LDH enzyme was deactivated at approximately the same treatment levels for both tips, even though, the cooling and heating times and intensities were different (Karl Pope, Thermage, Inc., personal communication).

These reliable LDH and HSP heating depth results confirm the heating profile postulated by Zelickson et al., who used transmission electron microscopy to evaluate ex vivo bovine tendon immediately after treatment with the ThermaCool TC[TM] at various energy and cooling settings (9). Results showed collagen fibrils with increased diameter and loss of distinct borders as deep as 6 mm. Higher energy settings produced deeper and more extensive collagen changes (Fig. 4).

In a clinical study involving in vivo human skin, a similar pattern of immediate collagen fibril contraction was observed, an acute effect that has not been associated with nonablative lasers (9). In this same study of intact abdominal tissue, northern blot analysis demonstrated increased steady-state expression of collagen type I mRNA in treated tissue, an evidence that wound healing is initiated by the single treatment. The secondary collagen synthesis in response to collagen injury is purported to occur over several (2–6) months. Kilmer noted fibroplasia and signs of increased collagen formation in the papillary dermis and, less frequently, in the reticular dermis (10). Histology specimens taken four months after

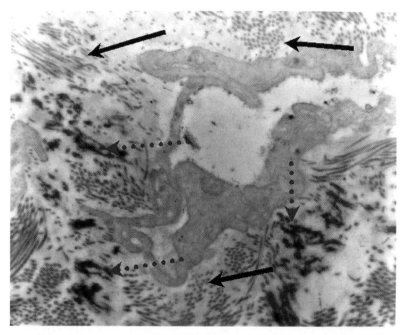

Figure 4
Transmission electron microscopy of human skin 4 to 5 mm below the surface immediately post-treatment with the ThermaCool TC™, 181 J with cooling. Large arrows show scattered diffuse changes in collagen fibril architecture, areas of increased size, and loss of distinct borders compared to normal fibrils noted by small arrows. Original magnifications × 8,640. *Source*: Courtesy of Thermage.

treatment demonstrate epidermal and papillary dermal thickenings as well as shrinkage of sebaceous glands (Fig. 5).

CLINICAL SCIENTIFIC DATA

To obtain FDA clearance for the aesthetic application of the ThermaCool TC™, researchers undertook a six-month study to evaluate the device's efficacy and safety (11). Eighty-six subjects received a single treatment with the ThermaCool TC™ on the forehead and temple area. On an average, patients were treated on 68 cm² of tissue with a single pass at settings ranging from 65 to 95 J/cm². Twenty-two patients received a nerve block just superior to the eyebrows immediately before or shortly after initiation of treatment. Independent scoring of blinded photographs taken six months after treatment resulted in Fitzpatrick wrinkle score improvement of at least one point in 83.2% (99/119) of treated periorbital areas. Additionally, 14.3% (17/119) of treated areas

(A)

(B)

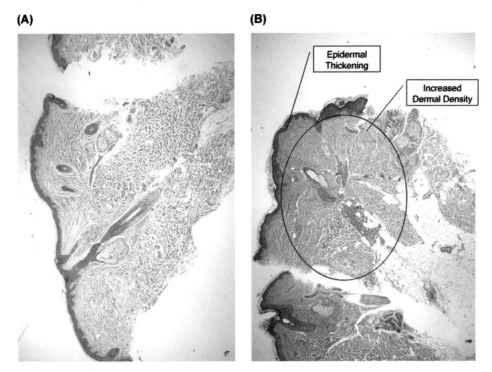

Epidermal Thickening

Increased Dermal Density

Figure 5
Human skin: (**A**) before, and (**B**) four months after treatment with the Therma-Cool TC™, showing epidermal thickening as well as increased dermal density. *Source*: Courtesy of Thermage.

had no change, and 2.5% (3/119) worsened (Table 2). Photographic analysis revealed an eyebrow lift of at least 0.5 mm in 61.5% (40/65) of patients after six months (Fig. 6). Fifty percent (41/82) of subjects were satisfied or very satisfied with their treatment outcome. Incidence of side effects was low and consisted of edema (13.9% immediately) and erythema (36% immediately). By one month, no subject had signs of edema, and only three (3.9%) had lingering signs of erythema. Rare second-degree burns occurred in 21 firings of 5858 radiofrequency exposures, indicating a burn risk of 0.36% per application. Three patients had small areas of residual scarring six months after treatment. The authors concluded that a single treatment with the ThermaCool TC™ reduced periorbital wrinkles, produced lasting brow elevation, and improved eyelid aesthetics. They also concluded that the safety profile of this device, used by physicians with no previous experience in its operation, was impressive.

In another study, Hsu and Kaminer evaluated 16 patients treated with a single pass on the cheeks, jawline, and/or upper neck. Treatment levels averaged 113.8 J/cm² on the cheeks, decreasing to 99.7 J/cm² on the neck. In post-treatment follow-up phone interviews, 36% of patients who

Table 2
The FWCS

Class	Wrinkling	Score	Degree of elastosis
I	Fine	1–3	Mild (fine textural changes with subtly accentuated skin lines)
II	Fine to moderate depth; moderate number of lines	4–6	Moderate [distinct popular elastosis (individual papules with yellow translucency under direct lighting) and dyschromia]
III	Fine to deep; numerous lines; with or without redundant skin folds	7–9	Severe [multipapular and confluent elastosis (thickened yellow and pallid) approaching or consistent with cutis rhomboidalis]

Abbreviation: FWCS, Fitzpatrick Wrinkle Classification System.

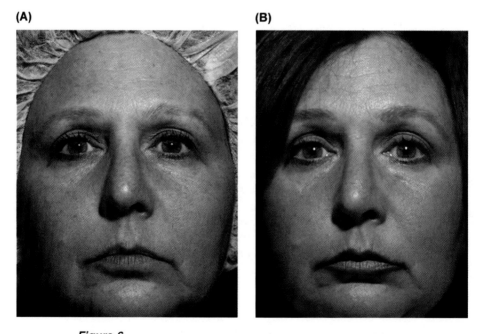

(A)   **(B)**

Figure 6
Example of brow lift after RF treatment: (**A**) pretreatment, (**B**) four weeks post-treatment: average lift = 3.42 mm (*right*) and 3.41 mm (*left*). *Source*: Courtesy of Thermage.

were treated at all three sites reported satisfactory results compared to 25% of patients who were treated at only one or two sites. Also, satisfied patients were those treated with higher energies (12).

This study had three important findings:

1. Treatment with higher fluences generally led to improved or more consistent results.
2. The greater the surface area treated, the better the results.
3. Younger age is a predictor of increased efficacy with the Thermage procedure.

These findings have direct implications for refining treatment algorithm guidelines. Guidelines should include treating a broad surface area and carefully selecting patients in their 40s, 50s, or early 60s, who have medium quality skin thickness and mild to moderate jawline and neck laxity. Treating areas on and adjacent to the described laxity may also improve response rate. Patients with advanced photoaging or more severe skin sagging may still benefit from ThermaCool TC^{TM} treatment, but possibly to a lesser extent.

Tanzi and Alster evaluated cheek laxity in 30 patients and neck laxity in 20 patients after a single treatment with the ThermaCool TC^{TM}. Patients were pretreated with 5 to 10 mg of oral diazepam and topical anesthetic cream (LMX-5% cream, Ferndale Laboratories, Inc., Fernadale, Michigan). The cheek treatment area extended from the nasolabial folds to the preauricular margin and down to the mandibular ridge. Treatment of the neck extended from the mandibular ridge to the mid-neck. Fluences ranged from 97 to 144 J/cm^2 on the cheeks and from 74 to 134 J/cm^2 on the neck. Mild post-treatment erythema was seen in all patients and persisted up to 12 hours after the procedure. Fifty-six percent of subjects complained of soreness at the treated sites; the soreness resolved with oral nonsteroidal anti-inflammatory medications. Erythematous papules that resolved after 24 hours were observed in three patients. One patient developed dysesthesia along the mandible that resolved over five days. No blistering or scarring was observed. A quartile grading system was used and independent assessment noted improvement in 28 of 30 patients who were treated on the cheeks and 17 of 20 patients who were treated on the neck. The five subjects who demonstrated no clinical improvement were all more than 62 years of age. At six months, the mean clinical improvement score was 1.53 on the cheeks and 1.27 on the neck (scale of 1 = 25–50% improvement, 2 = 51–75% improvement). On a scale of 1 to 10, the average patient satisfaction score was 6.3 and 5.4 for cheek and neck treatments, respectively (13).

Finally, in a study by Ruiz-Esparza and Gomez, 15 patients, falling in the age range of 41 to 68 years, were treated with one pass on the preauricular area using investigational tip designs. Five patients were treated with a 0.25-cm bipolar electrode, eight with a "window frame" bipolar electrode, and two with a 1-cm monopolar electrode. Independent evaluators graded nasolabial softening to be at least 50% improved in half the patients. Cheek contour was 50% improved in 60% of patients, and

Table 3
Ideal Candidates for the ThermaCool TC™

Patient age	35–75 years
Skin laxity	Mild to moderate
Thickness of skin	Thin to normal
Facial adipose	Not excessive

marionette lines improved 50% or more in 65% of patients. And, the mandibular line improved 50% or more in only 27% of patients. One patient did not have any improvement. Results were typically seen after 12 weeks, but one patient developed results after one week (14).

TREATMENT PROTOCOLS

Patients who may benefit from treatment with the Thermacool TC™ are between the ages of 35 and 75 with mild to moderate skin laxity. Patients who are facelift candidates may benefit less from the use of the Thermacool TC™ than those with resilient but mildly photoaged skin (Table 3).

All areas to be treated are first covered with a thick layer of anesthetic cream (LMX-5% cream, Ferndale Laboratories, Inc., Ferndale,

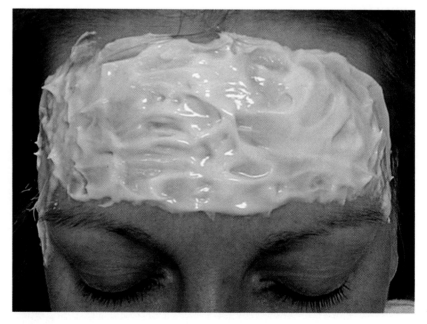

Figure 7
Pretreatment preparation of forehead and temples with anesthetic cream.

Michigan) and occluded with plastic wrap to create mild epidermal anesthesia and hydration (Fig. 7). After one hour, the cream is removed and a temporary ink grid is applied to the area to be treated. Or, the physician can create his/her own grid by using a red extra fine Sharpie™ marking pen (Fig. 8). The grid is used to ensure even

(A)

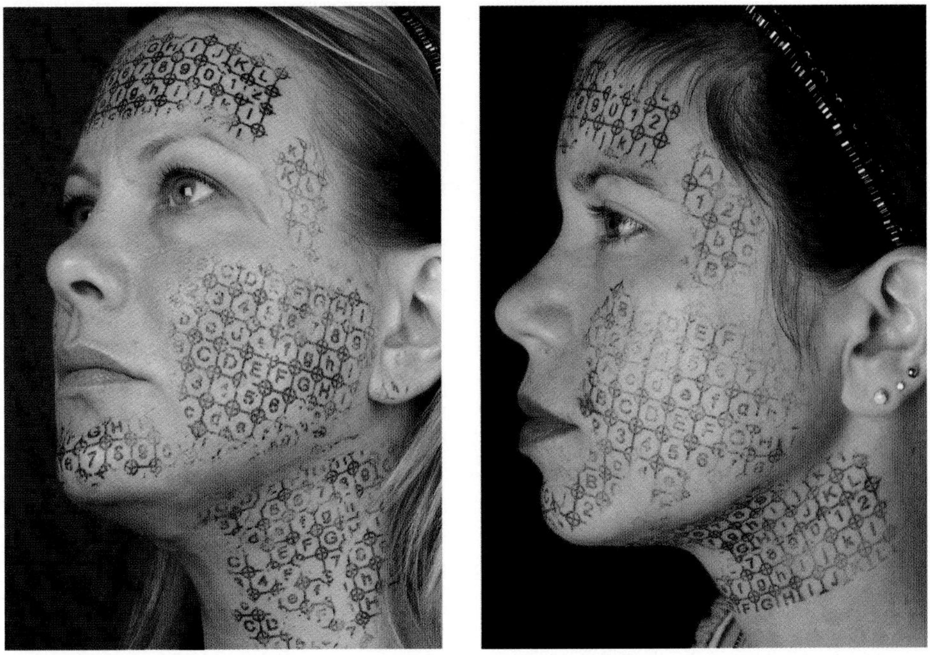

(B)

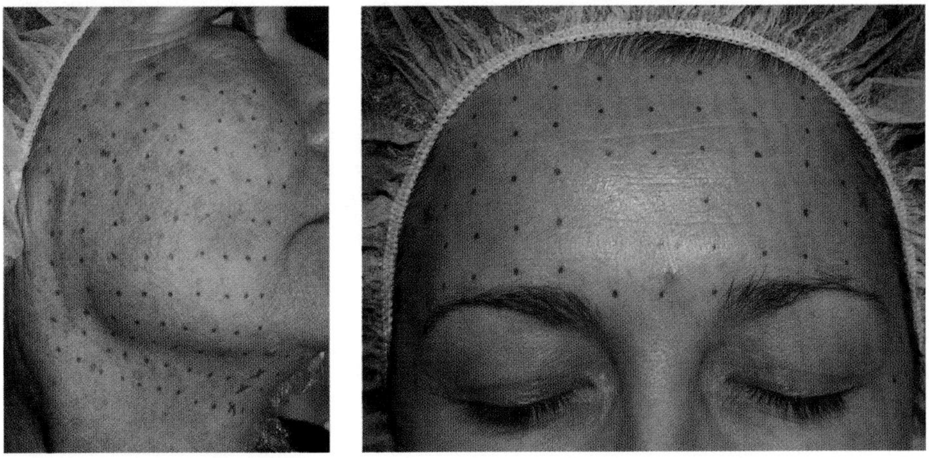

Figure 8
Placement of ink grid: (**A**) Thermage proprietary grid. *Source*: Courtesy of Thermage. (**B**) Hand-drawn grid.

placement of the treatment pulses and to prevent overlap, which could lead to excessive heat and epidermal or dermal injury. The adhesive return pad is applied to the patient's left flank to ensure a travel conduit for the RF energy and to complete the circuit. It is important that the return pad be placed in the location that is same as the one mentioned on all patients, has impedance readings can change when the pad is moved to other locations (Thermage, Inc., personal communication). The return pad is attached to the machine, and a new treatment tip is placed into the handpiece.

Anesthesia Alternatives

Owing to the potentially uncomfortable nature of the Thermage procedure a variety of pain control methods have been explored.

Many doctors prefer to use topical anesthetic for 60 to 90 minutes, usually under occlusion. Although the topical anesthetic affects only the surface of the skin, many physicians believe that it can provide substantial pain relief if its effect can be maximized. In contrast, some physicians treat without any topical anesthetic, presumably at somewhat lower settings. These doctors believe that patients are more comfortable because they are better able to feel the cooling that accompanies each pulse.

The challenge with pain control while heating the areas of deep dermis, and potentially subdermal structures, is that topical anesthetics do not typically penetrate to that depth. Therefore, adjunctive measures have been utilized to enhance patient comfort and to relieve anxiety caused by the deep heating sensation.

However, users are cautioned that complete elimination of pain feedback from the patient as a data point for energy adjustment may put the patient at risk of thermal injury. As pain perception can help the physician understand when the local tissue impedance is high, and therefore local heat build-up is high, complete blockage of pain feedback with local or nerve block anesthesia can carry significant risk.

This begs the question as to whether injectable local anesthesia can be used at all. Although local anesthesia can eliminate pain, it also adds a conductive fluid to the subdermal environment, which in turn reduces tissue impedance. This man-made alteration in tissue impedance can have negative effects on both patient outcomes and predictability. Until further study is undertaken to predict its effects, it is not recommended as a form of anesthesia.

For these reasons, physicians have turned to various forms of sedation to improve patient comfort. Complete general anesthesia or intravenous conscious sedation can be useful, but these measures eliminate patient feedback and are to be used with great caution and only by users who have experience in making equipment adjustments based on tissue thickness and patient variability. On the other hand, pain control options using oral and intramuscular (IM) medications seem to dramatically improve patient comfort during the procedure, and yet enable some feedback from the patients.

In practice, physicians use various combinations of medications including oral diazepam, lorazepam, triazolam, and oxycodone as well as IM meperidine, hydroxyzine, and butorphanol. The authors have developed a combination approach that has substantially improved the patient's tolerance of the procedure. Patients are given 1 mg of lorazepam orally upon arrival. Fifteen minutes before the procedure is to begin, patients are given meperidine 75 mg and hydroxyzine 25 mg intramuscularly. A second 1 mg dose of lorazepam is given sublingually at the start of the procedure, if patients are still uncomfortable.

It is clear that physicians will have their own comfort level with various oral and IM medications, and it is not suggested that the anesthesia algorithm is the only way to make patients comfortable. Performing the first 20 to 30 cases with topical anesthesia alone is a useful learning tool. Although patients may be uncomfortable, it teaches the physician how to manage different areas of the face and different pain perceptions from patient to patient. Once the doctor is experienced in using the Therma-Cool TC™, pain control can be expanded by utilizing sedating medications.

General Treatment Principles

Early treatments (2001–2002) with the Thermage device were done with a single pass at relatively high fluences. As the understanding of radiofrequency tissue physics has improved, so has the comfort level with decreasing the fluence per pulse. A key breakthrough seems to have occurred with the addition of selectively placed additional passes to the treatment algorithm (as many as 8 to 10 passes).

When a single pass is used, many patients will benefit from treatment. Adding multiple passes in selected lax areas appears to yield greater benefit, sometimes visible at the time of treatment. Rarely do we see any

---

Table 4
Treatment Fluences for Each Pass with the ThermaCool TC™

First and second passes
    62.5 central forehead
    62.5 cheeks and neck
    61.5 temples
Third pass
    62.0 central forehead
    62.0 cheeks and neck
Additional passes
    61.0–62.0 cheeks, submental, and jawline

immediate benefit after one pass, but we now see it almost routinely when multiple passes were employed (Table 4).

What has made this multiple-pass findings even more exciting is that patients who would not have had much improvement with one pass are achieving significant improvement with multiple passes. Thus, the population of patients who might benefit from the Thermage procedure has expanded considerably with the addition of multiple passes to the treatment algorithm. These changes in fluence and number of passes began in early 2003, and research into their true value is ongoing. Also, the role of multiple treatment sessions is under investigation.

The four variables that seem to determine how much benefit a patient will obtain from the ThermaCool TC^{TM} are:

1. The extent of photoaging as well as the age of the patient,
2. Treatment fluences,
3. Number of passes,
4. Number of treatments and interval between treatments.

Early data suggest that younger patients (under the age of 60–65) will do best, as will those with mild to moderate amounts of skin laxity. Lower fluences covering a broad surface area of skin also appear to promote better results, as does the use of multiple (2,3) carefully placed passes. The role of multiple treatments is not yet adequately understood.

Periorbital Rejuvenation

Treatment for periorbital improvement should extend across the entire forehead, down to the temples and the crow's feet area. Initially, a "fine tune" series of two to three treatment firings were performed to tune the device to the patient's skin. A generous amount of coupling gel is applied to ensure complete contact between the treatment tip and the skin. The gel can be added or reapplied as needed during the treatment session. After the fine-tuning, actual treatment firings may begin after choosing the energy level. With the 1.5 cm^2 treatment tip and a typical setting of 62.0–63.0 an initial single pass is delivered across the forehead. The temples and crow's feet are treated at levels 61.0–62.0 in this first pass (Fig. 9A). It is critical to reduce treatment fluences over the temporal region (lateral to the frontalis muscle), as there may be an increase in side effects (subcutaneous depressions or superficial burning) when settings over 62.0 are used in this thin tissue area. Extending treatment to the lateral periorbital region can have a significant impact on periorbital rhytides and can provide substantial local rejuvenation and tissue tightening that can affect adjacent areas (Fig. 10).

With the 1.5 cm^2 treatment tip, pain sensation is a crescendo of warmth, ending in a brief "spike" of heat. Differing patient tolerances to this sensation may inhibit higher treatment levels. The sensation appears to be stronger over the temporal area, where the frontalis muscle is absent, and this is yet another reason the treatment setting should be dropped to 61.0 to 62.0. Levels in all areas are adjusted to the patient's comfort.

(A)

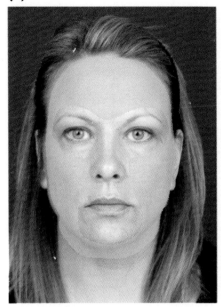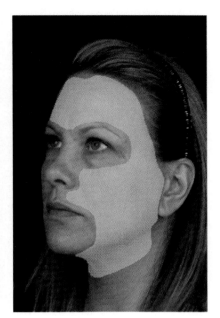

(B)

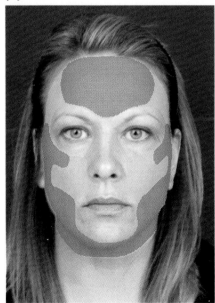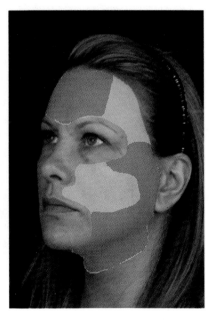

Figure 9
Multiple-pass treatment algorithm: (**A**) first pass (*in purple*), (**B**) second pass
(*in brown*), and (**C**) third pass (*in green*). (*Continued next page*)

(C)

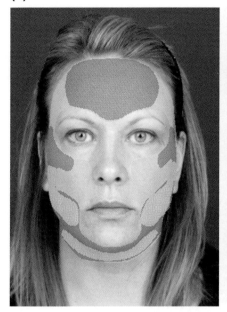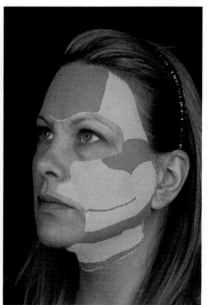

Figure 9 (*Continued*)

(A)   (B)   (C)

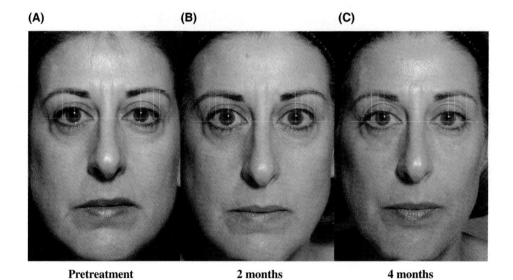

Pretreatment   2 months   4 months

Figure 10
Periorbital rejuvenation including brow lift. *Source*: Courtesy of Thermage.
(**A**) Pretreatment, (**B**) two months after treatment, and (**C**) four months after
treatment.

Newer treatment recommendations utilize a second pass on the forehead over the brows. The second pass is performed at a slightly lower setting than the first pass, and only over the central two-thirds of the forehead where there is frontalis muscle deep into the treatment tip (Fig. 9B). Placement of the second pass is critical over "lifting points," from the medial to lateral portion of the brow extending up to the hairline. When this is performed, the entire first pass should be completed before beginning the second pass, thereby allowing time for residual dermal heat from the first pass to dissipate before retreating the same area.

It is important to know that patient tolerance is an indicator of treatment levels, and treatment levels should not exceed 64.0 on the forehead because of the rare occurrence of temporary indentations on the forehead skin. This is thought to be because of heating of the adipose, but this observation has not been confirmed with histologic studies (C.I.J., personal experience) (Fig. 11). Typically 100 to 150 treatment pulses are required to cover the entire forehead and temples. This number may vary based on the size of the patient's forehead (men tend to have larger foreheads) and on the number of passes used.

After treatment, the ink grid is gently wiped off with the aid of coupling gel or a gentle cleanser. Alcohol swabs should be avoided as they may cause irritation to the newly treated skin. The patient is counseled to use sunblock containing a UVA block, such as zinc oxide or titanium dioxide, for 7 to 10 days and to avoid direct sun exposure as UV rays can

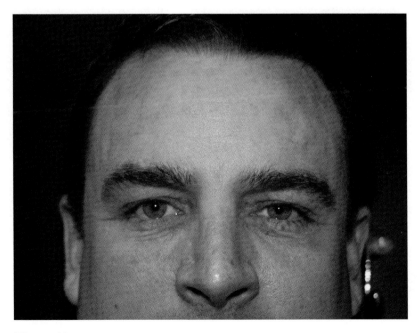

Figure 11
Subtle indentations four weeks after high-energy treatment on lateral forehead. These resolved spontaneously after five months.

increase the amount of metalloproteinases leading to potential collagen and elastic tissue degradation.

Treatment of the Lower Face

It is currently recommended to treat the entire cheek, jawline, and neck areas as one cosmetic unit, beginning at the malar prominence and peri-orbital/crow's feet areas, extending medially toward the nasolabial folds, laterally toward the preauricular area, and inferiorly to the mandible. The jawline, upper one-third of the neck, and submental regions are included as well (Figs. 12–14). One to two pulses on each side of the cutaneous upper lip may also be of benefit. It is recommended that treatment pulses be placed lateral and inferior to the bony orbital rim (Fig. 9A). One pass of the lower face may be sufficient if energy levels are set at 64.0 or above. However, results have improved substantially when as many as ten passes are used at lower settings (Table 4). The skin is made taut, creating a trampoline-like effect, by putting tension on the skin to be treated with the nontreating hand. It is important for the treatment tip to meet some resistance when it is placed on the skin to allow equal contact throughout the surface of the electrode. It can also be useful to gently pull the skin off of the jawline and neck upwards, superiorly to move this skin off the sensitive (and challengingly convex) mandibular region.

(A)   **(B)**

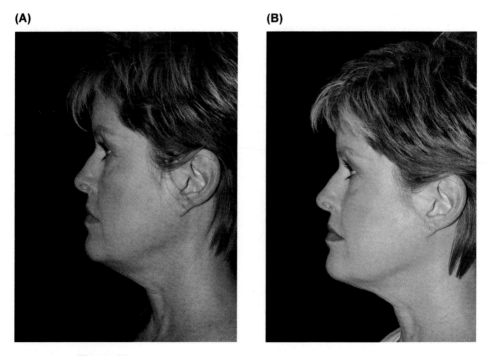

Figure 12
Lower face treatment with Thermage. *Source*: Courtesy of Thermage. (**A**) pretreatment, and (**B**) six months after one pass at 15.0.

(A) **(B)**

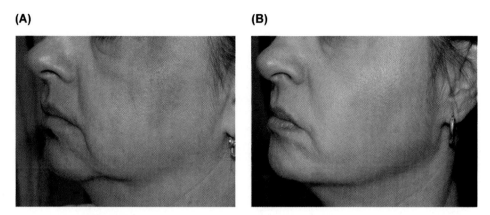

Figure 13
Lower face treatment with ThermaCool TC™. *Source*: Courtesy of Robert Weiss. (**A**) pretreatment, and (**B**) after two treatments, six months apart, with two passes each at setting of 15.0.

(A) **(B)**

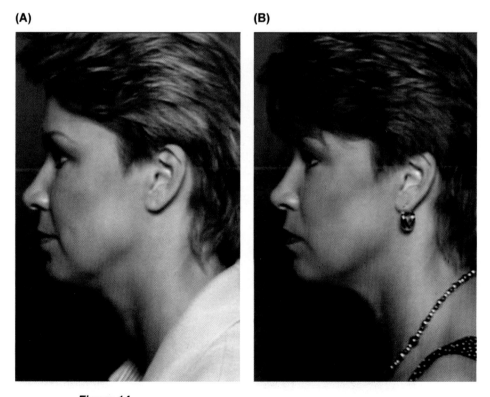

Figure 14
Lower face treatment with ThermaCool TC™. *Source*: Courtesy of Thermage. (**A**) Pretreatment, and (**B**) two weeks after one treatment at levels 13.5 to 15.5.

Treatment settings for the first pass are usually in the range of 62.5 to 63.0 for the entire lower face. A second pass at 62.0 to 63.0 is performed in the periorbital region, the lateral cheek, and preauricular region, as well as the jawline, submental region, and upper neck. The medial upper cheek is sometimes avoided with this second pass (Fig. 9B). The pulses of the second pass are spaced a bit farther apart than for the first pass. Additional passes can then be performed (Fig. 9C). There are differing theories as to the mechanism of action of the additional passes and they include:

1. Tissue tightening in the x (horizontal) and y (vertical) plane along the cutaneous surface,
2. Melting of fat and tissue tightening in the z-axis perpendicular to the skin which pulls tissue in, toward the bony underlying structures,
3. A combination of the two.

This z-axis effect appears to be an important element of the improved results seen recently in treatment of the lower face (Fig. 15). Whether this comes from additional tightening in the x (horizontal)

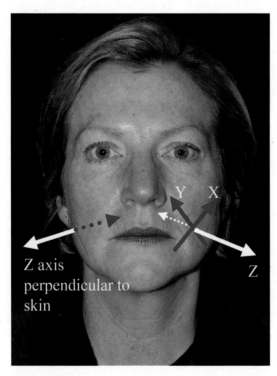

Figure 15
The *x*, *y*, and *z* planes of skin contraction.

(A)   **(B)**

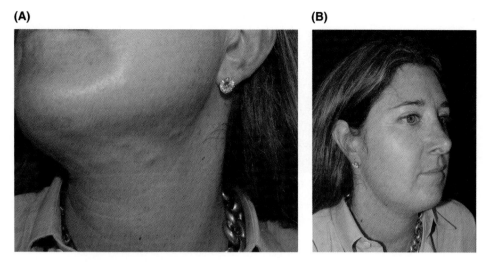

Figure 16
(**A**) Temporary nodules, and (**B**) swelling on the cheek one week after treatment.

and *y* (vertical) plane or from a direct third dimension effect on subdermal fat and collagen of the fibrous septae remains to be determined.

However, physicians can use these *z*-axis changes to their advantage. The third pass can therefore be carefully placed in areas where maximal *z*-axis improvement is needed. This would include the jowl and submental region. Additionally, further *x*- and *y*-axis changes can be produced with this third pass, and should include the preauricular region to create a "vector" of pull, laterally (Fig. 9C).

Treatment of the lower face can lead to mild to moderate edema of the jawline and neck, which usually resolves in 7 to 14 days, and occasional tenderness along the preauricular or mandibular area, which can be managed by ibuprofen. Small 0.5 to 1 cm nodules can also rarely be seen. These usually resolve without treatment or sequelae within two to four weeks (Fig. 16).

Other Sites and Acne

Off-the-face treatment sites under investigation include the lower abdomen for skin laxity (age related, postpregnancy, or postliposuction) (Fig. 17), tissue areas adjacent to the breasts for tightening and lifting, arms (Fig. 18), and others. Currently there are no validated treatment algorithms for these off-the-face sites, but typically one pass has been used at energy settings of 63.0 to 64.0, though multiple passes are also being evaluated. It should be noted that this is a very early experimental data, and treatment of these off-the-face areas is not recommended for inexperienced users until more data are available.

(A)   **(B)**

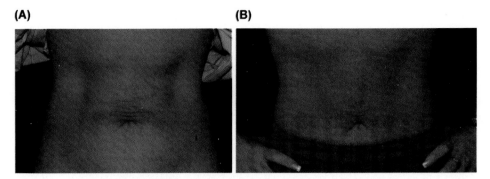

Figure 17
Tightening of abdominal skin with ThermaCool TC™. (**A**) Pretreatment, and
(**B**) one year after treatment at 15.5 with tumescent anesthesia.

One promising area of research involves use of the ThermaCool
TC™ for the treatment of active acne. A multicenter, FDA-monitored,
split-face comparison of no treatment versus radiofrequency treatment
is underway. This study has been initiated based on some early promising
results from pilot work done by several physicians (15).

DISCUSSION

The ThermaCool TC™ radiofrequency device for tissue tightening is the
latest and perhaps most distinctive treatment option in the quest for nonablative rejuvenation. Studies show that the device can lead to substantial
improvement in some patients. Because the treatment risks are extremely

(A)   **(B)**

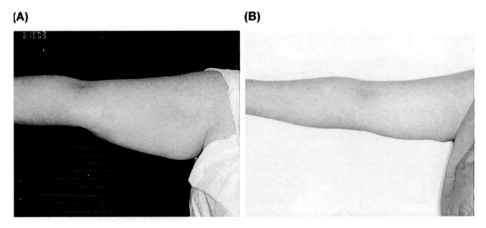

Figure 18
Improvement of arm contours with ThermaCool TC™. *Source*: Courtesy of
Thermage. (**A**) Pretreatment, and (**B**) four days post-treatment.

low, the Thermage device offers a relatively simple alternative for patients who do not want major surgery or who have moderate skin laxity that does not warrant an invasive surgical procedure.

One of the central questions is what the role of Thermage will be in the future of facial rejuvenation. It is clear that radiofrequency tissue tightening produces effects that are not achievable with other devices currently in the market. And although a facelift may be an option for some, many patients are reluctant to go through the expense and recovery of such a procedure. For these and other reasons, the Thermage procedure is likely to become a central part of facial rejuvenation.

In exploring the mechanisms and effects of photoaging, there are two basic components: (1) superficial (epidermal) and (2) deeper (dermal and subcutaneous) structural changes (sagging). Although the Thermage procedure may yet be determined to have some benefit on superficial epidermal changes, this would be a secondary effect. But it is clear that the technique has a direct and at times profound effect on dermal and subdermal tissues. This is where the uniqueness of the ThermaCool TC^{TM} becomes its greatest utility.

Other devices exist for treatment of epidermal changes (ablative resurfacing, chemical peels, pigment lasers, and photorejuvenation), and dermal remodeling can be achieved with several of the nonablative lasers. Yet, none of these techniques or devices is capable of producing nonablative tissue tightening, and that is clearly the niche for Thermage to fill. Because sagging of tissues is a fundamental part of the aging process, nearly all patients who are candidates for other forms of facial rejuvenation are also candidates for the Thermage procedure. Radiofrequency tissue tightening is not a substitute for the wide array of nonablative lasers, but rather a companion to them. There may be some overlap, for example, in remodeling of the dermis achieved by nonablative lasers and the Thermage device. However, only the ThermaCool TC^{TM} can produce tightening of dermal collagen in the x- and y-axis, and the z-axis changes discussed earlier are not seen with any of the other nonablative options available.

The future role of Thermage and radiofrequency tissue tightening is relatively clear. It is most useful for those patients who would benefit from dermal remodeling as well as from tissue tightening of the forehead, cheeks, jawline, and neck. When the Thermage technique is combined with other procedures that improve the more superficial changes associated with photoaging, patients are likely to experience results that were previously impossible to achieve in the absence of a more aggressive, invasive surgery.

REFERENCES

1. Goldberg DJ. Non-ablative dermal remodeling: does it really work? Arch Dermatol 2002; 138:1366–1368.
2. Capurro S, Fiallo P. Epidermal disepithelialization by programmed diathermosurgery. Dermatol Surg 1997; 23:600–601.
3. Grekin RC, Tope WD, Yarborough JM Jr, Olhoffer IH, Lee PK, Leffell DJ, Zachary CB. Electrosurgical facial resurfacing: A prospective multicenter study of efficacy and safety. Arch Dermatol 2000; 136:1309–1316.
4. Thermage company web site, www.Thermage.com.
5. Tunell JW, Pham L, Stern RA, Pope KA. Mathematical model of non-ablative RF heating of skin, publication in progress.
6. Nouri K, Singer L, Lodha R, Ruiz-Esparza J. Subsurfacing: a non-ablative approach to facial rejuvenation. Cosmet Dermatol 2003; 16(6):63–69.
7. Arnoczky SP, Aksan A. Thermal modification of connective tissue: basic science considerations and clinical impressions. J Am Acad Orthop Surg 2000; 8:305–313.
8. Hardaway CA, Ross EV. Non-ablative laser skin remodeling. Dermatol Clin 2002; 20:97–111.
9. Zelickson BD, Kist D, Bernstein E, Brown DB, Sergey K, Burns J, Kilmer S, Mehregan D, Pope K. Histological and ultrastructural evaluation of the effects of a radio-frequency-based non-ablative dermal remodeling device: a pilot study. Arch Dermatol 2004; 140(2): 204–9.
10. Kilmer SL. First human clinical trial of new non-ablative radiofrequency technology on abdominal skin. In press.
11. Fitzpatrick R, Geronemus R, Goldberg D, Kaminer M, Kilmer S, Ruiz-Esparza J. Multicenter study of noninvasive radiofrequency for periorbital tissue tightening. Lasers Surg Med 2003; 33(4):232–242.
12. Hsu TS, Kaminer MS. The use of non-ablative radiofrequency technology to tighten the lower face and neck. Semin Cutan Med Surg 2003; 22:115–123.
13. Tanzi El, Alster TS. Improvement of neck and cheek laxity with a non-ablative radio-frequency device: a lifting experience. In press.
14. Ruiz-Esparza J, Gomez JB. The medical face lift: a noninvasive, nonsurgical approach to tissue tightening in facial skin using non-ablative radiofrequency. Dermatol Surg 2003; 29(4):325–332.
15. Ruiz-Esparza J, Gomez JB. Nonablative radiofrequency for active acne vulgaris: the use of deep dermal heat in the treatment of moderate to severe active acne vulgaris (Thermotherapy): a report of 22 patients. Dermatol Surg 2003; 29:333–339.

Index